Image-Guided Diagnosis and Treatment of Cancer

Preface

Cancer detection and treatment have been greatly enhanced by advances in imaging technology during the last decade. *Image-Guided Diagnosis and Treatment of Cancer* aims to describe the past, current, and future applications of imaging in the diagnosis, staging, treatment, and outcome assessment of cancer of the prostate, central nervous system, and breast. Given the multitude of advances in image-guided biopsy and treatment, this book aims to be the first of its kind to introduce the field of minimally invasive image-guided surgery to the medical community.

Earlier detection using screening mammography has decreased breast cancer mortality (Chapter 3). Approaches to breast cancer detection using magnetic resonance imaging (MRI) are currently under study (Chapter 4). Improved visualization of the prostate gland first using transrectal ultrasound (Chapters 1 and 6) and later using MRI (Chapters 2 and 7) has provided the ability to diagnose prostate cancer and perform minimally invasive delivery of high-dose radiation to the tumor bearing region(s) of the prostate with minimal toxicity. MRI-guided resection of neoplasms and sites of functional disorders allows for minimally invasive biopsy (Chapter 5) and neurosurgery (Chapters 8 and 9) with maximum benefits.

As imaging technology has become increasingly sophisticated, the ability to assess response to chemotherapy (Chapter 10), map temperature profiles (Chapter 11), and visualize gene expression in vivo is becoming a reality (Chapter 12). *Image-Guided Diagnosis and Treatment of Cancer* outlines the current clinical applications of image guidance in the detection (Part I) and treatment (Part II) of carcinoma of the prostate, central nervous system, and breast in order to define the future paradigm of genetic-based imaging and its potential clinical applications (Part III).

Anthony V. D'Amico, MD, PhD

Jay S. Loeffler, MD

Jay R. Harris, MD

Contents

Contributors

HOOMAN AZMI, MD, *Department of Neurosurgery, Neurological Institute of New Jersey, New Jersey Medical School, Newark, NJ*

PETER M. BLACK, MD, PhD, *Department of Neurosurgery, Brigham and Women's Hospital and The Children's Hospital, Harvard Medical School, Boston, MA*

JOHN BLASKO, MD, *Seattle Prostate Institute and Department of Radiation Oncology, University of Washington School of Medicine, Seattle, WA*

AMAN U. BUZDAR, MD, *Department of Breast Medical Oncology, The University of Texas M. D. Anderson Cancer Center, Houston, TX*

PETER R. CARROLL, MD, *Department of Urology, UCSF/Mt. Zion Comprehensive Cancer Center, University of California, San Francisco, CA*

ROBERT CORMACK, PhD, *Department of Radiation Oncology, Brigham and Women's Hospital, Harvard Medical School, Boston, MA*

ANTHONY V. D'AMICO, MD, PhD, *Department of Radiation Oncology, Brigham and Women's Hospital, Dana Farber Cancer Institute, Harvard Medical School, Boston, MA*

TRACY M. DOWNS, MD, *Department of Urology, UCSF/Mt. Zion Comprehensive Cancer Center, University of California, San Francisco, CA*

PETER GRIMM, DO, *Seattle Prostate Institute, Seattle, WA*

GARY D. GROSSFELD, MD, *Department of Urology, UCSF/Mt. Zion Comprehensive Cancer Center, University of California, San Francisco, CA*

STEVEN HAKER, PhD, *Department of Radiology, Brigham and Women's Hospital, Harvard Medical School, Boston, MA*

HEDVIG HRICAK, MD, PhD, *Departments of Medical Physics and Radiology, Memorial Sloan-Kettering Cancer Center, New York, NY*

JOHN HUMM, MD, PhD, *Departments of Medical Physics and Radiology, Memorial Sloan-Kettering Cancer Center, New York, NY*

MARK D. HURWITZ, MD, *Department of Radiation Oncology, Brigham and Women's Hospital, Harvard Medical School, Boston, MA*

REVATHY B. IYER, MD, *Department of Diagnostic Radiology, The University of Texas M. D. Anderson Cancer Center, Houston TX*

FAROUC A. JAFFER, MD, PhD, *Center for Molecular Imaging Research, Massachusetts General Hospital, Charlestown, MA and Department of Medicine, Massachusetts Hospital, Harvard Medical School, Boston, MA*

FERENC JOLESZ, MD, *Department of Radiology, Brigham and Women's Hospital, Harvard Medical School, Boston, MA*

JASON KOUTCHER, MD, PhD, *Departments of Medical Physics and Radiology, Memorial Sloan-Kettering Cancer Center, New York, NY*

SANJAYA KUMAR, MD, *Department of Urology, Brigham and Women's Hospital, Harvard Medical School, Boston, MA*

OREN H. LIFSHITZ, MD, *Department of Diagnostic Radiology, The University of Texas M. D. Anderson Cancer Center and The University of Texas-Houston Medical School, Houston, TX*

C. CLIFTON LING, PhD, *Departments of Medical Physics and Radiology, Memorial Sloan-Kettering Cancer Center, New York, NY*

LYNN LOPES, RN, *Department of Radiation Oncology, Brigham and Women's Hospital, Boston, MA*

VASILIS NTZIACHRISTOS, PhD, *Center for Molecular Imaging Research, Massachusetts General Hospital, Harvard Medical School, Charlestown, MA*

SUSAN GREENSTEIN OREL, MD, *Department of Radiology, University of Pennsylvania School of Medicine, Philadelphia, PA*

MICHAEL SCHULDER, MD, *Department of Neurosurgery, Neurological Institute of New Jersey, New Jersey Medical School, Newark, NJ*

KATSUTO SHINOHARA, MD, *Department of Urology, UCSF/Mt. Zion Comprehensive Cancer Center, University of California, San Francisco, CA*

DARRELL N. SMITH, MD, MSc, *Department of Radiology, Brigham and Women's Hospital, Harvard Medical School, Boston, MA*

JOHN SYLVESTER, MD, *Seattle Prostate Institute, Seattle, WA*

ION-FLORIN TALOS, MD, *Department of Radiology, Brigham and Women's Hospital, Harvard Medical School, Boston, MA*

CLARE M. TEMPANY, MD, *Division of MRI, Department of Radiology, Brigham and Women's Hospital, Harvard Medical School, Boston, MA*

RALPH WEISSLEDER, MD, PhD, *Center for Molecular Imaging Research, Massachusetts General Hospital, Harvard Medical School, Charlestown, MA*

GARY J. WHITMAN, MD, *Department of Diagnostic Radiology, The University of Texas M. D. Anderson Cancer Center, Houston, TX*

KRISTIN VALENTINE, BS, *Department of Radiation Oncology, Brigham and Women's Hospital, Boston, MA*

I
IMAGE-GUIDED DIAGNOSIS

Transrectal Ultrasound-Guided Prostate Biopsy

Tracy M. Downs, MD**, Gary D. Grossfeld,** MD**,**
Katsuto Shinohara, MD**, and Peter R. Carroll,** MD

INTRODUCTION

Prostate cancer is a significant health care problem for American men. It continues to be the most commonly diagnosed malignancy in American men and the second leading cause of cancer deaths *(1)*. In 2002, the American Cancer Society estimated over 189,000 new cases of prostate cancer *(2)*. Based on the yearly incidence of new prostate cancer cases in the United States, it was estimated that more than a half-million transrectal ultrasound –guided prostate biopsies were performed in 2001.

Transrectal ultrasound (TRUS) of the prostate was first reported by Wild and Reid in 1955 and popularized by Watanabe and associates in 1971 *(3,4)*. TRUS-guided prostate needle biopsies were introduced a decade later in the early 1980s, and in 1989 Hodge et al. *(5)* proposed the sextant method of prostate biopsy. Technological developments that have improved TRUS and its role in prostate cancer detection include an automated spring-loaded prostate biopsy device, multi-axial planar imaging, and a better understanding of prostate zonal anatomy *(6–8)*.

Despite these technological advances, the standard sextant TRUS-guided prostate needle biopsy has limitations. This is evident clinically, in which approx 20% of patients with an initially negative biopsy will be found to have cancer on subsequent biopsies *(9)*. New refinements in biopsy location and the number of biopsies taken have been investigated to improve the performance of TRUS-guided prostate needle biopsy *(10–15)*. In addition improved ultrasound technology, including the introduction of power Doppler ultrasound *(16–18)*, contrast agents *(19,20)*, and new imaging techniques, such as three-dimensional image reconstruction *(21–23)* may improve the performance of TRUS in cancer detection and staging.

PROSTATE ZONAL ANATOMY

The diagnostic capabilities and limitations of TRUS are best understood by a complete understanding of prostatic zonal anatomy. McNeal *(24–27)* described the concept of zones rather than lobes, and his is the model of prostate anatomy that is most widely accepted. The urethra divides the prostate into an anteriorly located fibromuscular stroma and posteriorly located glandular tissue. The glandular tissue is further subdivided into a peripheral zone (PZ), central zone (CZ), and a transition zone (TZ) (Fig. 1).

From: *Image-Guided Diagnosis and Treatment of Cancer*
Edited by: A. D'Amico, J. S. Loeffler, and J. R. Harris © Humana Press Inc., Totowa, NJ

The peripheral zone (PZ) comprises the bulk of the normal adult prostate gland (70% of the glandular tissue) and is thought to derive embryologically from the urogenital sinus *(27)* The PZ comprises all of the prostatic glandular tissue at the apex and essentially all of the prostatic tissue located posteriorly near the capsule. Approximately 68% of prostatic cancers arise from this zone, and benign prostatic hypertrophy does not arise in this area *(28)*

The central zone (CZ) comprises 25% of the glandular tissue and is thought to arise embryologically from the Wolffian duct. *(27)* The CZ is cone-shaped with the apex of the cone surrounding the ejaculatory duct complex (ejaculatory ducts, specialized loose stroma and, sometimes, the utricle). The base of the cone surrounds the origin of the seminal vesicles and the ampulla of the vas deferens. Eight percent of prostate cancers arise from this zone *(28)*.

The transition zone (TZ) comprises 5–10% of the glandular tissue in young men and is derived from the urogenital sinus *(27)*. The TZ is the site of benign prostatic hyperplasia (BPH) development and exhibits significant growth with aging. The TZ is located anteriorly to the PZ and consists of two equal portions of glandular tissue lateral to the urethra in the midprostate just superior to the point at which the urethra angles anteriorly *(28)*. Twenty-four percent of prostatic carcinomas arise in this area.

TRUS-GUIDED PROSTATE BIOPSY

Indications

TRUS alone should not be used as a first-line screening study because it lacks acceptable specificity, is relatively expensive when compared with digital rectal examination (DRE) and prostate-specific antigen (PSA) testing, and adds little information to that already gained by the use of serum PSA and DRE *(29,30)*. The most important role for TRUS is to provide visual guidance for systematic biopsy templates as well as precise biopsy of abnormal areas. In general, most agree that TRUS-guided prostate needle biopsy should be performed in men with an abnormal DRE, an elevated PSA (>4.0 ng/mL), or PSA velocity (rate of PSA change) >0.75 ng/mL/yr *(31)*. Also, men who were diagnosed with high-grade prostatic intraepithelial neoplasia (PIN) or atypia on a previous prostate needle biopsy should undergo a repeat biopsy 3 to 12 mo later *(32–34)*. Less commonly agreed upon recommendations for TRUS-guided prostate needle biopsy include age-specific PSA elevation, ethnicity-specific PSA parameters, a low percentage of free PSA (<25%), elevated human glandular kallikrein-2 levels, and a PSA density >0.15 (35), which is a measure of the amount of PSA relative to the overall prostatic volume (PSA divided by theprostate volume in cubic centimeters). Table 1 shows the age-adjusted PSA reference ranges for Caucasian and African-American men. In patients previously treated with curative intent for prostate cancer (i.e., radical prostatectomy, radiation therapy, and cryotherapy) relative indications for TRUS-guided prostate needle biopsy include a palpable abnormality on DRE or a rising PSA suggestive of local, rather than distant, recurrence.

TRUS, although not a perfect staging tool, may allow one to estimate the risk of extracapsular extension in those who might be candidates for a nerve sparing approach at the time of radical prostatectomy.

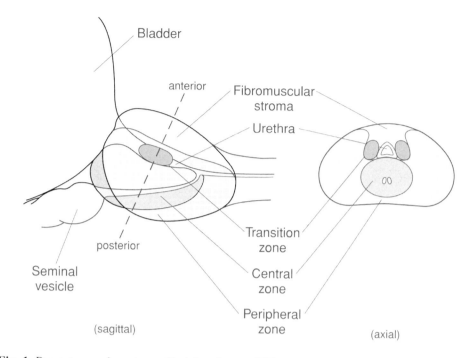

Fig. 1. Prostate zonal anatomy. Peripheral zone (PZ), central zone (CZ), and transition zone (TZ).

Table 1
Age-Adjusted PSA (111–114)

Age range (years)	African-American (ng/mL)	Specificity (%)	Caucasian (ng/mL)	Specificity (%)	Asians (ng/mL)	Specificity (%)
40–49	0.0–2.0	93	0.0–2.5	95	0.0–2.0	95
50–59	0.0–4.0	88	0.0–3.5	95	0.0–3.0	95
60–69	0.0–4.5	81	0.0–4.5	95	0.0–4.0	95
70–79	0.0–5.5	78	0.0–6.5	95	0.0–5.0	95

Patient Preparation

Shandera et al. *(36)* analyzed surveys from 568 US urologists regarding their preprostate needle biopsy patient preparation. He reported that although there was significant variability in the type and duration of antibiotic prophylaxis, 93.3% of urologists prescribed antibiotics before the procedure. The most commonly used antibiotic was an oral quinolone used by 91.6% of urologists. Seventy-eight percent of urologists prescribed antibiotics ranging from 1 to 3 d *(36)*.

Another issue in prebiopsy patient preparation is whether a rectal-cleansing enema should be given before the procedure. Shandera et al. *(36)* reported that 81% of urologists used a rectal-cleansing enema. Carey and Korman *(37)* recently reported their experience with patients treated with identical antibiotic prophylaxis who underwent TRUS-guided prostate needle biopsy with or without an enema before the biopsy. In this retrospective review, 225 patients received enemas before prostate biopsy and 185 patients received no bowel preparation. Overall, clinically significant complications developed in 4.4% of patients who had an enema compared to 3.2% of those who did not. The difference in complication rates was not statistically significant, and the authors concluded that TRUS-guided prostate biopsy with appropriate antibiotic prophylaxis can be performed safely without the use of a cleansing enema. Lindert and colleagues *(38)* investigated the incidence of bacteremia and bacteriuria after prostate biopsy and analyzed the value of a prebiopsy enema. Fifty men undergoing TRUS-guided prostate biopsy were randomized to receive a prebiopsy enema (25 patients) or no enema (25 patients). Postbiopsy bacteriuria was noted in 44% of patients in both groups. Bactermeia occurred in seven participants (28%) who did not receive an enema before biopsy and in one patient (4%) who was given an enema before TRUS-guided prostate needle biopsy. The authors concluded that a prebiopsy enema could significantly reduce the incidence of postbiopsy bacteremia. Although no clear consensus exists in the literature regarding the impact of a cleansing enema before TRUS-guided prostate needle biopsy, the most common practice pattern among United States urologists is to prescribe a rectal-cleansing enema *(36)*.

At our institution, we routinely use a 3-d course of an oral fluoroquinolone starting the day before the biopsy is performed. We instruct the patient to perform a self-administered cleansing enema (sodium phosphate and dibasic sodium phosphate) the morning before the biopsy to eliminate gas and remove feces. We also recommend that aspirin and nonsteroidal anti-inflammatory drugs be discontinued for 7 and 3 d, respectively, before the scheduled prostate needle biopsy. Patients on anticoagulation therapy are not biopsied until the anticoagulant dosage is adjusted or held to allow the coagulation status to normalize.

TRUS Procedure

The patient is positioned in either the right or left lateral decubitus position. This allows for easier insertion of the rectal probe. A DRE is performed to familiarize the examiner with the location of any palpable nodularity or extracapsular disease extension. The authors apply Hurricaine® gel (Beutlich L.P., Waukegan, IL), a topical anesthetic ointment to the index finger before performing the DRE. We believe this provides some local anesthesia to the rectal mucosa, which diminishes the pain associated with TRUS probe insertion. The TRUS probe is covered with a latex condom sheath and generously lubricated. Once the probe is positioned in the rectum, the balloon surrounding the tip of the probe is inflated with water (i.e., 30 to 50 mL) and the examination is begun in the transaxial plane. A 5.0- to 7.5-mHz transducer is used for transrectal imaging of the prostate. Contemporary equipment has either a biplanar probe or an end-firing probe to obtain transverse and sagittal images. In general, lower-frequency transducers have better tissue penetration but poorer image resolution. In contrast, higher-frequency transducers have greater image resolution but have decreased ability to penetrate distally (anterior portion of the prostate).

After insertion of the probe, the ultrasound console settings are adjusted so that the peripheral zone has a uniform midgray image. This is important because the echogenicity in the peripheral zone will be the standard by which other areas in the prostate are classified as hyperechoic, isoechoic, and hypoechoic. The probe is gently advanced cephalad to the base of the bladder until the seminal vesicles are visualized. Transverse images are then obtained as the probe is moved caudad from the prostate base to the prostate apex. Hardcopy images are made at the level of the seminal vesicles, base, midprostate, and apex. After completion of transverse imaging, the probe is repositioned (end-fire probe) or the console setting selected (biplanar probe) to provide sagittal imaging. Sagittal imaging is typically begun on the right side of the gland and the transducer is rotated medially through the midsagittal section. The left side of the gland is scanned in a similar fashion. Hardcopy images are taken in a parasagittal location bilaterally. With the transducer at the largest cross-sectional image in the transverse plane and in the mid-sagittal plane, prostate volume can be calculated. A simple pro-rated ellipsoid formula is commonly used to calculate prostate volume: (anterior–posterior diameter) × (transverse diameter) × (superior–infereior diameter) × (Π/6 (approx 0.52) is accurate and reproducible *(39)*.

TRUS Findings

During TRUS, the prostate is routinely assessed for any abnormal echogenicity and for integrity of the prostatic capsule. In addition, the junction between the seminal vesicle and the prostatic capsule and the trapezoidal area bordered by the prostatic apex, membranous urethra, rectourethralis muscle, and rectum are assessed for any evidence of irregularity or obliteration. Lee et al. *(40)* has denoted these areas as possible sites of local cancer spread.

The PZ has a homogeneous medium echogenicity, which is a useful background for the depiction of abnormal lesions, which might represent prostate cancer. In general, in the normal prostate gland, the PZ and CZ appear isoechoic and the TZ appears slightly hypoechoic *(41)*.

TRUS echogenic patterns can be classified as anechoic, hypoechoic, isoechoic, and hyperechoic. Anechoic lesions are classically fluid-filled cysts. Hypoechoic areas result in less reflection of the sound images than the normal peripheral zone. Isoechoic areas have a sonographic appearance indistinguishable from the normal PZ. Hyperechoic lesions have echo reflection far greater than the normal PZ. Some hyperechoic lesions may have virtually all of the sound energy being reflected (i.e., prostatic calcifications), resulting in an acoustic shadow. Among these various echogenic patterns, the most important finding is a hypoechoic PZ lesion.

Several investigators have correlated the ultrasound images with pathologic findings on radical prostatectomy specimens *(42,43)* Lee et al. *(44)*, in the pre-PSA era, investigated tumor echogenicity and demonstrated that the most common appearance for cancer is a hypoechoic lesion in the peripheral zone. A clear understanding of normal sonographic anatomy can be helpful in assessing nonmalignant hypoechoic areas (Fig. 2, Table 2) as well as sonographic findings suggestive of malignancy (Fig. 3, Table 3).

With PSA-based screening and earlier cancer detection, a significant stage migration has occurred, resulting in lower stages and smaller tumor volumes at the time of diagnosis. This has translated into fewer overt abnormal sonographic findings at the time of TRUS-guided biopsy. The sonographic finding of the classic hypoechoic PZ lesion has a sensitivity of cancer detection of 85.5%, specificity of 28.4%, positive predictive value of 29%, negative predictive value of 85.2%, and overall accuracy of

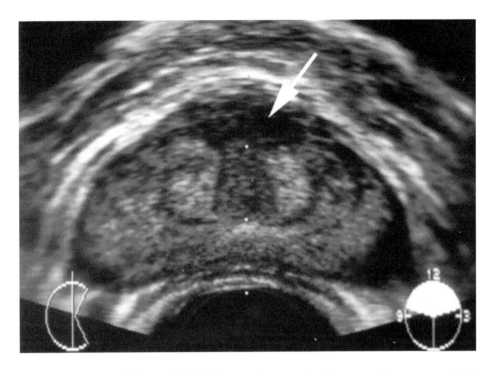

Fig. 2. TRUS. The solid arrow (white) denotes the anterior fibromuscular stroma, which is a normal anatomic structure that can appear hypoechoic.

Table 2
Conditions That May Produce Hypoechoic
Areas in the Prostate

Normal anatomical structure
  Urethra
  Anterior fibromuscular stroma
  Ejaculatory duct complex
  Prostate capsule
  Seminal vesicles ampullae
  Periprostatic veins
  Neurovascular bundle

Benign conditions
  Hyperplasia
  Granulomatous nonspecific prostatitis
  Cysts
  Hematoma

Artifacts
  Inappropriate use of distance gain control adjustment
  Acoustic shadowing
  Edge effect (reflection refraction)
  Reverberation artifact

Prostate cancer

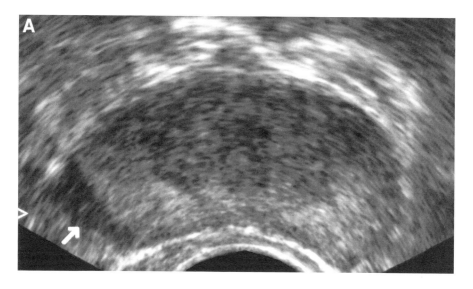

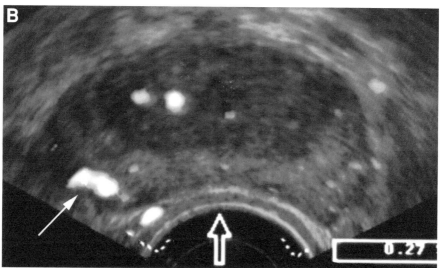

Fig. 3. (A) TRUS. Hypoechoic lesion within the PZ is a concern for prostate cancer (*see* white circled area). **(B)** Hypervascular area seen with color Doppler imaging corresponds to the hypoechoic area seen on the gray-scale ultrasonography.

43% *(45)*. Shinohara et al. and other investigators *(46–48)* have reported the prevalence of isoechoic or nearly invisible prostate cancers on TRUS to range from 25 to 42%. To date, no biologic differences have been noted between isoechoic and hypoechoic prostate cancers.

Color flow Doppler imaging (CDI) is another tool that may be used to improve biopsy performance. Most agree that CDI should not be used alone as a single screening instrument because it misses cancers that would otherwise be detected with systematic TRUS-guided biopsies *(49)*. When CDI is used in combination with gray-scale transrectal ultrasonography, it can enhance prostate cancer detection by 7% to 13%

Table 3
Sonographic Appearance of Confined (Stage A,B or T1: T2)
Not Confined (Stage C or T3:T4) Prostate Cancer

Sonographic appearance

Features	Confined	Not confined
Prostate shape	Symmetrical	Asymmetrical
	Semilunar	Distorted
	Concave posterior outline	Convex posterior outline
Echogenicity	Homogeneous	Diffusely heterogeneous
	± focal hypoecoicity	Large hypoechoic area
Internal anatomy	Preserved	Distorted
Prostate boundary	Clear	Fuzzy
	Smooth	Irregular
	Round	Bulging
		Loss of roundness
		Disruption
Seminal vesicles	Symmetrical	Asymmetrical in shape and echogenicity
	Clear appreciation of ampullae	Unclear ampullae
		Thickened base
	Concave shape	Convex shape
	Fat plane between prostate seminal vesicle	Loss of fat pane between prostate and seminal vesicle
		Abnormal tissue posterior to the ampullae

(50). Shigeno and colleagues *(51)* have shown CDI plus gray-scale ultrasonography to have a sensitivity of 81.2%, specificity of 93%, positive predictive value of 63.7%, and a negative predictive value of 97%. Power Doppler imaging (PDI) is presumably more sensitive than standard CDI because of its ability to detect slow- and low-flow lesions. (17,52) PDI has been reported to have a sensitivity from 74% to 98%, and specificity from 78% to 96% *(17,18,53)*. However, not all investigators have found that PDI is useful in detecting prostate cancer, as evidenced by Halpern and Strup *(49)*, who reported PDI to have a sensitivity of 27% with a specificity of 77.1%.

Intravenous contrast agents are being administered before color or gray-scale to enhance cancer detection with color and gray-scale ultrasonography *(54)*. These microbubble agents have the ability to increase the strength of detected ultrasound echoes by several orders of magnitude and also depict tumor vasculature better than conventional contrast agents *(50,55,56)*. Frauscher and colleagues *(19)* compared CDI plus contrast agent–enhanced targeted biopsy to systematic biopsy performed with gray-scale ultrasonography and found that the overall cancer detection rate was not statistically different (24.4% contrast enhancement vs 22.6% systematic biopsy).

However, when comparing the likelihood of detecting cancer with an individual core biopsy, the contrast enhanced targeted biopsy was 2.6-fold more likely to detect cancer than the systematic biopsy. Also, the cancer detection rate with the contrast-enhanced method was higher if there was only one hypervascular area noted and if multiple biopsies opposed to a single biopsy was taken of the hypervascular area.

Prostate Biopsy

An 18-gage biopsy needle loaded in a spring-action automatic biopsy device is commonly used to procure multiple 1.5-cm prostate biopsy specimens. After the prostate images are obtained, a biopsy reference line is placed onto the suspicious lesion or targeted region (Fig. 4). If the biplanar probe is used, the biopsy is performed in the sagittal view whereas the biopsy can be performed in either the transverse or sagittal view with the end-firing probe. Once the biopsy reference line is positioned, the needle is inserted into the guide and biopsies are then performed. When a biopsy is directed at a suspicious lesion, it is important for the needle tip to be placed precisely at the boundary of the lesion before activating the biopsy gun. This technical point can improve sampling accuracy. If the prostate capsule is "tented up" by the needle tip, tissue may be taken too deep inside the gland and a tumor located in the PZ may be missed. The excursion of the needle tip during a biopsy is approx 2.5 cm and the biopsy notch, which procures the tissue, is approx 1.5 cm. These parameters should be taken into account when performing a prostate needle biopsy.

Complications

Modern TRUS-guided prostate needle biopsy is associated with frequent minor (range 60–79%) and rare major (range 0.4–4.3%) complications, and the need for hospitalization ranges from 0.4 to 3.4% *(57–62)*. Rodriguez and Terris *(63)* performed a prospective study to evaluate the morbidity associated with TRUS-guided prostate needle biopsy. One hundred and twenty-eight patients were enrolled in the study and underwent a TRUS-guided prostate needle biopsy. A procedure questionnaire and a telephone interview (3 to 7 d after biopsy) were used to analyze the immediate and delayed complication rates associated with TRUS-guided prostate biopsy. In their cohort, 135 minor complications occurred in 77 patients and 63.6% of patients had at least one complication. The only major complication, which did require hospitalization, was a vasovagal episode and seizure, which occurred in the same patient during the actual prostate biopsy. The most common complication was persistent hematuria in 47.1% of patients, which lasted 3 to 7 d after the biopsy. Immediate complications of TRUS-guided prostate needle biopsy included a vasovagal episode (5.3%), rectal bleeding (8.3%), and hematuria (70.8%). Delayed complications of TRUS-guided prostate needle biopsy at 3 to 7 d postbiopsy included dysuria (9.1%), vague pelvic discomfort (13.2%), persistent hematuria (47.1%), hematochezia (9.1%), and hematospermia (9.1%).

ANESTHESIA

Systematic sextant TRUS-guided prostate biopsies have traditionally been performed with no form of anesthesia and have been relatively well tolerated *(64–68)*. Recent studies have reported that 65 to 95% of men report some level of discomfort during TRUS-guided prostate needle biopsy *(65,69–71)*. Specifically 10 to 25% of patients undergoing sextant biopsy experience moderate to severe pain *(64,66,72,73)* Pain during a TRUS-guided prostate biopsy predominantly occurs when the needle

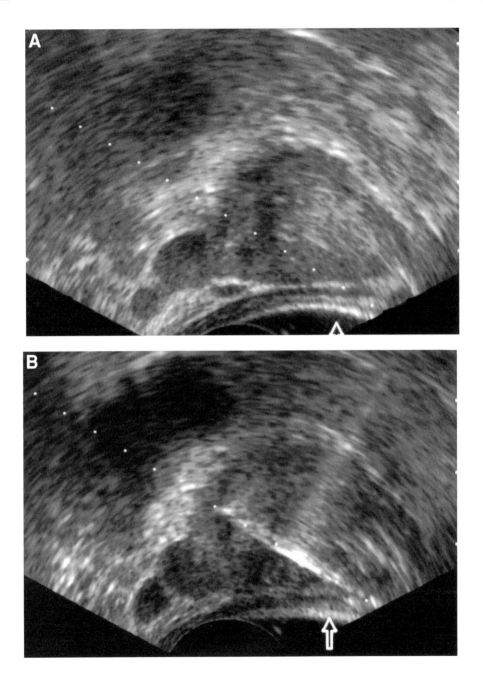

Fig. 4. (A) TRUS image displays the reference guide used during prostate needle biopsy.
(B) Prostate biopsy needle alongside the reference guide after biopsy.

penetrates the prostatic capsule and stroma, which has a rich innervation of autonomic
fibers *(74)* These fibers ramify in the prostatic plexus and course posterolaterally to the
prostate along with the prostatic vascular pedicles. Positioning and maintenance of the
ultrasound probe in the rectum may also contribute to the discomfort generated by the
procedure. Several studies have been performed to evaluate whether local anesthesia is

needed before TRUS-guided prostate needle biopsy. These studies can be categorized as comparing intrarectal lidocaine gel vs no anesthesia, periprostatic anesthesia vs placebo injection, and periprostatic anesthesia vs intrarectal lidocaine gel (Table 4). The visual analog scale (VAS) is commonly used to assess a patient's pain level before and after prostate needle biopsy. The visual analog scale can be marked (numbers) or unmarked. In general, marks toward the right end of the line and higher numbers represent higher amounts of overall pain.

Intrarectal Lidocaine Gel vs No Anesthesia

Desgrandchamps et al. *(72)* performed a prospective randomized placebo-controlled study comparing the efficacy of rectal administration of lidocaine gel vs placebo in the tolerance of TRUS-guided prostate biopsy. Patients were age-matched and had never undergone a previous prostate biopsy. Fifty-six patients were in the lidocaine group and 53 patients in the placebo group. Fifteen milliliters of 2% lidocaine was administered intrarectally by a nurse 15 min before the biopsies were taken in the lidocaine group. Both groups underwent a total of six biopsies with an 18-gage Tru-cut needle. Using a self-administered verbal rating system to report the severity of discomfort, they found no statistically significant difference between the groups pertaining to the severity of pain in those who did and did not receive intrarectally administered lidocaine (moderate to severe pain: 11% placebo group vs 12.5% lidocaine group). Chang et al. *(68)* in a double-blind randomized prospective trial compared the pain level associated with intrarectal 2% lidocaine gel vs a nonanesthetic lubricant gel in men undergoing TRUS-guided prostate needle biopsy. Both groups had a minimum of eight biopsy cores (range 8–13). Using an unmarked horizontal VAS without numbers, they reported no difference in the mean pain scores (lidocaine gel 28.3 vs 28.9 lubricant).

Conversely, Issa et al. *(75)* published the Emory University experience with the administration of intrarectal lidocaine gel vs no anesthesia before prostate needle biopsy. Twenty-five patients were randomized to each group. The anesthesia group received 10 mL of 2% lidocaine gel administered intrarectally. Sextant biopsies were performed in both groups and a 10-point linear VAS was used to assess pain. The lidocaine group had lower mean pain scores (2.5) compared with the control group (4.4). Also, the percentage of patients having a score of 5 (moderate to severe pain) was more frequent in the control group (52%) than the lidocaine group (4%). One potential bias in this study is that although patients were blinded before the biopsy, they were told they received lidocaine after the biopsy and before completing the questionnaire.

Periprostatic Anesthesia vs Placebo

Nash and colleagues *(74)* in 1996 performed a prospective randomized placebo-controlled study evaluating prostatic nerve blockade before TRUS-guided prostate needle biopsy. Thirty-four patients received a periprostatic unilateral injection of 1% lidocaine (5 mL) and 30 patients received a placebo injection of 5 mL of saline. Mean pain scores were significantly lower in the lidocaine group (1.6 ± 0.9) compared with 2.9 ± 1.2 in the placebo group ($p < 0.0001$). Also, 68% of patients who received lidocaine injection reported that they would prefer to receive lidocaine before prostate biopsy.

Table 4
Prospective Randomized Control Studies: Utility of Anesthesia to Reduce Pain in Patients Undergoing TRUS-Guided Prostate Needle Biopsy

Study	Patients (N)	Groups compared	Biopsies (N)	Anesthesia (site of injection)	Pain analog	Benefit to anesthesia
Desgrandchamps et al. (1999) (72)	108	No anesthesia vs intrarectal anesthesia	6	Lidocaine gel 2%(15 mL)	Verbal rating system	No
Chang et al. (2001) (68)	108	Lubricant vs intrarectal anesthesia	8–13	Lidocaine gel 2% (10 mL)	Visual Analog scale	No
Issa et al. (2000) (75)	50	No anesthesia vs intrarectal anesthesia	6	Lidocaine gel 2%(10 mL)	10-point linear VAS	Yes
Nash et al. (1996) (74)	64	Saline vs periprostatic anesthesia	2–6	Lidocaine 1% (5 mL) lateral to the junction between the prostate and seminal vesicle	NA	NA
Wu et al. (2001) (73)	40	Placebo injection vs periprostatic anesthesia	12	Lidocaine 1% (5 mL) lateral to the tip of the seminal vesicle	VAS	No
Pareek et al. (2001) (115)	132	Placebo vs periprostatic anesthesia	6	Lidocaine 1% (2.5 mL) inferolateral to the prostate	10-point linear scale and outpatient questionnaire	Yes
Alavi et al. (2001) (69)	150	Intrarectal anesthesia vs periprostatic anesthesia	6–14 (mean 6.7)	Lidocaine gel 2% (10 mL) vs Lidocaine 1% (10 mL) lateral aspect of the prostate	11-Point Wayne State University VAS	Yes

VRS, verbal rating system; VAS, visual analog scale.

Soloway and Obek *(71)* in 2000 reported his results with a pilot study looking at the ability of local anesthesia injected before prostate biopsy to decrease patient discomfort.

Fifty men were injected with 1% lidocaine without epinephrine before prostate biopsy. A modified technique of Nash and Shinohara was used and 1% lidocaine was injected at three locations along the lateral aspect of the prostate in the region of the neurovascular bundle. In this group of 50 men, all men who had undergone a previous biopsy, a significant reduction in pain was noted in patients that received the anesthetic before biopsy. The authors concluded that this technique had little morbidity and dramatically improved patient comfort associated with prostate biopsy *(74)*.

Wu et al. *(73)* performed a prospective randomized double-blinded study comparing the effect of local anesthetic injected before TRUS-guided prostate needle biopsy. One group received a 5-mL injection of 1% lidocaine directly lateral to the tip of the seminal vesicles on each side and the other group (placebo) received a 5-mL injection of sterile normal saline. A VAS for pain at rest and with activity was obtained at three time points: preprocedure, immediately after the procedure (representing intraprocedural pain level), and at 30 min postprocedure. They found no significant differences between the groups with regard to VAS pain scores at rest or activity over each time point. Although not statistically significant ($p = 0.16$) the placebo group did have a higher intraprocedure VAS score associated with activity (2.3 ± 2.6) compared with the local anesthetic group (1.5 ± 1.7). They concluded that lidocaine injection before prostate needle biopsy did not diminish biopsy-associated VAS pain at rest or with activity during and immediately after the procedure. Their results were similar to Naughton et al. *(67)*, who noted a mean pain score of 3 of 10 in 80 men undergoing either 6- or 12-score prostate biopsies. In contrast, their results were different than Nash et al. *(74)* and Soloway et al. *(71)*, who concluded that periprostatic injection of local anesthesia did result in lower pain associated with prostate needle biopsy.

Periprostatic Anesthesia vs Intrarectal Lidocaine Gel

Alvavi and Soloway et al. prospectively compared the efficacy of periprostatic lidocaine injection under ultrasound guidance with instillation of lidocaine gel in the rectum before TRUS-guided prostate biopsy.

Group 1 received 10 mL of 1% lidocaine injected bilaterally into the periprostatic nerve plexus, located along the lateral aspect of the prostate. Group 2 received 10 mL of 2% turboject lidocaine gel (IMS, El Monte, CA) intrarectally 10 min before the procedure. Each group received 6 to 14 biopsies (mean 6.8 for group 1 and 6.6 for group 2). Seventy-five equally matched patients were randomized into each group and the 11-point Wayne State University visual analog scale (0, no discomfort to 10, the most severe discomfort) was used to evaluate the overall pain scale. There was a statistically significant difference favoring group 1 (mean pain score 2.4 group 1 vs 3.7 group 2). Also, the percentage of patients having a pain score less than 5 (mild pain) occurred more frequently in group 1 (85.3%) than group 2 (61.3%).

At our institution, we apply a topical anesthetic Hurricaine® gel as lubricant at the time of the DRE. Clinically, this seems to make the transrectal probe insertion less painful for the patient. After the prostate gland has been completely imaged (transaxial and sagittal planes) and the prostate volume has been calculated, we then inject a total of 10 mL of 1% lidocaine into the prostate gland at the lateral edge and anesthetize the gland on each side from the base to the apex.

Although no consensus regarding the use of anesthesia before prostate biopsy has been reached, possible explanations for the discrepancies seen in the various studies include different prebiopsy pain levels (e.g., VAS scale), different sites of anesthetic injection (tip of seminal vesicle vs length of the periprostatic nerve plexus), and the amount of anesthetic injected.

PROSTATE NEEDLE BIOPSY SCHEMES: SEXTANT AND ALTERNATE BIOPSY TEMPLATES

Before the widespread use of TRUS, DRE-guided prostate needle biopsy was performed to make the diagnosis of prostate cancer. In an attempt to improve the efficacy of prostate cancer detection, TRUS and eventually TRUS-guided prostate needle biopsy was instituted as a part of the urologic evaluation for prostate cancer.

Lee et al. *(76)* in a screening cohort of 784 men noted that TRUS-guided biopsy was twice as sensitive as DRE-guided biopsy for detecting prostate cancer. Hodge and associates *(77)* reported data on 43 patients who had an abnormal DRE and had a negative DRE-guided prostate biopsy. In this cohort, a repeat TRUS-guided prostate biopsy was performed and cancer was detected in 53% of the patients with previously negative DRE-guided biopsies. It was concluded from this study that TRUS-guided biopsy sampled malignant areas of palpably abnormal prostates that would have been missed with DRE-guided biopsy alone. Likewise, the Mayo Clinic series included 347 patients who were referred for an abnormal DRE. TRUS-guided prostate biopsy detected cancers in 25% of patients who had negative DRE-guided prostate biopsies *(78)*.

Sextant Biopsy Template

Hodge et al. *(5)* in 1989 proposed a systematic prostate biopsy technique to improve the diagnostic yield of TRUS-guided prostate biopsy. TRUS-guided biopsies were performed in the parasagittal plane and bilateral peripheral zone biopsies were obtained from the base, midgland, and the apex (sextant biopsy template)

In this study, Hodge and colleagues performed directed biopsies of specific hypoechoic areas and systematic sextant biopsies in 136 patients with abnormal DREs. Sixty-eight percent of patients had a clinical stage stage B (T2) and PSA values were not reported. In 79 patients at least one and usually several of the systematic biopsies were in close proximity to hypoechoic areas. Prostate cancer was detected in 83 of 136 patients (62%). The systematic biopsy method detected 96% of the cancers, and the lesion directed method detected only 4% of unique cancers. In 57 patients, a suspicious hypoechoic area was located outside of the midlobe parasagittal plane of systematic biopsy. Both systematic and lesion directed biopsies were performed in this group of patients. Nine percent of cancers detected by the systematic method were missed by the lesion directed biopsy method, and 5% of cancers detected by the lesion directed method were missed by the systematic biopsies *(5)*.

Clinically, the sampling error of the sextant biopsy template has been evident by the 20% to 30% cancer detection rate in men undergoing a repeat transrectal ultrasound guided biopsy *(9,79)*. This has lead investigators to question the sampling adequacy of the sextant prostate biopsy template and to propose alternate biopsy schemes to improve prostate cancer detection. The alternate prostate biopsy templates aim to improve sampling of the prostate by either increasing the number of core biopsies taken and/or by

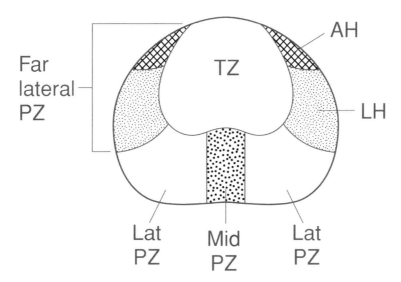

Fig. 5. Cross-sectional view of commonly biopsied zones. TZ, transition zone; PZ, peripheral zone; Mid PZ, midperipheral zone; Lat PZ, lateral peripheral zone; AH, anterior horn; LH, lateral horn.

directing the biopsies more laterally to better sample the anterior horn (the far lateral regions of the peripheral zone) as recommended by Stamey *(10)*.

Computer Models for Prostate Biopsy Optimization

Chen et al. *(80)* developed a stochastic (Monte-Carlo) computer simulation model of ultrasound guided biopsies using mathematically reconstructed radical prostatectomy specimens. Simulated biopsies were analyzed for 180 prostates and cancer detection by biopsy was considered reliable if 90% of the simulation runs for each prostate were positive for cancer. In prostate models with tumor volume >0.5 cc, 27.2% of cancers were not reliably detected with sextant biopsy (fewer than 90% of the simulations were positive). The areas that were inadequately sampled by sextant biopsy were the anterior TZ, midline PZ, and the inferior portion of the anterior horn of the PZ (laterally directed biopsies) (Fig. 5). If the biopsy template was expanded to include these areas, then cancers >0.5 cc volume could be reliably detected in 70% of the cases. Based on these findings they recommended a 10-biopsy template that sampled two cores each from the apex, the base, the inferior portion of the anterior horn, the midline PZ, and two cores from the anterior TZ. The biopsies from the apex and base are identical to the routine sextant biopsies and the inferior portion of the anterior horn biopsies replaced the sextant midlobar biopsies. With the 10-biopsy template cancer detection increased to 96% in tumors with volumes >0.5 cc compared with 73% with the sextant biopsy scheme.

Egevad et al. *(81)* compared the sextant biopsy template to a 10-biopsy template using a computer program for three-dimensional (3D) modeling of prostate cancer. Eighty-one men (57% with abnormal DRE) were found to have prostate cancer after a TRUS-guided prostate needle biopsy and subsequently underwent radical prostatectomy. The biopsy template used to establish the 3D prostate cancer model included the routine sextant TRUS biopsy protocol in addition to biopsies targeting the midlateral and the TZ. After step-sectioning radical prostatectomy specimens, a 3D reconstructed prostate with prostate cancer was developed using previously described 3D computer software program *(82)*. A virtual sextant and 10-biopsy template was compared for cancer detection and tumor volume. The simulated 10-biopsy template detected 82.7% of cancers.

Twenty-four percent (16 of 67) of cancers that were detected with the 10-biopsy template would have gone undetected with the sextant biopsy template. In all 16 cases, at least one of the midlateral biopsies was positive, and in seven, a TZ biopsy was also positive. Thus, few additional cancers were detected exclusively with TZ biopsies. Additionally, 14 of 16 of the missed cancers were larger than 1 mL, indicating that sextant biopsies could miss clinically significant cancers. Although the simulated 10-biopsy template outperformed the sextant biopsy method, it missed 14 cancers. Ten of these cancers were <1.5 mL, and four were located in the TZ.

Extensive Biopsy Protocols

Not all extensive biopsy templates are the same. Therefore, it is not surprising that some authors have reported improved cancer detection with extensive biopsy templates whereas others have not (Table 5). Another consideration when interpreting the literature is whether overall cancer detection rates are reported or if a subgroup analysis of the percentage of cancers detected (sensitivity) that were diagnosed by the new biopsy template is reported.

Extensive biopsy templates can be categorized in the following ways: 1) increasing the number of biopsies only or 2) directing peripheral zone biopsies more laterally. Additionally, several different lateral PZ-extensive biopsy protocols have been evaluated to optimize prostate biopsy strategies.

Increasing the Number of Biopsies Only

Hodge originally suggested that three biopsies be obtained from each lobe at points 1 cm apart.

The biopsy template used did not sample the TZ and was not optimal for sampling the PZ. This template in its original presentation had an overall cancer detection rate of 62%. However, no PSA values were reported in this study and the higher overall cancer detection rate in this series is most likely secondary to the high percentage of patients with palpable (T2) disease (68%). In the PSA era, multiple studies have shown the sextant biopsy template to have an overall cancer detection rate of 20% to 36% *(13,83–88)* Levine and colleagues *(86)* investigated the role of performing two consecutive TRUS-guided sextant biopsies in a single office visit. A total of 137 patients undergoing their first prostate needle biopsy were enrolled in this study. No modifications were made in the standard sextant biopsy template and the mid-PZ was the area sampled. The overall cancer detection rate was 31%. The second set of sextant biopsies exclusively detected 13 cancers, which improved the cancer detection rate by 30%.

Naughton and colleagues *(87)* randomized 244 patients to receive 6 or 12 TRUS-guided prostate needle biopsies to analyze whether doubling the number of sextant biopsies improved cancer detection. The biopsy template used in this study included the standard sextant biopsy (six-biopsy arm) compared to a 12-biopsy template. The

Table 5
Clinical Studies Comparing Different Biopsy Templates Prostate Cancer Detection in Patients Undergoing Their First Prostate Needle Biopsy

Study	Patients (N)	Biopsy category	Biopsies (N)	Overall caner detection rate	% cancer detection (sextant biopsy)	Additional cancers detected by extended biopsy template (%)
Hodge et al. (1989) (5)	136	Mid PZ	6–11	Sextant: 61%[a]	96%	NA
Levine et al. (1998) (86)	137	Increase biopsy number	12	Sextant: 22%	70%	Twelve: 30%
				Twelve: 31%		
Naughton et al. (2000) (87)	244	Increase biopsy number	6 vs 12	Sextant: 26%	79%	Twelve: 21%
				Twelve: 27%		
Ravery et al. (2000) (83)	303	Lateral PZ	10–12	Sextant: 32%	83%	Extensive:17%
				Extensive: 39%		
Gore et al. (2001) (85)	104	Lateral PZ	10–12	Sextant: 31%	71%	Eight: 25%
				Eight: 41%		Ten: 29%
				Ten: 43%		Twelve: 29%
				Twelve: 43%		
Chang et al. (1998)	273	Lateral PZ	10	Sextant: 36%	82%	Ten: 14%
				Ten: 43%		
Eskew et al. (1997) (11)	119	Lateral PZ	18[b]	Sextant: 26%	65%	5-Region: 35%
				5-Region: 40%		
Presti et al. (2000) (13)	483	Lateral PZ	6–10	Sextant: 33%	80%	Eight: 15%
				Eight: 40%		Ten: 16%
				Ten: 40%		
Babian et al. (2001) (88)	362[c]	Lateral PZ	11	Sextant: 20%	67%	Eleven: 33%
				Eleven: 30%		

[a]All patients had abnormal palpable DRE.
[b]Mean number of biopsies.
[c]Study included patients undergoing an initial repeat prostate needle biopsies.

additional six biopsies in the 12-core biopsy template were directed slightly more later-ally than the original sextant biopsies. In this template the "far" lateral PZ and TZ were not sampled. In these two matched groups, the overall cancer detection rate was not significantly different between the two groups (26% for the six-core group vs 27% for the 12-core group). Although the 12-core biopsies did not improve overall cancer detec-tion, the additional biopsies in this group exclusively detected 7 of 33 cancers (21%). One possible explanation for the equivalent cancer detection rates, as mentioned by the authors, is that inadvertently the original sextant biopsies may have been directed more laterally. It is also possible that the extra biopsies, although being laterally directed, were not targeting the anterior horns in the PZ.

Ravery and colleagues *(89)* analyzed the diagnostic value of ten systematic TRUS-guided prostate needle biopsies. (89) One hundred and sixty-two patients underwent five biopsies from each side of the prostate. All biopsies were performed in the same plane as the standard sextant biopsy, and no changes were made in the angle of the biopsy needle. The overall cancer detection rate was 40% but the overall improvement in cancer detection with the additional biopsies was only 3.1%. The authors concluded that increasing the number of biopsy cores alone did not improve overall cancer detec-tion and that additional alterations such as zones sampled and biopsy angle are needed to improve cancer detection.

Laterally Directed PZ Biopsy Templates

Detailed histologic studies have shown that approx 68% of prostate cancers arise from the PZ. By performing prostate biopsies in the midlobe parasagittal plane (sextant method), the needle trajectory often passes through both the PZ and TZ. Laterally directed PZ zone biopsy templates are modifications of the original sextant biopsy template to increase sampling of the lateral aspect of the PZ.

Stamey *(10)* reported that prostate cancer tends to spread in a transverse direction more than a posterior–anterior extension. PZ tumors (94%) spread transversely along the prostatic capsule. In 1995, Stamey recommended that the original sextant biopsies be moved more laterally to improve TRUS-guided prostate cancer detection.

Ravery et al. *(83)* prospectively performed an extensive biopsy protocol in 303 patients. The mean PSA in this group of patients was 11.3 ng/mL (monoclonal Tosoh assay, Foster City, CA). At least 10 biopsies were performed in each patient. The biopsy template included a standard sextant biopsy template, performed at a 45° angle, plus lateral peripherally directed biopsies. The peripherally directed biopsies were modified based upon the size of the prostate gland. In cases of prostate volume <50 cm^3 a peripheral biopsy at a 30-degree angle was obtained on each side at the base and middle of the lobe. In cases of prostate volume >50 cm^3 an additional biopsy was ob-tained at the periphery of the apex bilaterally, increasing the total number of biopsies to 12. Using this biopsy protocol, prostate cancer was detected in 118 cases (38.9%). The extensive biopsy protocol detected 20 additional cancers, which improved the cancer detection rate by 17%. The performance of this extensive biopsy protocol was also analyzed in its ability to improve cancer detection in patients with PSA <10 ng/mL. In this subgroup, the cancer detection rate was increased by 21.7%. Also, in patients with a prostate volume >50 cm^3, the cancer detection rate was improved by 29.4%. The authors concluded that an extensive biopsy protocol improves cancer detection in men with PSA <10 ng/mL, with a normal DRE, and in men with a prostate gland exceeding 50 cc in size.

Gore and colleagues *(85)* reported their experience with laterally directed prostate needle biopsies to improve overall prostate cancer detection. Three hundred and ninety six patients underwent systematic sextant biopsy with additional laterally directed biopsies. In this study 66.7% (*n*=264) patients had not been previously biopsied, 28% (*n*=111) had previously undergone at least one biopsy, and 5.3% (*n*=21) patients had previously diagnosed prostate cancer and were undergoing a staging biopsy. The biopsy template included a standard sextant biopsy plus four laterally directed PZ biopsies (base and midgland) in 396 patients. A subset of 178 patients underwent a total of 12-core biopsies, which added two additional laterally directed biopsies (apex) to the biopsy template. The overall cancer detection rate in this group of 178 patients using the standard sextant biopsy template was 26.4% compared with 37.6% and 38.2% for the 10-core and 12-core biopsy methods, respectively. In patients undergoing their first prostate needle biopsy the overall cancer detection rate was higher with the extensive biopsy templates (30.8% for sextant and 43.3% for 10- or 12-core biopsies). An analysis of the percentage of cancer detected by specific core biopsy sites showed the highest cancer detection rates in cores taken from the lateral apex and lateral base. The sextant midgland biopsy had the lowest cancer detection rate. The authors emphasized the importance of adequately sampling the prostatic apex and base in any biopsy template, as well as performing laterally directed prostate needle biopsies in this area.

Chang and colleagues *(84)* prospectively evaluated the addition of four laterally directed PZ biopsies to improve prostate cancer detection. Two hundred and seventy-three patients were biopsied with this template and the overall cancer detection rate was 44%. Sextant biopsy detected 99 of the 121 diagnosed cancers for a sensitivity of 82%. The laterally directed biopsies had a sensitivity of 70% alone, and when both templates were combined the sensitivity was increased to 96%. Four percent of cancers were detected exclusively in the transition zone. The authors concluded that laterally directed biopsies have a higher sensitivity and emphasized the importance of biopsy location opposed to strictly increasing the number of biopsies alone.

Strategies to Optimize Prostate Biopsy Templates

It is known from the work of McNeal and colleagues that most prostate cancers arise from the PZ and, therefore, contemporary biopsy templates are being modeled to sample this area more effectively.

Some of the pitfalls in terms of cancer detection by biopsy site can be explained by the prostatic zonal anatomy. For example, at the prostate base lateral biopsies will sample the PZ, whereas medially directed biopsies are more likely to sample the CZ, a zone that rarely develops prostate cancer. In the midgland, especially in patients with significant benign prostatic hypertrophy, a medially directed biopsy in this area can traverse the PZ and predominantly sample the TZ. If biopsies in this area are directed laterally, the so-called anterior horns of the PZ are more likely to be sampled because they wrap around the TZ in this area. Biopsies directed at the prostatic apex have a higher detection rate for prostate cancer because this area is composed entirely of PZ.

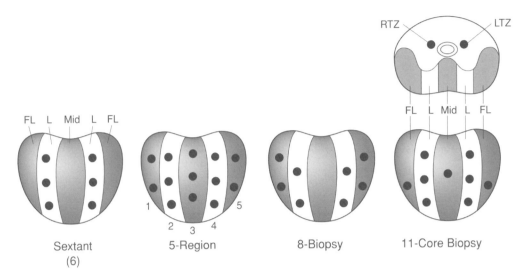

Fig. 6. Popular biopsy strategies to optimize prostate cancer detection. Contemporary sextant biopsy template, five-region biopsy template, right-systematic biopsy template and the 11-core multisite-directed biopsy template. FL, far lateral PZ; L, lateral PZ; Mid, mid-PZ; RTZ, right TZ; LTZ, left TZ. Gary D. Grossfeld MD: Transrectal ultrasound guided prostate biopsy.

Carefully directed apical biopsies can also sample the distal aspect of the TZ. Three popularized methods for optimizing the number and location prostate needle biopsies are the five-region, eight systematic-core template and the 11-multisite biopsy protocol (Fig. 6).

Five-Region Systematic Prostate Biopsy Template

Eskew et al. *(11)* prospectively evaluated a five-region prostate biopsy template for its ability to increase the detection of prostate cancer *(11)*. One hundred nineteen patients underwent the five-region biopsy template. The biopsies were taken from the standard sextant locations (zones 2, 4), from the midline (zone 3), and from the far lateral peripheral zone (zones 1, 5). The average number of biopsies taken was 18 (minimum of 13). The overall cancer detection rate was 40%. The additional region 1, 3, and 5 biopsies detected 35% of cancers that would have been missed with the sextant biopsy template alone. Interestingly, 88% of the additionally detected cancers with the region 1, 3, and 5 biopsies were in regions 1 and 5 (far lateral lobes). A total of 28 cancers (59%) were detected in the two different zones (zones 2, 4 and zones 1, 3, 5) simultaneously. The five-region technique appeared most effective for patients with a serum PSA level <10 ng/mL. In these patients, 54% of cancers were diagnosed with the five-region technique and not the standard sextant biopsies. In contrast, for patients with a serum PSA level >10 ng/mL, only 10% of cancers were diagnosed exclusively with the five-region technique. Similarly, Ravery and colleagues *(83)* found that an extensive biopsy template improved overall cancer detection less significantly in patients with a PSA >10 ng/mL than in patients with PSA <10 ng/mL (12.7% vs 21.7%) *(83)*. The findings of each group of investigators is consistent with other reports of improved cancer detection rates with increasing PSA levels and suggests that the routine sextant biopsy methods may miss fewer cancers when the PSA level is >10 ng/mL.

Eight Systematic Prostate Biopsy Template

Presti et al. *(13)* in a prospective clinical trial compared the cancer detection efficacy of the standard sextant biopsy template with a 10-core biopsy template. Four hundred eighty-three patients with a PSA 4.0 ng/mL and/or an abnormal DRE who had never undergone a previous TRUS-guided prostate needle biopsy were studied. The 10-core biopsy template included the standard sextant biopsy plus two laterally directed PZ biopsies on each side (lateral midlobar and lateral base lobar). This method was similar to the five-region biopsy template with the exception that midline biopsies were eliminated. Forty-four percent of patients had positive biopsies for prostate cancer. Various sextant and extended (>6) biopsy templates were analyzed for their overall cancer detection ability. The routine sextant biopsies detected 79.7% of all cancers compared with 88.6% when a laterally directed sextant biopsy template was used (lateral mid- and lateral-base biopsies). In the extended biopsy templates, multiple eight-biopsy templates were compared with the 10-biopsy template. The best performing eight-biopsy template included biopsies directed at the apex, midgland, lateral midgland, lateral base, and excluded the midbase biopsies. The overall cancer detection rate with this eight-biopsy template was 94.6% compared with 96% with the 10-biopsy template. In this study, the standard midlobar base biopsy had the lowest unique cancer detection rate (1%) and was excluded from their optimal eight-biopsy template. One explanation for the low detection rate in this area is that this biopsy may be sampling the CZ, which has a low incidence of prostate cancer. The authors concluded that six systematic biopsies of the PZ were inadequate and that a minimum of eight biopsies with more extensive sampling of the lateral aspects of the PZ should routinely be performed. Interestingly, in a subgroup analysis among the different sextant biopsy templates, the cancer detection rates were significantly higher in the laterally directed biopsy templates in patients with PSA <10 ng/mL (89.6 vs 74.8%) and/or prostate volumes >50 cc (80 vs 65.4%).

Eleven-Core Multisite-Directed Biopsy Template

Babian and colleagues *(88)* reported their experience with an 11-core multisite-directed biopsy strategy. The idea and design for the study was a result of the findings reported by Chen et al. *(80,90)* in which a stochastic computer simulation model was used to improve the accuracy of prostate biopsy to detect prostate cancer. The 11-core multisite-directed biopsy strategy was evaluated at two medical centers: M.D. Anderson and Toronto General Hospital. A total of 362 men underwent this prostate biopsy template, 183 at M.D. Anderson (mean PSA 8.3 ng/mL) and 179 at Toronto General Hospital (mean PSA 12.0 ng/mL). In this group of patients, 277 were undergoing a repeat prostate needle biopsy. The biopsy template included the standard sextant biopsies as well as a midline biopsy, TZ, and anterior horn biopsies on each side. The anterior horn biopsy represents extreme lateral and anterior PZ tissue. The 11-core multisite biopsy template had a higher overall cancer detection rate than the standard sextant biopsy template (30 vs 20%). The 11-core multisite biopsy template detected 33% additional cancers. The anterior horn was the most common positive alternate biopsy site followed by the TZ and midline biopsy site. The 11-core biopsy template showed statistically significant improvement in cancer detection over the standard sextant biopsy template when the patient had a PSA 4–10 ng/mL, normal digital rectal exam, a normal transrectal ultrasound and a PSA density 0.16.

Insignificant vs Significant Cancer Detection in Extensive Biopsy Templates

In the literature, up to 31% of all nonpalpable prostate cancers (stage T1c) that are diagnosed with needle biopsy and treated with radical prostatectomy are so-called insignificant tumors with volumes less than 0.5 cc *(91–93)*. Therefore, a justifiable concern as the numbers of biopsies are increased is whether the incidence of insignificant tumors will be increased. Chan et al. *(94)* specifically addressed this question in a recent study *(94)*. They retrospectively reviewed the number of "insignificant" prostate cancers detected in 297 patients who had a different number of biopsy cores taken during TRUS-guided prostate needle biopsy. Patients were classified as having six cores or less (17.1%), eight cores or less (36%), nine cores or greater (64%), and 12 cores or greater (48.8%). Overall, 75.6% of the tumors detected were clinically significant. When the results were analyzed by the number of biopsies taken no significant difference in the percentage of insignificant tumors detected was noted (six cores or less, 27.5%; eight cores or less, 22.6%; nine cores or greater, 25.4%; and 12 cores or greater, 27.8%.

Repeat Prostate Needle Biopsy

Clinicians are commonly faced with the dilemma of how to manage the patient who has a negative prostate needle biopsy but whose clinical history is suggestive of prostate cancer. Ellis and Brawer *(95)* specifically addressed the issue of who benefits from a repeat prostate needle biopsy. They retrospectively reviewed the records of 100 consecutive repeat prostate needle biopsies after an initial negative prostate biopsy to develop indications for repeat prostate needle biopsy. Cancer was detected in 20% of repeat biopsies. The main indications for repeat prostate needle biopsy were glandular atypia or high-grade prostate intraepithelial neoplasia on the initial biopsy. Other indications included a change in DRE, persistently elevated PSA, and/or PSA velocity >25%/yr or median increase >0.72 ng/mL/yr.

Djavan et al. *(96)* performed a prospectively designed study to evaluate predictors of prostate cancer detection on repeat prostate biopsy. Eight hundred twenty patients with a PSA ranging from 4–10 ng/mL had an initial negative prostate needle biopsy and were rebiopsied 6 wk later. The repeat biopsy template included the standard sextant biopsy template plus two transition zone biopsies. Overall cancer detection in this repeat biopsy cohort was 10%. The optimal predictors to help determine whether a patient should undergo a repeat prostate needle biopsy included percent-free PSA <30% and TZ PSA density 0.26 ng/mL/cc. The authors concluded that using these two parameters could increase the number of men in whom rebiopsy could be safely avoided.

The overall cancer detection rates for patients undergoing repeat prostate needle biopsy with various biopsy templates ranges from 10 to 38% *(9,79,88,95–99)*. Stewart and colleagues *(97)* retrospectively analyzed 224 patients that underwent a repeat biopsy using the saturation biopsy technique. An inward radial step biopsy method was used, and a mean of 23 core biopsies were obtained at each biopsy. Patients required intravenous or general anesthesia, and the overall cancer detection rate was 34%. The overall complication rate was 12%, and 5% of patients required overnight hospitalization for hematuria. The incidence of insignificant cancer at radical prostatectomy detected by saturation biopsy increased from 11.1 to 15.4 to 22.2% in patients with one, two, or three or more previous negative biopsies, respectively. In contrast with other studies, the incidence of cancer detection with the saturation biopsy technique did not decrease based upon the total number of previous sextant biopsies. Keetch et al. *(9)* interestingly looked at the number of cancers detected in 1136 men who underwent serial prostate needle biopsies every 6 mo. Four to six core biopsies were taken in this study. They found that 96% of the cancers diagnosed were detected within the first or second prostate needle biopsy setting.

Park and colleagues *(34)* analyzed clinical variables to predict prostate cancer detection on repeat biopsy in 88 patients with high-grade PIN or atypia on initial biopsy *(34)*. Fifty-one percent of men in this study were found to have cancer on rebiopsy. Multivariate analysis demonstrated that an abnormal digital rectal examination and increasing patient age were independent predictors of cancer in patients previously diagnosed with atypia. The authors were unable to identify significant predictors of cancer for those initially diagnosed with high-grade PIN. For patients with atypia or high-grade PIN, the rebiopsy strategy should focus on the site of the initial abnormal biopsy area. However, the yield of cancer detection is improved by sampling adjacent areas and remote sites (10 to 12% of cancer discovered at remote sites).

Value of TZ Biopsies

Although the majority of prostate cancer arises in the PZ, approx 24% of prostate carcinomas originate in the TZ. Lui et al. *(100)* performed six TZ biopsies in addition to the standard sextant biopsy template in four different categories of men undergoing prostate needle biopsy. The transition zone biopsies exclusively detected 26% of cancers in patients undergoing repeat prostate needle biopsy. This cancer-specific detection rate is higher than most series and may be related to the higher PSA levels in this group of patients. Fleshner et al. *(101)* retrospectively reviewed the indications for TZ biopsies in 185 patients. TZ biopsies were performed in three groups of patients: patients with PSA elevation only, patients with hypoechoic TZ lesions, and patients with a previously negative TRUS-guided prostate needle biopsy. The TZ biopsies exclusively detected no cancers in the first two groups but detected 16% of cancers in the repeat biopsy group. The authors concluded that men with previously negative PZ biopsies and persistently elevated PSA would be the best candidates to undergo TZ biopsies in addition to standard PZ biopsies. Keetch and Catalona *(102)* reported that 89% of cancers originated in the PZ. They concluded that undetected cancer in the TZ is seldom the cause of a persistently elevated PSA. Bazinet and colleagues *(103)* prospectively evaluated the value of TZ biopsies for the detection of early prostate cancer. The overall cancer detection rate was 32.9%. They found that although a substantial amount of patients harbor disease in the transition zone (24.4%), the majority of these patients have coexistent disease in the PZ that is detected with PZ biopsies. There were only a small number of cancers (2.9%) detected in TZ biopsies alone. Because of such a low detection rate, the authors recommended that TZ biopsies be omitted in the early detection of prostate cancer.

Chang et al. *(84)* prospectively evaluated the performance of TZ biopsies in prostates > 50 cc in volume. In this group of patients undergoing an initial prostate needle biopsy, a total of 12-core biopsies (six TZ–core biopsies) were performed. In 30

Table 6
Clinical Studies Comparing the Prostate Cancer Diagnostic Yield of TZ Biopsies

Study	Patients (*N*)	TZ biopsies (*N*)	Overall cancer detection rate	% cancer detection (PZ biopsy) (%)	Additional cancers detected by TZ biopsy
Lui et al. (1995) *(100)*	187	6	39%	74%	26%
Fleshner et al. (1997) *(101)*	185	2–6	31%	86%	14%
Keetch et al. (1995) *(102)*	166	4	11%	89%	11%
Bazinet et al. (1996) *(103)*	847	2	33%	97%	3%
Chang et al. (1998) *(84)*	213	6	26%	87%	13%
Terris et al. (1997) *(106)*	161	1–3	34%	98%	2%

patients with positive TZ biopsies, the individual sector results of the PZ biopsy were compared with the TZ biopsy. The PZ biopsy was positive in 43 of the 66 sectors in which the TZ biopsy was positive. Therefore, the PZ biopsy was positive 65% of the time in detecting prostate cancer in the sectors in which the TZ biopsy was positive. One explanation for this phenomenon is that the distal excursion of the needle during PZ biopsy may be sampling the TZ as well. Table 6 summarizes the diagnostic yield of transition zone biopsies among contemporary series.

In a computer model, Chen et al. *(90)* found that the cancer detection rate from TZ biopsies was the highest when the biopsy needle was inserted to a depth of 3 cm before firing the biopsy gun.

The use of transurethral resection of the prostate (TURP) to diagnose prostate carcinoma in patients with a persistently elevated PSA and a previously negative TRUS-guided prostate biopsy is controversial. Rovner et al. *(104)* retrospectively analyzed 71 patients with a previous negative prostate needle biopsy who underwent transurethral biopsy in conjunction with repeat TRUS-guided prostate needle biopsy. A four-quadrant transurethral sampling of the prostatic fossa was performed followed by repeat sextant prostate needle biopsies (mean number of biopsies = 12.3). They resected an average of 1.47 g of tissue and cancer was detected in two patients using the transurethral biopsy method, for an overall detection rate of 2.8%. Both patients also had prostate cancer detected using the TRUS-guided prostate needle biopsy and the authors concluded that transurethral biopsy was of minimal value and not warranted.

Niesel et al. *(105)* analyzed the utility of peripheral zone biopsies to exclude prostate cancer in 132 patients undergoing a TURP for obstructive voiding symptoms. This group of patients had not undergone previous prostate needle biopsy and their mean prostate volume was 80 cc. Before TURP, a minimum of six core needle biopsies was obtained. As a secondary analysis, the authors looked at the cancer detection ability of TURP compared with systematic biopsies. The overall cancer detection rate was 20.5%. Of the 27 cancers detected, 15 cancers were detected by both TURP and needle biopsy methods whereas TURP alone detected 11 cancers. The authors concluded that although TRUS-guided needle biopsy remains the standard to diagnose prostate cancer, they would consider performing a TURP to diagnose and relieve obstructive voiding symptoms in patients with two previously negative TRUS-guided prostate needle biopsies that sampled both the peripheral and transition zones.

In summary, the overall increase in cancer detection using TZ biopsies ranges from 0.9% to 4.3% *(84,100–103,106)*. Therefore, there is little data supporting the routine use of TZ biopsies in the initial prostate biopsy template. The highest yield in prostate cancer detection was in men with persistently elevated PSA undergoing repeat prostate needle biopsy. Thus, TZ biopsies may be beneficial in this subgroup of patients.

Prostate Cancer Detection and the Impact of Prostate Gland Size

Alternate biopsy schemes, as mentioned previously have been implemented to improve sampling of the prostate gland and to improve the cancer detection rate of TRUS-guided prostate needle biopsy. An additional factor that can impact on TRUS-guided prostate cancer detection is the size of the prostate gland.

Uzzo and colleagues *(107)* retrospectively reviewed the TRUS-guided sextant biopsy cancer detection rate in 1021 patients to determine whether cancer detection was varied based on prostate size. Patients were categorized based upon prostate size >50 cc volume (large gland) and <50 cc volume (small gland). The overall cancer detection rate in this cohort was 33%. The cancer detection rate was 38% in the small gland group compared with 23% in the large gland group ($p < 0.01$). A secondary analysis in patients with very large glands (>100 cc) and smaller glands (<25 cc) had a cancer detection rate of 14 and 49%, respectively.

Epstein and colleagues *(108)* retrospectively analyzed the relationship between prostate gland volume and the frequency of previous negative prostate needle biopsies in patients who eventually underwent surgery for prostate cancer. Of 395 men who underwent radical prostatectomy for T1c disease, 74 patients had at least one previous negative prostate needle biopsy. In this group of patients, the likelihood of a previous negative biopsy was 32.5% in men with a prostate volume of 75 cc compared with 15.2% in patients with a prostate volume < 75 cc.

Letran and colleagues *(109)* reviewed the impact of prostate gland volume on prostate cancer detection in 1057 patients The overall cancer detection rate was 30.8% in this cohort. The authors found no relationship between cancer yield and prostate size in glands less than 55.6 cc. In patients with total gland size >55.6 cc and peripheral zone size >33.61 cc, there was a statistically significant decrease in cancer detection. The authors concluded that although the cancer detection rate is lower in larger glands that no optimal number of biopsies has been established for larger glands.

Vashi and colleagues *(110)* developed a mathematical model to determine the appropriate number of cores per prostate biopsy based on patient age and gland volume (Table 7). Life-threatening tumor volumes were based on patient age at diagnosis (life expectancy) as well as prostate cancer doubling time, with different cancer doubling times taken into account, ranging from 3 to 6 yr. The authors concluded that the standard sextant prostate needle biopsy was optimal in only a minority of patients and in the majority of cases it provided under sampling for the detection of clinically significant prostate cancer.

Table 7
**Recommended Number of Cores Per Prostate Biopsy Based
on Patient Age and Gland Volume (110)**

Prostate size (cc)	Patient age (years)					
	50	55	60	65	70	75
10	8	5	4	3	2	2
20	15	10	7	5	4	3
30	23	15	10	7	5	4
40		20	13	9	7	5
50			17	11	8	6
60			20	13	10	7
80				18	13	9

CONCLUSIONS

The introduction of TRUS of the prostate as an imaging and diagnostic tool has lead to significant improvements over nonvisually guided biopsy techniques, such as DRE-guided prostate biopsy. Modifications in the biopsy template based on zonal anatomy and detailed histologic studies have been made to increase overall cancer detection. Likewise, modifications in the prebiopsy regimen using local anesthesia has been analyzed in an attempt to minimize patient discomfort. PSA-based screening has lead to earlier detection of prostate cancer, and this has translated into fewer sonographic abnormalities. Continued refinements in technique, biopsy templates, and technology are needed to further improve cancer detection rates.

REFERENCES

1. Greenlee R, Murray T, Bolden S, Wingo P. Cancer Statistics, 2000. *CA Cancer J Clin* 2000;50:7–33.
2. Jemal A, Thomas A, Murray T, Thun M. Cancer Statistics. *CA Cancer J Clin* 2002;52:23–47.
3. Wild J, Reid J. Echographic tissue diagnosis. *Fourth Annual Conference on Ultrasound Therapy*, Philadelphia, PA; 1955.
4. Watanabe H, Kaiho H, Tanaka M. Diagnostic application of ultrasonography of the prostate. *Invest Urol* 1971;8:548.
5. Hodge KK, McNeal JE, Terris MK, Stamey TA. Random systematic versus directed ultrasound guided transrectal core biopsies of the prostate. *J. Urol.* 1989;142:71–74; discussion 74–75.
6. Klein EA, Zippe CD. Transrectal ultrasound guided prostate biopsy—defining a new standard. *J Urol* 2000;163:179–180.
7. Torp-Pedersen ST, Lee F. Transrectal biopsy of the prostate guided by transrectal ultrasound. *Urol Clin North Am* 1989;16:703–712.
8. Torp-Pedersen S, Lee F, Littrup PJ, et al. Transrectal biopsy of the prostate guided with transrectal US: longitudinal and multiplanar scanning. *Radiology* 1989;170:23–27.
9. Keetch D, Catalona W, Smith D. Serial prostatic biopsies in men with persistently elevated serum prostate specific antigen values. *J Urol* 1994;151:1571–1574.
10. Stamey T. Making the most out of six systematic sextant biopsies. *Urology* 1995;45:2–12.
11. Eskew LA, Bare RL, McCullough DL Systematic 5 region prostate biopsy is superior to sextant method for diagnosing carcinoma of the prostate. *J Urol* 1997;157:199–202; discussion 202–203.
12. Karakiewicz P, Aprikian A, Meshref A, Bazinet M. Computer-assisted comparative

analysis of four-sector and six-sector biopsies of the prostate. *Urology* 1996;48:747–750.

13. Presti J, Chang J, Bhargava V, Shinohara K. The optimal systematic prostate biopsy scheme should include 8 rather than 6 biopsies: results of a prospective clinical trial. *J Urol* 2000;163:163–167.

14. Norberg M, Egevad L, Holmberg L, Sparen P, Norlen BJ, Busch C. The sextant protocol for ultrasound-guided core biopsies of the prostate underestimates the presence of cancer. *Urology* 1997;50:562–566.

15. Beurton D, Barthelemy Y, Fontaine E. Twelve systematic prostate biopsies are superior to sextant biopsies for diagnosing carcinoma: a prospective randomized study. *Br J Urol* 1997;80:239–245.

16. Cornud F, Hamida K, Flam T. Endorectal color Doppler sonography and endorectal MR imaging features of nonpalpable prostate cancer: Correlation with radical prostatectomy findings. *Am J Roentgenol* 2000;175:1161–1168.

17. Cho J, Kim S, Lee S. Peripheral hypoechoic lesions of the prostate: evaluation with color and power Doppler ultrasound. *Eur Urol* 2000;37:443–448.

18. Franco OE, Arima K, Yanagawa M, Kawamura J. The usefulness of power Doppler ultrasonography for diagnosing prostate cancer: histological correlation of each biopsy site. *Br J Urol Int* 2000;85:1049–1052.

19. Frauscher F, Klauser A, Volgger H, et al. Comparison of contrast enhanced color doppler targeted biopsy with conventional systematic biopsy: impact on prostate cancer detection. *J Urol* 2002;167:1648–1652.

20. Halpern E, Verkh L, Forsberg F. Initial experience with contrast-enhanced sonography of the prostate. *Am J Roentgenol* 2000;174:1575–1580.

21. Feleppa E, Fair W, Liu T. Three-dimensional ultrasound analyses of the prostate. *Mol Urol* 2000;4:133–139; discussion 141.

22. Campani R, Bottinelli O, Calliada F. Three-dimensional imaging II (in process citation). *Eur J Radiol* 1998;27(suppl 2):S183.

23. Tong S, Downey D, Cardinal H. A three-dimensional ultrasound prostate imaging system. *Ultrasound Med Biol* 1996;22:735.

24. McNeal J. Regional morphology and pathology of the prostate. *Am J Clin Pathol* 1968;49:347.

25. McNeal J. Anatomy of the prostate: an historical survey of divergent views. *Prostate* 1980;1:3–13.

26. McNeal J. Normal and pathologic anatomy of prostate. *Urology* 1981;17:11–16.

27. McNeal J. Normal histology of the prostate. *Am J Surg Pathol* 1988;12:619–633.

28. McNeal J. Zonal distribution of prostatic adenocarcinoma: correlation with histologic pattern and direction of spread. *Am J Surg Pathol* 1988;12: 897.

29. Coley C, Barry M, Fleming C. Should Medicare provide reimbursement for prostate-specific antigen testing for early detection of prostate cancer? Part II: early detection strategies. *Urology* 1995;46:125–141.

30. Grossfeld G, Carroll P. Prostate cancer early detection: a clinical perspective. *Epidemiol Rev* 2001;23:173–180.

31. Carter H, Pearson J. PSA velocity for the diagnosis of early prostate cancer: a new concept. *Urol Clin North Am* 1993;20:665–670.

32. Davidson D, Bostwick D, Qian J, et al. Prostatic intra-epithelial neoplasia is a risk factor for adenocarcinoma: predictive accuracy in needle biopsies. *J Urol* 1995;154:1295–1299.

33. Bemer A, Danielsen H, Pettersen E, Fossa S, Reith A, Nesland J. DNA distribution in the prostate. Normal gland, benign and pre-malignant lesions and subsequent adenocarcinomas. *Anal Quant Cytol Histol* 1993;15:247–252.

34. Park S, Shinohara K, Grossfeld G, Carroll P. Prostate cancer detection in men with prior high grade prostatic intraepithelial neoplasia or atypical prostate biopsy. *J Urol* 2001;165:1409–1414.

35. Benson M, Whang I, Pantuck A. Prostate specific antigen density: a means of distinguishing benign prostatic hypertrophy and prostate cancer. *J Urol* 1992;147: 815–816.

36. Shandera K, Thibault G, Deshon G. J. (1998) Variability in patient preparation for prostate biopsy among american urologists. *Urology* 1998;52:644–646.

37. Carey J, Korman H. Transrectal ultrasound guided biopsy of the prostate. Do enemas decrease clinically significant complications? *J Urol* 2001;166: 82–85.

38. Lindert KA, Kabalin JN, Terris MK. Bacteremia bacteriuria after transrectal ultrasound guided prostate biopsy. *J Urol* 2000;164:76–80.

39. Terris M, Stamey T. Determination of prostate volume by transrectal ultrasound. *J Urol* 1987;145:984.

40. Lee F, Torp-Pedersen S, Siders D, Littrup P, McLeary R. Transrectal ultrasound in the diagnosis staging of prostate carcinoma. *Radiology* 1989;170:609–615.

41. Rifkin M. Normal sonographic anatomy, in Ultrasound of the Prostate. Raven Press, New York, 1998; pp. 51–93.

42. Lee F, Gray J, McLeary R. Transrectal ultrasound in the diagnosis of prostate cancer: location, echogenicity, histopathology, staging. *Prostate* 1985;7:117–129.

43. Shinohara K, Wheeler T, Scardino P. The appearance of prostate cancer on transrectal ultrasonography: correlation of imaging pathological examinations. *J Urol* 1989;142: 76.

44. Lee F, Gray J, McLeary R. Prostatic evaluation by transrectal sonography: criteria for diagnosis of early carcinoma. *Radiology* 1986;158:91–95.

45. Brawer M. Chetner M. Ultrasonography of the prostate biopsy, in *Campbell's Urology* (Walsh P, Retik A, Vaughan EJ, Wein A, eds.), W. B. Saunders Company, Philadelphia, 1998; pp. 2506–2518.

46. Ellis WJ, Brawer MK. The significance of isoechoic prostatic carcinoma. *J Urol* 1994;152:2304–2307.

47. Carter H, Hamper U, Sheth S. Evaluation of transrectal ultrasound in the early detection of prostate cancer. *J Urol* 1989;142:1008–1010.

48. Shinohara K, Scardino P, Carter S, Wheeler T. Pathologic basis of the sonographic appearance of the normal malignant prostate. *Urol Clin North Am* 1989;16:675–691.

49. Halpern E. Strup S. Using gray-scale color power Doppler sonography to detect prostatic cancer. *Am J Roentgenol* 2000;174:623.

50. Ornstein D. Kang J. How to improve prostate biopsy detection of prostate cancer. *Curr. Urol Rep* 2001;2:218–223.

51. Shigeno K, Igawa M, Shiina H, Wada H, Yoneda T. The role of colour Doppler ultrasonography in detecting prostate cancer. *BJU Int* 2000;86:229–233.

52. Downey D. Fenster A. Three-dimensional power Doppler detection of prostatic cancer. *Am J Roentgenol* 1985;165:741.

53. Okihara K, Kojima M, Nakanouchi T. Transrectal power Doppler imagin in the detection of prostate cancer. *Br J Urol Int* 2000;85:1053–1057.

54. Ismail M, Gomella LG Ultrasound for prostate imaging biopsy. *Curr. Opin. Urol.* 2001;11: 471–477.

55. Unal D, Sedelaar J, Aarnik R. Three dimensional contrast-enhanced power Doppler ultrasonography conventional examination methods: the value of diagnostic predictors of prostate cancer. *Br J Urol Int.* 2000;86:58–64.

56. Cosgrove D, Kiely P, Williamson R. Ultrasonographic contrast media in the urinary tract. *Br J Urol In.* 2000;86(suppl):11–17.

57. Cooner W, Mosley B, Rutherford C. Prostate cancer detection in a clinical urological practice by ultrasonography, digital rectal exam prostate specific antigen. *J Urol* 1990;143:1146.

58. Rodriguez L. Terris M. Risks compications of transrectal ultrasound guided prostate needle biopsy. *J Urol* 1998;160:2115.

59. Rietbergen JB, Kruger AE, Kranse R, Schroder FH. Complications of transrectal ultra-

sound-guided systematic sextant biopsies of the prostate: wvaluation of complication rates risk factors within a population-based screening program. *Urology* 1997;49:875–880.

60. Aus G, Ahlgren G, Bergdahl S. Infection after transrectal core biopsies of the prostate: risk factors antibiotic prophylaxis. *Br J Urol* 1996;77: 851.

61. Desmond P, Clark J, Thompson I. Morbidity with contemporary prostate biopsy. *J Urol* 1993;150:1425.

62. Norberg M, Holmberg L, Haggman M, Magnusson A. Determinants of complications after multiple transrectal core biopsies of the prostate. *Eur Radiol* 1996;6:457–461.

63. Rodriguez LV, Terris MK. Risks complications of transrectal ultrasound guided prostate needle biopsy: a prospective study review of the literature. *J Urol* 1998;160: 2115–2120.

64. Aus G, Hermansson CG, Hugosson J, Pedersen KV. Transrectal ultrasound examination of the prostate: Complications acceptance by patients. *Br J Urol* 1993;71:457–459.

65. Collins GN, Lloyd SN, Hehir M, McKelvie G. B. Multiple transrectal ultrasound-guided prostatic biopsies—true morbidity patient acceptance. *Br J Urol* 1993;71: 460–463.

66. Rani J, Fournier F, Bon D, Gremmo E, Dore B, Aubert J. Patient tolerance of transrectal ultrasound-guided biopsy of the prostate. *Br J Urol* 1997;79: 608–610.

67. Naughton CK, Ornstein DK, Smith DS, Catalona WJ. Pain morbidity of transrectal ultrasound guided prostate biopsy: a prospective randomized trial of 6 versus 12 cores. *J Urol* 2000;163:168–171.

68. Chang SS, Alberts G, Wells N, Smith JA Jr, Cookson MS. Intrarectal lidocaine during transrectal prostate biopsy: Results of a prospective double-blind randomized trial. *J Urol* 2001;166:2178–2180.

69. Alavi AS, Soloway MS, Vaidya A, Lynne CM, Gheiler EL. Local anesthesia for ultrasound guided prostate biopsy: A prospective randomized trial comparing 2 methods. *J Urol* 2001;166:1343–1345.

70. Clements R, Aideyan OU, Griffiths GJ, Peeling WB. Side effects patient acceptability of transrectal biopsy of the prostate. *Clin Radiol* 1993;47:125–126.

71. Soloway M. S. Obek C. Periprostatic local anesthesia before ultrasound guided prostate biopsy. *J Urol* 2000;163:172–173.

72. Desgrandchamps F, Meria P, Irani J, Desgrippes A, Teillac P, Le Duc A. The rectal administration of lidocaine gel tolerance of transrectal ultrasonography-guided biopsy of the prostate: a prospective randomized placebo-controlled study. *Br J Urol Int* 1999;83:1007–1009.

73. Wu CL, Carter HB, Naqibuddin M, Fleisher LA. Effect of local anesthetics on patient recovery after transrectal biopsy. *Urology* 2001;57:925–929.

74. Nash PA, Bruce JE, Indudhara R, Shinohara K.Transrectal ultrasound guided prostatic nerve blockade eases systematic needle biopsy of the prostate. *J. Urol.* 1996;155: 607–609.

75. Issa M, Bux S, Chun T, et al. A randomized prospective trial of intrarectal lidocaine for pain control during transrectal prostate biopsy: the Emory University experience. *J Urol* 2000;164:397–399.

76. Lee F, Littrup P, Torp-Pedersen S, et al. Prostate cancer: comparison of transrectal US DRE for screening. *Radiology* 1998;168:389–394.

77. Hodge KK, McNeal JE, Stamey TA. Ultrasound guided transrectal core biopsies of the palpably abnormal prostate. *J Urol* 1989;142:66–70.

78. Wilson T. Guthman D. Current status of transrectal ultrasonography in the detection of prostate cancer. *Oncology* 1991;5:73–76.

79. Borboroglu PG, Comer SW, Riffenburgh RH, Amling CL. Extensive repeat transrectal ultrasound guided prostate biopsy in patients with previous benign sextant biopsies. *J Urol* 2000;163:158–162.

80. Chen, ME, Troncoso P, Johnston D, Tang K, Babaian R. Optimization of prostate biopsy strategy using computer based analysis. *J Urol* 1997;158:2168–2175.

81. Egevad L, Frimmel H, Norberg M, et al. Three-dimensional computer reconstruction of

prostate cancer from radical prostatectomy specimens: evaluation of the model by core biopsy simulation. *Urology* 1999;53:192–198.

82. Loughlin M, Carlbom I, Busch C. Three-dimensional modeling of biopsy protocols for localized prostate cancer. *Comput Med Imaging Graph* 1998;22:229–238.

83. Ravery V, Goldblatt L, Royer B, et al. Extensive biopsy protocol improves the detection rate of prostate cancer. *J Urol* 2000;164:393–396.

84. Chang JJ, Shinohara K, Hovey RM, Montgomery C, Presti JC Jr. Prospective evaluation of systematic sextant transition zone biopsies in large prostates for cancer detection. *Urology* 1998;52:89–93.

85. Gore JL, Shariat SF, Miles BJ, et al. Optimal combinations of systematic sextant laterally directed biopsies for the detection of prostate cancer. *J Urol* 2001;165:1554–1559.

86. Levine MA, Ittman M, Melamed J, Lepor H. Two consecutive sets of transrectal ultrasound guided sextant biopsies of the prostate for the detection of prostate cancer. *J Urol* 1998;159:471–475; discussion 475–476.

87. Naughton CK, Miller DC, Mager DE, Ornstein DK, Catalona WJ. A prospective randomized trial comparing 6 versus 12 prostate biopsy cores: impact on cancer detection. *J Urol* 2000;164:388–392.

88. Babaian RJ, Toi A, Kamoi K, et al. A comparative analysis of sextant an extended 11-core multisite directed biopsy strategy. *J Urol* 2000;163:152–157.

89. Ravery V, Billebaud T, Toublanc M, et al. Diagnostic value of ten systematic TRUS-guided prostate biopsies. *Eur Urol* 1999;35:298–303.

90. Chen M, Troncoso P, Tang K. Comparison of prostate biopsy schemes by computer simulation. *Urology* 1999;53:951.

91. Epstein J, Chan D, Sokoll L. Nonpalpable stage T1c prostate cancer: prediction of insignificant disease using free/total prostate specific antigen levels needle biopsy findings. *J Urol* 1998;160:2407.

92. Eskew L, Woodruff R, Bare R. Prostate cancer diagnosed by the 5 region biopsy method is significant disease. *J Urol* 1998;160:794.

93. Carter H, Savageot J, Walsh P, Epstein J. Prospective evaluation of men with stage T1c adenocarcinoma of the prostate. *J Urol* 1997;157:2206.

94. Chan T, Chan D, Lecksell K, Stutzman R, Epstein J. Does increased needle biopsy sampling of the prostate detect a higher number of potentially insignificant tumors? *J Urol* 2001;166:2181–2184.

95. Ellis W. J. Brawer M. K. Repeat prostate needle biopsy: who needs it? *J Urol* 1995;153:1496–1498.

96. Djavan B, Zlotta A, Remzi M, et al. Optimal predictors of prostate cancer on repeat prostate biopsy: A prospective study of 1:051 men. *J Urol* 2000;163:1144–1148; discussion 1148–1149.

97. Stewart CS, Leibovich BC, Weaver AL, Lieber MM. Prostate cancer diagnosis using a saturation needle biopsy technique after previous negative sextant biopsies. *J Urol* 2001;166:86–91; discussion 91–92.

98. Fleshner NE, O'Sullivan M, Fair W. R. Prevalence predictors of a positive repeat transrectal ultrasound guided needle biopsy of the prostate. *J Urol* 1997;158:505–508; discussion 508–509.

99. Epstein J, Walsh P, Sauvageot J. Use of repeat sextant transition zone biopsies for assessing extent of prostate cancer. *J Urol* 1997;158:1886.

100. Lui PD, Terris MK, McNeal JE, Stamey TA. Indications for ultrasound guided transition zone biopsies in the detection of prostate cancer. *J Urol* 1995;153:1000–1003.

101. Fleshner NE, Fair WR. Indications for transition zone biopsy in the detection of prostatic carcinoma. *J Urol* 1997;157:556–558.

102. Keetch D. Catalona W. Prostatic transition zone biopsies in men with previous negative

biopsies persistently elevated serum prostate specific antigen values. *J Urol* 1995;154:1795–1797.

103. Bazinet M, Karakiewicz P, Aprikian A, et al. Value of systematic transition zone biopsies in the early detection of prostate cancer. *J Urol* 1996;155:605–606.
104. Rovner ES, Schanne FJ, Malkowicz SB, Wein AJ. Transurethral biopsy of the prostate for persistently elevated or increasing prostate specific antigen following multiple negative transrectal biopsies. *J Urol* 1997;158:138–141; discussion 141–142.
105. Niesel T, Breul J, Hartung R. Diagnostic value of additional systematic prostate biopsies in patients undergoing transurethral resection of the prostate. *Urology* 1997;49:869–874.
106. Terris MK, Pham TQ, Issa MM, Kabalin JN. Routine transition zone seminal vesicle biopsies in all patients undergoing transrectal ultrasound guided prostate biopsies are not indicated. *J Urol* 1997;157:204–206.
107. Uzzo RG, Wei JT, Waldbaum RS, et al. The influence of prostate size on cancer detection. *Urology* 1995;46:831–836.
108. Epstein J, Walsh P, Akingba G, Carter H. The significance of prior benign needle biopsies in men subsequently diagnosed with prostate cancer. *J Urol* 1999;162:1649–1652.
109. Letran JL, Meyer GE, Loberiza FR, Brawer MK. The effect of prostate volume on the yield of needle biopsy. *J Urol* 1998;160:1718#1721.
110. Vashi A, Wojno K, Gillespie B, Oesterling J. A model for the number of cores per prostate biopsy based on patient age prostate gland volume. J Urol 1998;159:920–924.
111. Polascik T, Oesterling J, Partin A. Prostate specific antigen: a decade of discovery—what we have learned where we are going. *J Urol* 1999;162:293–306.
112. Oesterling J, Jacobsen S, Chute C. Serum prostate-specific antigen in a community-based population of healthy men: establishment of age-specific reference ranges. *JAMA* 1993;270:860–864.
113. Morgan T, Jacobsen S, McCarthy W. Age-specific reference ranges for prostate-specific antigen in black men. *N Engl J Med* 1996;335:304–310.
114. Oesterling J, Kumamoto Y, Tsukamoto T. Serum prostate-specific antigen in a community-based population of healthy Japanese men: lower values than for similarly aged white men. *Br J Urol* 1995;75:347–353.
115. Pareek G, Armenakas NA, Fracchia JA. Periprostatic nerve blockade for transrectal ultrasound guided biopsy of the prostate: a randomized, double-blind, placebo controlled study. *J Urol* 2001;166:894–897.

2

Magnetic Resonance-Guided Prostate Biopsy

Clare M. Tempany, MD, and Steven Haker, PhD

INTRODUCTION

The goal of a cancer detection program is to detect and diagnose cancer at an early, treatable stage. Prostate cancer is routinely diagnosed by needle biopsy after the detection of either an abnormal prostate-specific antigen (PSA) level or a palpable nodule in the gland. The current standard method to obtain the tissue diagnosis is to sample the prostate gland using transrectal ultrasound (TRUS) imaging guidance. Although this method is the standard clinical approach, this chapter will describe a novel diagnostic method using magnetic resonance imaging guidance that is currently being evaluated in a prospective National Cancer Institute clinical trial.

Prostate Cancer Diagnosis and Treatment

Prostate cancer is the most common noncutaneous malignancy diagnosed in American men. It is estimated that approx 189,000 men were diagnosed in 2002 with prostate cancer *(1)*, although it is also estimated that this figure may be low because of inadequate methods of detection. Currently, either TRUS-guided biopsy or sampling during transurethral prostatectomy are the two most common methods used to diagnose prostate cancer. In the presence of high PSA levels, current biopsy methods are significantly limited by a false-negative rate estimated to be as high as 15 to 31%. TRUS biopsies are specifically limited by low sensitivity of 60%, with only 25% positive predictive value. Studies have shown, moreover, that in more than 20% of cases in which cancer was suspected, at least two biopsy sessions were required to diagnose the tumor *(2,3)*. The TRUS approach does not target focal lesions in the gland; rather, it samples the gland in a sextant manner: bilaterally at the base, the midgland, and the apex. A randomized study of the efficacy of six vs twelve cores in 160 patients showed no difference in cancer detection, thus suggesting that it is the location or target that is actually biopsied, rather than the actual number of samples that matters *(4)*.

Clearly, the difficulty in reaching a definitive diagnosis is not resolved by simply increasing the number of samples taken.

Many men are faced with a dilemma after they have had a negative transrectal prostate biopsy prompted by an abnormal PSA level. Should the patient and his physician

From: *Image-Guided Diagnosis and Treatment of Cancer*
Edited by: A. D'Amico, J. S. Loeffler, and J. R. Harris © Humana Press Inc., Totowa, NJ

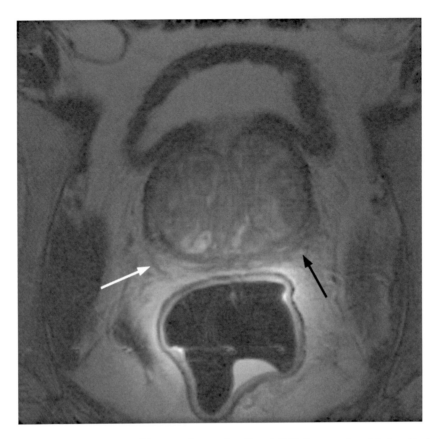

Fig. 1. Axial T2W image with an endorectal coil at 1.5 T. Lower signal intensity in the left PZ (black arrow) compared with right (white arrow) indicates a tumor.

have confidence in the results of the original biopsy in the presence of abnormal PSA levels? In the context of this question, we present a novel biopsy method in such a way that abnormal tissue is depicted in advance of the actual procedure. Then using this information, a targeted and sampling biopsy can be performed. We hypothesis that by using magnetic resonance imaging (MRI), the more precise target definition will improve both the speed and accuracy with which a diagnosis is reached. More timely diagnosis and treatment, in turn, should be to the benefit of the patient in terms of prognosis and quality of life.

MRI OF THE PROSTATE

Significant advances have been made in MRI of the prostate gland in the past decade. It is now clearly established that a combination of T1- and T2-weighted (T1W and T2W) images in multiple planes provide a comprehensive set of images of the entire prostate and its substructure, including the central gland and the peripheral zone. MRI can provide full visualization of the rectum, bladder, seminal vesicles, and neurovascular bundles *(5,6)*. The technology behind MRI has improved significantly, with current state-of-the-art images acquired with an endorectal coil/phased array coil combination

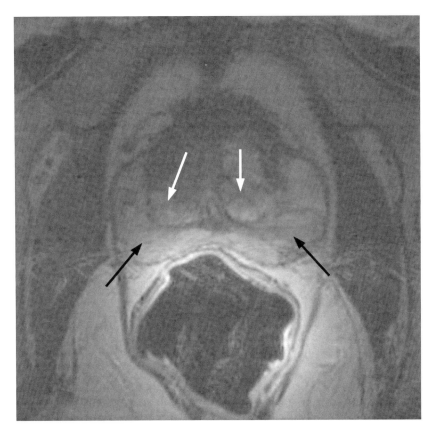

Fig. 2. Axial T2W image with an endorectal coil at 1.5 T showing normal prostate substructure. Specifically, high-signal intensity PZ (black arrows) typical CG heterogeneous signal BPH (white arrows).

at 1.5 T. The combination of the endorectal and multicoil array has been shown to provide the most accurate imaging technique for visualizing and staging the patient's tumor *(7)*. The T2W images allow clear visualization of the peripheral zone (PZ) of the prostate, where over 75% of cancers arise. MRI can detect suspicious lesions in the PZ of the gland on T2W images. Focal (low-signal) lesions in the PZ are suspicious for tumor, especially when located posteriorly in the gland. The sensitivity of MRI for the detection of cancer is relatively high, but the specificity for diagnosis of cancer is not as high. We and others have previously shown that the detection of tumor foci on MRI is, in part, a function of size, with 89% of foci greater than 10 mm and 62% of foci less than 5 mm being detected *(8,9)*. Because PZ is the most common site of origin of prostate cancer among the three prostate zones (PZ, central zone [CZ], and transitional zone [TZ]), localizing and targeting PZ and tumor foci in prostate biopsy may increase the cancer detection rate. For these reasons and those related to the problems of TRUS, we, and others have sought alternative biopsy approaches. We can now perform MR-guided biopsies in an open, interventional MRI unit, which allows for MR-guided needle placement and sampling of biopsy sites *(10–13)* (Figs. 1–6).

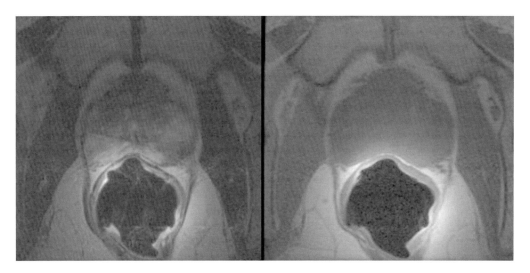

Fig. 3. Axial images with endorectal coil at 1.5 T. On the left, a T2W image, on the right, a T1W image. The same craniocaudial postion is presented.

CURRENT TECHNIQUES TO IMPROVE MR CANCER DETECTION

In an effort to provided greater tumor detection and characterization, there are several new noninvasive imaging techniques currently being tested. These include MR spectroscopy, T2 mapping, diffusion imaging, and intravenous contrast enhancement with gadolinium.

PROSTATE MR SPECTROSCOPY

Several groups have shown the utility of 1H spectroscopy to detect biochemical markers in the prostate that can be used to differentiate prostate cancer from normal tissue or from benign prostatic hyperplasia (BPH) in vivo *(14,15)*. The primary metabolite signal from normal tissue and BPH is the citrate resonance at 2.6 ppm. The primary metabolite signal from prostate cancer is the choline resonance at 3.2 ppm. The ratio of the areas under these two resonances has proven to be a statistically significant indicator for the presence or absence of cancer. Other metabolites that can be detected and quantified with 1H spectroscopy include myo-inositol, creatine, and lipid resonances. Quantification of these resonances and the subsequent formation of various metabolite ratios should further enhance the likelihood of localizing regions where prostate cancer will be encountered with MR-guided biopsies.

T2 MAPPING OF THE PROSTATE GLAND

A British group has produced intriguing results that suggest a positive correlation between the concentration of citrate, as determined by 1H spectroscopy, and the water T2 value, as mapped with multi-echo imaging methods. Because citrate is the so-called good metabolite of the prostate gland, presenting the strongest metabolite signal in normal tissue and BPH *(16–19)*, a decrease in the citrate signal provides an indirect indication of potential PC. Thus, if the correlation between citrate concentration and water T2 values can be independently established, we will improve the spatial resolu-

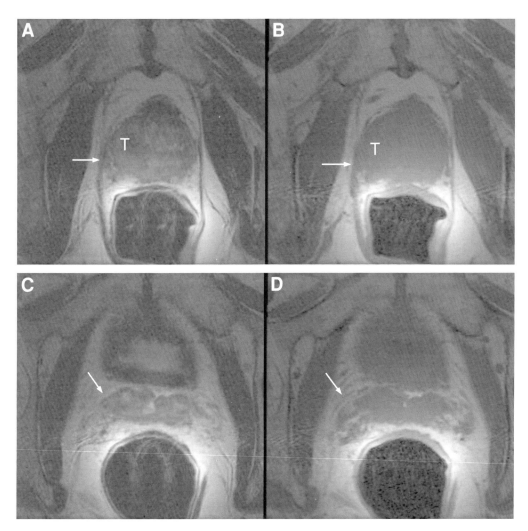

Fig. 4. Axial T2W **(A, C)** T1W **(B, D)** images with an endorectal coil at 1.5 T acquired at the midgland seminal vesicles levels. Images demonstrate a large extensive tumor arising on the right side (T), which invades both the capsule and the seminal vesicles (white arrows).

tion with which suspicious regions of the prostate can be identified for biopsy. Hence, we perform high spatial resolution imaging with fast spin echo sequences at multiple effective echo times to generate quantitative T2 maps of the prostate gland. From these maps, we will identify regions corresponding to spectroscopically interrogated voxels. Currently, we are seeking a correlation between the T2 values of these regions and the metabolite ratios obtained from the two dimensional chemical shift imaging studies, which are currently the best differential indices for prostate cancer vs normal tissue or BPH.

DIFFUSION IMAGING OF THE PROSTATE GLAND

MRI methods for obtaining tissue contrast reflecting water molecular diffusion have become essential for assessing acute stroke in the brain. More recently, evidence has been presented that suggests diffusion imaging may also play a role in the early detec-

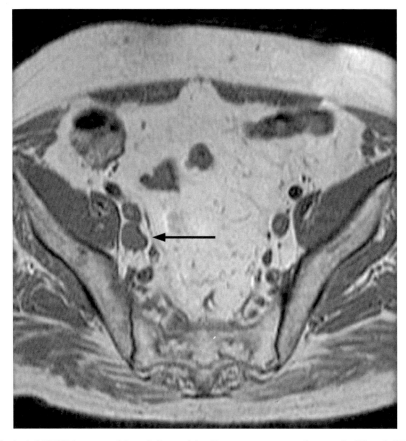

Fig. 5. Axial T1W image with pelvic multicoil array, same patient as in Fig. 4. This image shows an enlarged metastatic lymph node in the right external iliac chain (arrow).

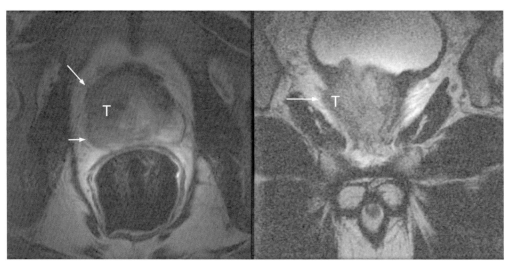

Fig. 6. Axial (left) and coronal (right) T2W images, with an endorectal coil at 1.5 T. Patient is a 56-yr-old man with prostate cancer. This staging MRI shows a large right-sided tumor (T). This tumor involves both the PZ and TZ on the right. Both images show extra-capsular extension of disease (white arrows). Thus, this patient has T3 disease.

tion of brain tumor response to therapy *(20)*. Such successes have encouraged the pursuit of diffusion imaging for characterizing pathology in the prostate. However, technical limitations have largely confined diffusion studies to the brain with only very limited studies of other organs. As a result a technique that overcomes these limitations has been developed and so opens up the possibility of making meaningful water diffusion studies of the prostate possible. To measure tissue water diffusion or the so-called apparent diffusion coefficient (ADC), strong, nonimaging gradient pulses are incorporated that cause a signal reduction related to the overall motion of the water molecules within an imaged pixel. The primary motion of interest for tissue characterization is the microscopic diffusive motion, which is sensitive to the local environment, for example, stroke or tumor environments having different ADCs from that of the surrounding normal tissue. Of course, other artifactual motions may occur during measurement, including respiratory, cardiac, and peristaltic, which will also lead to signal reductions that confound ADC measurements, particularly outside of the brain. Snapshot echo-planar imaging techniques are used to overcome these problems by effectively "freezing" macroscopic motion.

To overcome both the macroscopic motion problem and the inherent limitations of echo-planar imaging diffusion imaging, a new diffusion imaging technique has been developed called line scan diffusion imaging. The technical advantages of line scan diffusion imaging will allow us to make high-quality, high spatial resolution, quantitative diffusion imaging of the prostate *(20)*. This may allow for a meaningful assessment of the prostate tissue ADC parameter as an indicator of cancer and guide for biopsy localization.

Intravenous Contrast Agents

Recent work suggests that by giving intravenous gadolinium T1W images can show different enhancements patterns between cancer and benign tissue. The intravenous contrast is given as a rapid bolus, with multiphase acquisitions, before and after the bolus obtained, using fat suppression. This is preliminary work and may along with the above techniques add further to improve our specificity.

IMAGE-GUIDED PROSTATE INTERVENTIONS

Image-guided therapy has become an important approach for many forms of cancer treatment. The ability to identify the target ahead of time and deliver the maximum therapy to the target is the ultimate goal. The three critical components of any imageguided therapy method are navigation, control, and monitoring of therapy delivery. Precise navigation requires clear identification of the target. To control the delivery of treatment, one needs to accurately identify the target and all adjacent tissues while controlling the intervention or procedure.

Over the past decade, a broad multidisciplinary field of image-guided therapy has evolved from image-guided neurosurgery. At our institution, the image-guided therapy program uses advances in imaging, high-performance computing, and highly evolved new therapy delivery systems to move forward the image-guidance concept into multiple clinical applications *(21,22)*. Image-guided surgery brings powerful technologies into the operating room by taking advantage of advances in computer science and engineering. The simultaneous combination of direct vision and imaging is possible within a unique environment of intraoperative MRI, which incorporates both the operating room and an imaging system. Open configuration MRI systems are currently in use in several centers in the United States and around the world to guide many types of procedures ranging from diagnostic biopsies of the breast, liver, bone, and other organs to guiding neurosurgical procedures *(11)*. These systems also guide treatment and follow-up treatment effects, in brain and spinal surgery, laser and cryo-ablation of liver tumors and prostate *(23–27)* and breast cancer.

We have developed a computerized software environment for interactive multiplanar three-dimensional (3D) imaging, multimodal visualization, and display. The 3D Slicer is a software program developed in-house by Hata and Gering *(28)*. This system allows for the integration of several facets of image guidance into a single integrated environment. It provides capabilities for automatic registration (aligning data sets), semiautomatic segmentation (extracting structures such as vessels and tumors from the data), generation of 3D surface models (for viewing the segmented structures), and 3D visualization and quantitative analysis (measuring distances, angles, surface areas, and volumes) of various medical scans. The 3D Slicer, now in routine clinical use, has been integrated with the open MRI scanner to augment intraoperative imaging with a full array of preoperative data. The same analysis previously reserved for preoperative data can now be applied to exploring the anatomical changes as the surgery or intervention progresses. The trajectories of the surgical instruments are tracked. By switching the display mode, the real-time scans are visualized in the same 3D view along with the preoperative slices and surface models. The utility of this image-guidance system has been tested for MRI-guided neurosurgery and now under implementation for other image-guided procedures and for several diagnostic applications.

In prostate cancer, it is important to maximize the local treatment effect and to minimize the undesired effects on the normal structures close to the target, thus reducing complication rate. This is the fundamental principle underlying most modern radiation treatment programs for prostate cancer. In 1997, we introduced an MR-guided brachytherapy program for the treatment of localized prostate cancer. We use the MRI in place of ultrasound imaging to delineate the prostate gland and most importantly use the MRI in near-real time to monitor the treatment delivery and radiation dosimetry *(23–27)*.

The ability to use MR to guide biopsies of prostate lesions only detected on MRI is a powerful and useful application of this imaging technology. We are currently using this approach, along with others, in routine clinical practice. A recent pilot study of 33 patients by Perrotti et al. *(10)* showed that MRI could accurately localize tumor foci, with an accuracy of 67%, in patients with previous negative biopsy and elevated serum PSA. They used MRI to identify lesions/targets (based only on signal and not size) and then performed TRUS-guided biopsies attempting to directly biopsy the most suspicious MRI-identified lesions. Prospective evaluation of endorectal MRI to detect tumor foci in men with prior negative prostatic biopsy is described in a pilot study.

MRI-GUIDED BIOPSY

The experience we gained from the MR-guided brachytherapy program led us to believe that by adapting this approach we could perform MR-guided percutaneous prostate biopsies. The brachytherapy procedure demonstrated that it is feasible to place needles into specific targets in the prostate under intraoperative MRI guidance. Among

Table 1
MR-Guided Prostate Biopsy Patient Population

Eligibility criteria

- Either an abnormal serum PSA level (>4 ng/mL) or a palpable nodule in the prostate on digital rectal examination.
- Either previous negative biopsy or no transrectal access for biopsy sampling.
- MRI of the prostate gland, with or without a focal lesion.
- Age >30 yr.
- Informed consent.
- No contraindication to MR-induced anesthesia, that is, no risk of silent ischemia.

Exclusion criteria

- Inability to give informed consent.
- Contraindications to MRI cardiac pacemaker, inner ear implants, non-MR-compatible intracranial aneurysm clips.
- Contraindications to MR-induced anesthesia-epidural or general anesthesia.

the goals of our work is to answer the question of whether improved detection of clinically significant prostate cancers can occur if the biopsy is guided by MRI. As our brachytherapy program developed, it became apparent that this approach had the potential to allow MR-guided prostate biopsies. Thus, in response to a clinical demand, we adapted our system to perform MR-guided biopsies. We anticipate that biopsies based on MRI localization and needle guidance compared with random sextant sampling will be more effective in detecting localized prostate cancer.

BIOPSY PATIENT POPULATION

Our patients are all men with abnormal PSA levels (>4 ng/mL; Hybritech method) from one for the following two groups: 1) Men who have had previous abdomino-perineal resection (APR) of the rectum who cannot undergo a TRUS-guided biopsy and 2) Men who have abnormal PSA and have had more than one negative TRUS biopsy. All patients have a prebiopsy MR exam with either the multicoil-phased array alone or a multicoil array and endorectal coil, at 1.5 T. These images provide planning information for the biopsy both for target definition and depiction of the peripheral zone. We exclude from biopsy patients who have any of the standard exclusion criteria for MRI, for example, cardiac pacemakers. We also exclude men with significant cardiac ischemia. All men are evaluated by the anesthesia service, as they do of all men undergoing MR-guided brachytherapy, for the induction of anesthesia in an MR environment. Men with significant cardiac ischemia are excluded because they cannot be adequately monitored in the intraoperative MRI unit.

After patients have the initial MR exam, the biopsy procedure is discussed with them and informed consent is obtained (Table 1).

On the day of the procedure, the patient comes to the intraoperative MRI suite and is prepared for the biopsy. He is positioned in the lithotomy position, with the side entry position of the table. The patient receives either a general or spinal anesthesia, as selected by the anesthesiologist, to keep him from pain and discomfort and to immobilize his pelvis and provide a fixed target that will not move during the procedure. The external MR transmits and receive coil are wrapped around his pelvis, and initial images confirm a good position.

The skin of the perineum is prepared and draped after a Foley catheter has been placed in the bladder. Then a Plexiglas template is fixed up against the patient's perineum. If the rectum is normal, a stiff obturator is placed to allow for clear delineation of the anterior rectal wall and posterior prostate. Then, the prebiopsy images are obtained.

For biopsy localization, each sextant of the prostate gland can be targeted as they are under ultrasound guidance. We image the prostate in the coronal plane and divide the gland into three areas: apex, base, and midgland. We believe we are able to increase the likelihood that the samples are taken from the PZ for the following reasons: we have real-time MRI guidance and we use the 3D Slicer software, which allows for T2W images to be displayed in the operating room. Thus allowing for visualization of the PZ/central gland (CG), as the needle is inserted. As the approach is transperineal, the needles enter the posterior gland and travel in a vertical trajectory through the PZ, increasing the probability that all samples will be taken from the PZ. The real-time imaging with fast gradient recalled (FGR) imaging sequences, the 3D Slicer, and the T2W images are be used to confirm that the samples are being taken from the PZ.

An axial T2W volumetric sequence acquired in the 0.5 T Signa SP Magnetic Resonance Therapy (MRT) System (GE Medical Systems, Milwaukee, WI) at the start of the biopsy procedure is incorporated into the 3D Slicer to provide "virtual" guidance into the PZ of the prostate (Figs. 7 and 8).

As each real-time FGR image is obtained, this T2W sequence is resampled so as to match the spatial position of the FGR image. We alternate the display of the real-time FGR image with the corresponding resampled T2W image to provide the observer with information on the location of the needle, its position within the PZ, and its relation to targets visible on the T2W image. The 18-gage (MR-compatible) biopsy guns are placed into the gland under MR guidance. The real-time imaging sequences are FGRs, which are rapidly acquired and clearly depict the needle; they can be acquired in the axial, sagittal, and coronal planes. The needle artifact is clearly seen on these FGR images. Using the 3D Slicer, we can alternate the image on the in-bore monitor. Thus allowing the radiologist to see both the needle and the prostate substructure simultaneously.

We perform sextant sampling of the gland under MRI guidance in a way similar to TRUS, that is, we target the six locations on the gland. We use 18-gage biopsy guns, the same size used in routine clinical practice, to take the tissue samples. We sample the PZ at the apex, base, and midgland bilaterally. All specimens are labeled, sent to pathology, and handled in the standard clinical fashion (Fig. 9).

INTERVENTIONAL MRI TECHNIQUES

As described earlier, the current state of the art for imaging the prostate requires 1.5-T field-strength MR techniques using a combined endorectal and pelvic array coils. This is routinely performed on all patients in our brachytherapy program. In the development of the MRI-guided brachytherapy program, which uses a 0.5-T filed strength system, we felt that it was important to ensure that the MR sequences and coils would provide adequate images of the prostate. Thus, we compared the image quality in a subset of 20 patients, evaluating each of the studies for ease of identification of the gland, its substructure, and abnormal foci from the endorectal coil 1.5 T images and the 0.5 T images. The total score of conspicuity of normal structures was 27.95 for the 1.5 T images and 26.5 for the 0.5 T images. The mean signal-to-noise ratios (SNRs) for the PZ were 11.1 ± 4.7 at 1.5 T and 10.3 ± 3.8 at 0.5 T ($p = 0.40$). However, the contrast-to-

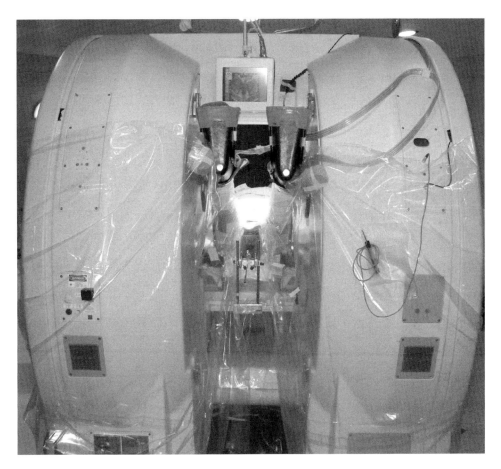

Fig. 7. General Electric Signa SP 0.5 T system with patient in lithotomy position.

noise ratios of the PZ vs the CG were significantly different ($p = 0.002$), being 7.0 ± 4.4 for 1.5T and 4.1 ± 2.2 at 0.5 T. In almost all aspects the 0.5 T images compared very favorably with the 1.5 T images. The only area where a difference was found was in the identification of focal lesions, in 12 of 20 men suspicious foci were seen at 1.5 T and not at 0.5 T *(27)*. This may be explained in part by the difference in field strength, SNR, and the imaging parameters, which are adapted for the lower field strength and the field of view; the imaging coil used is an external wrap-around coil, not an endorectal coil.

Image Analysis

Multiple biopsy locations are planned from the two image data sets, the 1.5 T data and the 0.5 T data. The latter, obtained on the day of the biopsy, after induction of anesthesia. All the 1.5 T MR images and the 0.5 T images are analyzed by the radiologist for the presence of any focal lesion, defined as any focal area of low T2W signal intensity in the PZ. Any and all lesions are identified, measured, and localized. These are thus the image-based "targets," and at least six sextant locations are also identified, which comprise the list of sites to be sampled.

Also under development is the ability to integrate 1.5 T images into the 0.5 T image display system and into the 3D Slicer visualization program to allow for improved

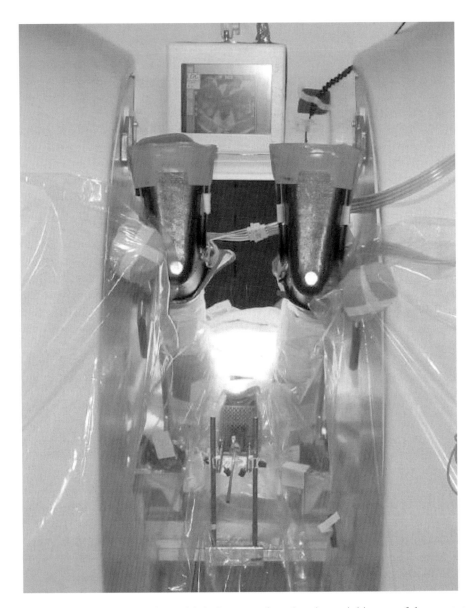

Fig. 8. Close-up of patient position, with in-bore monitor showing axial image of the prostate.

target definition. Our goals in this area are to achieve automated registration and segmentation for intraoperative treatment planning and to provide preoperative image data in the operating room for navigation to ultimately improve the accuracy and efficiency of the procedure.

3D VISUALIZATION

The real-time imaging sequences are gradient echo sequences, which are excellent for delineating the gland, the rectum, the catheter, and bladder but not the internal zones of the prostate. Therefore, the availability of T2W images provided by the 3D Slicer is critical in targeting the PZ during prostate biopsies.

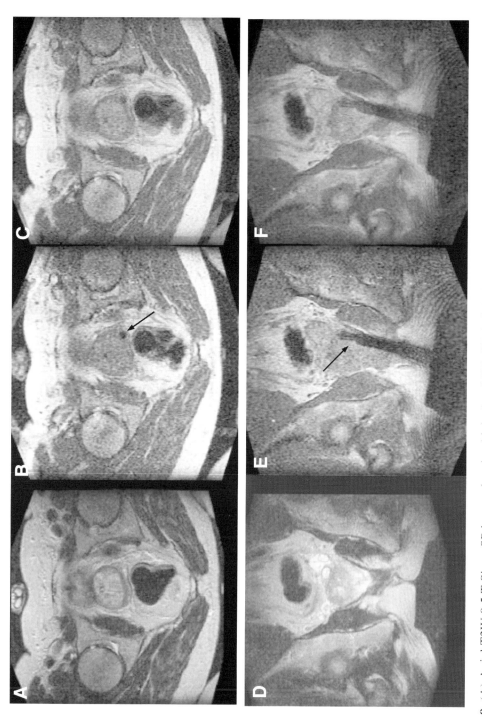

Fig. 9. (A) Axial T2W 0.5 T Signa SP image showing high-signal PZ. (B) Axial FGR real-time image shows needle artifact (arrow). (C) Fused image shows combining axial T2 FGR data. (D) Coronal T2W 0.5 T Signa SP image showing high-signal PZ. (E) Coronal FGR real-time image shows needle artifact (arrow). (F) Fused image shows combining coronal T2 FGR data.

IMAGE INTEGRATION AND FUSION

Image Registration and Segmentation

In performing prostate image segmentation, we are attempting to provide classification of the prostate substructure, which will allow automated definition of the PZ and CG. It will also allow for accurate definition of the prostate boundary and location of adjacent structures.

Segmentation

With the aim of integrating preoperative images into the intraoperative image dataset for navigation, control, and planning, we are working to develop an automated MRI segmentation program to analyze prostate gland, its boundary, and substructure. This approach, which is based on our preliminary investigations, will use the combined data from the pre- and intraprocedural MR images and allow the treatment plan to be based upon the full data set. We follow these steps:

1. Segment the PZ and the CZ/TZ in the 1.5 T preoperative PD/T2W MR images. This segmentation will also yield the outline of the prostate (i.e., the prostate capsule).
2. Deform the segmenting curves in accordance with how the prostate deforms as the patient moves from the supine to the lithotomy position, and
3. Segment the prostate capsule in the 0.5 T intraoperative MR images.
4. Apply rigid registration to match the capsule of the 1.5 T preoperative MR images to the capsule of the 0.5 T intraoperative MR images.

Once the pre- and intraoperative capsule segmentations are aligned, the PZ and the CZ/TZ segmentation of the 1.5 T MR images obtained can be overlaid on top of the 0.5 T MR images to provide the information needed for biopsy, namely, the differentiation of PZ and CZ/TZ in the procedural room. The important structures to be treated, or spared, are segmented by the method described above. These structures include the central and peripheral parts of the prostate, the urethra, and the anterior wall of the rectum. After this segmentation process, the treatment is designed and the dosimetry evaluated and refined as necessary. For rigid registration, a cost functional using similarity measures, such as mutual information, can be designed to capture the essence of a good alignment. By minimizing the cost functional, the two capsules will be aligned. Alternatively we may use an approach based on volume of overlap. Both of these methods have been used extensively in our laboratory in other applications.

Preliminary studies have shown that as the body moves from the supine position to the lithotomy position, the prostate has the tendency to shorten longitudinally, with the upper half of the prostate tilting slightly forward pivoting about the center of the organ. The different zones of the prostate are clearly visible in 1.5 T diagnostic MR images, and the challenge is to integrate this information into the 0.5 T interventional MR images obtained intraprocedurally during biopsy, while the patient is in the lithotomy position. To this end we have investigated methods for segmenting the prostate and simulating its deformation. Our segmentation approach uses a variant of the curve–evolution approach, and incorporates models of the intensity characteristics of the tissues. Previous work in these flows has demonstrated good results in segmenting images that may be differentiated by regions that have different intensity statistics, for example, different vegetations in synthetic aperture radar images *(29–31)*. We have demonstrated the feasibility and performance of these flow algorithms on preoperative prostate MR images. Curves are superimposed on top of each image slice to show the locations of the PZ and CG obtained by applying the algorithm. These contours appear to accurately outline the correct boundaries of the prostate structures. The remaining challenge is to increase the information content of the 0.5 T intraoperative MR images, which have two fundamental problems:

1. In both 1.5 T and 0.5 T MR images, the prostate gland is textured with weak or diffused boundaries that make the segmentation process challenging.
2. It is difficult to capture the nonrigid deformation of the prostate as the patient moves from a supine position to a lithotomy position.

REGISTRATION

The goal is the registration of 1.5 T images into the 0.5 T images, by mapping and deformation of the images. Much of this work is based on our experience with rigid and deformable registration in neurosurgery. Initially, a diagnostic staging MRI is obtained with an endorectal coil, which provides excellent SNR characteristics in the region of the prostate.

Registration techniques are useful when the organ or target of interest moves, changes shape, or has characteristics that vary at different points in time. Our experience in rigid and deformable registration is mostly from neurosurgery. Viola and Wells *(30–32)* have developed a fully automatic rigid registration method for multimodal medical image registration. The method is based on a formulation of the mutual information between the model and the image. The method is intensity based instead of feature based, which has the advantage of not requiring presegmentation of the data. Registration of MR to MR, MR to computed tomography, MR to single-photon emission computed tomography and positron emission tomography, and video to 3D models has be en successfully performed on test data sets and has been used in many cases *(33)*.

In deformable registration, Warfield, Dengler, and Robatino *(34)* implemented Dengler's optical flow-based deformable registration in our high-performance computing setting.

This method constructs and minimizes an energy function in which two terms control goodness-of-matching and elasticity of deformation. The deformation model is a continuous 3D vector field generalization of a controlled continuity functional. Our first major application of the technique was to use nonlinear registration for template driven segmentation. A method to measure spatial and temporal brain deformation from sequential intraoperative MRI has also been developed. Deformation is estimated with a volumetric optical flow measurement based on local intensity differences. The method demonstrated a good capability of intra-operative surface, subsurface and midline shift measurement.

Therefore, a manual and interactive matching tool may be helpful for matching the leg-up and leg-down images. Using this tool, we can start the registration from a better initial guess and thus can expect the more accurate matching in shorter time. Because of the close proximity and the anterior placement of the obturator relative to the prostate, the prostate also displaces posteriorly. In preliminary experiments, this deformation model has been based on physical principles associated with the soft tissue deformation under external force. The external force, in our case, is the obturator. We model this external force as a point source located in the rectum having a displacement force that falls off at the rate of $1/r$, with r being the distance from the point source. Under the influence of this external force, the soft tissue (i.e., the prostate) deforms. However, as with all soft tissues, the prostate deforms with resistance. The more the prostate deforms, the more it resists the change. Thus many steps have been integrated to allow a detailed and precise registration and segmentation of the prostate imaging data sets.

ACKNOWLEDGMENT

Funding for this research has been provided by NIH grant R01 AG19513.

SUMMARY

As our imaging techniques improve, the role of image guided interventions has increased. We will need tissue sampling for validation and pathological confirmation of disease activity. More importantly, we will need new and noninvasive methods to deliver therapy with image guidance to precise targets.

REFERENCES

1. American Cancer Society website: www.cancer.org. American Cancer Society Inc., Surveillance Research 2002.
2. Terris MK. Sensitivity and specificity of sextant biopsies in the detection of prostate cancer: preliminary report. *Urology* 1999;54:486–489.
3. Keetch DW, McMurtry JM, Smith DS, Andriole GL, Catalona WJ. Prostate specific antigen density versus prostate specific antigen slope as predictors of prostate cancer in men with initially negative prostatic biopsies. *J Urol* 1996;156:428–431.
4. Naughton CK, Smith DS, Humphrey PA, Catalona WJ, and Keetch DW. Clinical and pathologic tumor characteristics of prostate cancer as a function of the number of biopsy cores: a retrospective study. *Urology* 1998;52(5):808–813.
5. Tempany CM, Rahmouni AD, Epstein JI, Walsh PC, Zerhouni EA. Invasion of the neurovascular bundle by prostate cancer: evaluation with MR imaging. *Radiology* 1991;181:107–112.
6. Carter HB, Brem RF, Tempany CM, et al. Nonpalpable prostate cancer: detection with MR imaging. *Radiology* 1991;78:523–525.
7. Hricak H, White S, Vigneron D, et al. Carcinoma of the prostate gland: MR imaging with pelvic phased-array coils versus integrated endorectal–pelvic phased-array coils. *Radiology* 1994;193:703–709.
8. Ellis JH, Tempany C, Sarin MS, Gatsonis C, Rifkin MD, McNeil BJ. MR imaging sonography of early prostatic cancer: pathologic imaging features that influence identification diagnosis. *AJR Am J Roentgenol* 1994;162:865–872.
9. Ikonen S, Karkkainen P, Kivisaari L, et al. Magnetic resonance imaging of clinically localized prostatic cancer. *J Urol* 1998;159:915–919.
10. Perrotti M, Han, K-R, Epstein RE, et al. Prospective evaluation of endorectal magnetic resonance imaging to detect tumor foci in men with prior negative prostastic biopsy: a pilot study. *J Urol* 1999;162:1314–1317.
11. Silverman SG, Collick BD, Figueira MR, et al. Interactive MR-guided biopsy in an open-configuration MR imaging system [see comments]. *Radiology* 1995;197:175–181.
12. D'Amico AV, Cormack RA, Tempany CM. MRI-guided diagnosis treatment of prostate cancer. *N Engl J Med* 2001;344:776–777.

13. Hata N, Jinzaki M, Kacher D, et al. MRI-guided prostate biopsy with surgical navigation software: device validation feasibility. *Radiology* 2001;220:263–268.

14. Kurhanewicz J, Swanson MG, Nelson SJ, Vigneron DB. Combined magnetic resonsnce imaging spectroscopic imaging approach to molecular imaging of prostate cancer. *J Magn Reson Imaging* 2002;16:463.

15. Kaji Y, Kurhanewicz J, Hricak H, et al. Localizing prostate cancer in the presence of postbiopsy changes on MR images: role of proton MR spectroscopic imaging. *Radiology* 1998;206:785–790.

16. Liney GP, Knowles AJ, Manton DJ, Turnbull LW, Blackband SJ, Horsman A. Comparison of conventional single echo multi-echo sequences with a fast spin-echo sequence for quantitative T2-mapping: application to the prostate. *J Magn Reson Imaging* 1996;6: 603–607.

17. Lowry M, Liney GP, Turnbull LW, Manton DJ, Blackband SJ, Horsman A. Quantification of citrate concentration in the prostate by proton magnetic resonance spectroscopy: zonal age related differences. *Magn Reson Med* 1996;36:352–358.

18. Liney GP, Lowry M, Turnbull LW, et al. Proton MR T2 maps correlate with the citrate concentration in the prostate. *NMR Biomed* 1996;9:59–64.

19. Liney GP, Turnbull LW, Lowry M, Turnbull LS, Knowles AJ, Horsman A. In vivo quantitation of citrate concentration water T2 relaxation time of the pathologic prostate gland using ¹H MR MRI. *Magn Reson Imaging* 1997;15:1177–1186.

20. Maier SE, Bogner P, Bajzik G, et al. Normal brain brain tumor: multicomponent apparent diffusion coefficient line scan imaging. *Radiology* 2001;219:842–849.

21. Schenck JF, Jolesz FA, Roemer PB, et al. Superconducting open-configuration MR imagingsystem for image-guided therapy. *Radiology* 1995;195:805–814.

22. Jolesz FA. 1996 RSNA Eugene P. Pendergrass New Horizons Lecture. Image-guided procedures the operating room of the future. *Radiology* 1997;204:601–612

23. D'Amico AV, Cormack R, Tempany CM, et al. Real-time magnetic resonance image-guided interstitial brachytherapy in the treatment of select patients with clinically localized prostate cancer. *Int J Radiat Oncol Biol Phys* 1998;42:507–515.

24. Tempany C, D'Amico A, Cormack R, Kumar S, Silverman S, Jolesz F. MR guided prostatebrachytherapy: a new approach to seed implantation. in NE-AUA. 1999;

25. Cormack R, Kooy H, Tempany C, D'Amico A. (1998) A clinical method for real-time dosimetric guidance of transperineal 125I prostate implants using interventional magnetic resonance imaging. *Int J Radiat Oncol Biol Phys* 2000;46(1): 207–214.

26. Hurwitz MD, Cormack R, Tempany CM, Kumar S, D'Amico AV. Three-dimensional real-time magnetic resonance-guided interstitial prostate brachytherapy optimizes radiation dose distribution resulting in a favorable acute side effect profile in patients with clinically localized prostate cancer. *Tech Urol* 2000;6(2):89–94.

27. McTavish J, D'Amico A, Cormack R, Jolesz F, Tempany C. Evaluation of interventional MRI images (0.5T) of the prostate gland compared to endorectal coil MRI images (1.5T) in men undergoing MR guided brachytherapy (abstr), in *Proceedings of the Seventh Meeting of the International Society for Magnetic Resonance in Medicine*, Philadelphia, PA, 1999, p. 1972.

28. Hata N, Wells WM III, Warfield S, Kikinis R, Jolesz FA. Computer assisted intraoperative MR-guidedtherapy: pre- intra-operative image registration, enhanced three-dimensional display, deformable registration, in 7th Annual meeting Japan Society of Computer Aided Surgery. Sapporo, Japan; 1997.

29. Richard WD. Keen CG. Automated texture-based segmentation of ultrasound images of the prostate. *Comput Med Imaging Graph* 1996;20:131–140.

30. Wells WM III, Viola P, Atsumi H, Nakajima S, Kikinis R. Multi-modal volume registration by maximization of mutual information. *Med Image Anal* 1996;1:35–51.

31. Viola P. Wells W. Alignment by maximization of mutual information. *Int J Comp Vision* 1997;24:137–154.
32. Wells WM III, Viola P, Atsumi H, Nakajima S, Kikinis R. Multi-modal volume registration by maximization of mutual information. *Med Image Anal* 1996;1:35–51.
33. Kagawa K Lee WR, Schultheiss TE, Hunt MA, Shaer AH, Hanks GE. Initial clinical assessment of CT–MRI image fusion software in localization of the prostate for 3D conformal radiation therapy. *Int J Radiat Oncol Biol Phys* 1997;38:319–325.
34. Warfield SW, Robatino A, Dengler J, et al. Nonlinear registration and template driven segmentation, in *Brain Warping* (Toga AW, ed.), Academic Press, San Diego, CA, 1999, pp. 67–84.

3

Image-Guided Needle Biopsy of Nonpalpable Breast Lesions

Darrell N. Smith, MD, MSc

INTRODUCTION

The decline in mortality from breast cancer seen in the United States beginning in 1989 appears to be correlated with the increased use of screening mammography programs. Data from the Swedish Two County Study show that the implementation of a screening program decreased mortality by 60% *(1)*.

Before 1970, breast biopsies were performed most commonly because of abnormalities discovered by physical examination. Screening mammography changed the presentation of breast cancer from large palpable masses detected by physical examination to small nonpalpable invasive carcinomas and preinvasive lesions (ductal carcinoma *in situ*).

Even in the presence of a palpable breast mass, mammography is essential in the evaluation of palpable lesions to determine extent of disease and the presence of calcifications associated with nonpalpable disease. The most valuable and readily used adjunct to mammography is breast ultrasound. Not only useful in the evaluation of palpable abnormalities, ultrasound is an indispensable tool for interrogating masses detected by mammography. Both mammography and ultrasound are routinely used to guide the various interventional procedures used to diagnosis breast cancer. Currently, approx 1 million breast biopsies are performed in the United States each year, of which at least 300,000 (30%) are for nonpalpable lesions. This number is expected to increase steadily as the women of the baby-boom population continue to enter the pool of women recommended to undergo screening mammography.

WIRE LOCALIZATION FOR EXCISIONAL SURGICAL BIOPSY

The acceptance by the general public of breast cancer screening with mammography resulted in the increased detection of suspicious nonpalpable breast abnormalities that warranted tissue sampling. A review in 1997 of 12,563 breast biopsies from 49 studies showed positive predictive value to range from 0–63% but was 26% overall *(2)*. This means that up to 75% of breast biopsies will yield benign findings *(3)*. Accordingly, an accurate technique for sampling suspicious areas while sparing as much normal breast tissue as possible was needed. Mammographic wire localization of nonpalpable breast lesions became readily available in the 1980s *(4,5)*. For this procedure, the diagnostic

From: *Image-Guided Diagnosis and Treatment of Cancer*
Edited by: A. D'Amico, J. S. Loeffler, and J. R. Harris © Humana Press Inc., Totowa, NJ

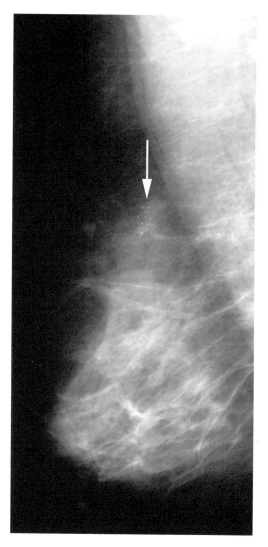

Fig. 1. The baseline mammogram in a 52-yr-old woman detected a nonpalpable 15-mm soft tissue mass with associated suspicious calcifications in the mid-upper left breast (arrow).

mammograms are reviewed to plan the approach of the localizing wire (Fig. 1). The procedure is explained to the patient. Although pneumothorax is a potential risk of this technique, it is extremely unlikely to occur with the grid localization technique that maintains a needle path parallel to the chest wall. The shortest distance from skin to lesion (mass or calcification cluster) is determined. This surface is positioned against the compression paddle. A compression paddle with an alphanumeric grid and an open window is used. The patient's breast remains in compression while the film is developed and the alphanumeric coordinates are determined (Fig. 2). The advent of digital imaging has significantly decreased the overall amount of time spent in compression by the patient (images are displayed instantaneously on a computer monitor rather than waiting for the film image to develop). The coordinates determined from the image are

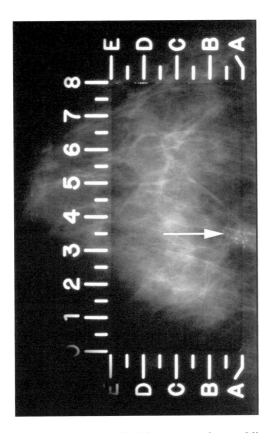

Fig. 2. Targeting mammogram obtained with compression paddle and alphanumeric grid positioned over the lesion (arrow).

use to mark the skin insertion site with ink. The skin overlying the needle insertion site is cleansed with povidone soap and alcohol. Local anesthetic is administered to the skin and deeper tissues along the expected path of the localizing needle. The localizing needled is placed perpendicular to the skin. The shadow of the hub of the needle is used to assess for any unwanted angulation of the needle's trajectory, that is, the shadow of the hub should directly overlie the insertion site. Mammographic images are obtained to confirm the needle position over the lesion (Fig. 3). Compression is released and the orthogonal plane image is obtained to assess the needle tip's location in relationship to the targeted lesion (Fig. 4). Depth adjustments are made as necessary. Ideally, the needle tip extends 1 cm beyond the lesion. A flexible localizing wire is placed through the localizing needle. The needle is withdrawn, leaving the hook wire behind (Fig. 5). Final images of the wire in orthogonal planes are obtained and annotated as a guide for the surgeon in the operating room. To facilitate the removal of extensive areas of involvement, two or more wires can be used to bracket the abnormality *(6)*. After surgical removal of the localizing wire(s) and lesion, it is important to radiograph the specimen (Fig. 6) to insure that the targeted lesion was removed *(7)*.

Subsequently, ultrasound-guided wire localization of masses was also reported in the 1980s *(8)*. The mass is identified by ultrasound (calcifications without an associ-

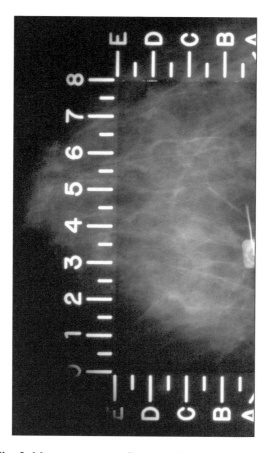

Fig. 3. Mammogram confirms needle position over the lesion.

ated soft tissue mass are not reliably visualized by ultrasound) (Fig. 7). The patient's breast is positioned to allow for an approach to the mass that is tangential to the chest wall. A skin entry site is marked with ink. Povidone soap and alcohol are used to cleanse the skin and the ultrasound transducer. Local anesthetic is used to make a skin wheal. A syringe with local anesthetic can be loaded onto the localizing needle. Direct ultrasound visualization of the needle is used to guide the needle tip to the targeted mass. Anesthesia is administered along the path of the needle as needed. As in mammographically guided localizations, the needle tip is advanced to at least 1 cm beyond the lesion (Fig. 8). The localizing wire is placed inside the needle and the needle is withdrawn over the wire. Although the wire with its hook can be visualized with ultrasound (Fig. 9), mammograms in orthogonal planes should be obtained as a guide for the surgeon in the operating room. Additionally, this can confirm that the ultrasonographic lesion correlates with a mammographic finding (if any). After the surgical excision, ultrasound should be used to image the biopsy specimen to insure that the targeted lesion has been removed *(9)*. The surgical specimen is placed in a clear plastic resealable bag with as much as possible of the surrounding air compressed out of the bag. The bag is placed on a firm surface. Ultrasound gel is applied over the outside of the plastic bag to provide an adequate coupling surface between the transducer and the specimen. Typically, the lesion and the localizing wire are readily visible.

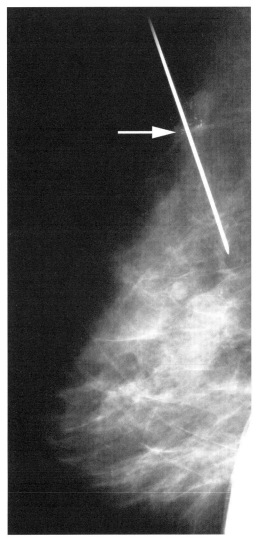

Fig. 4. Orthogonal mammographic projection shows that the localizing needle traverses the lesion (arrow).

FINE-NEEDLE ASPIRATION

The widespread use of this technique has been limited by several factors. Fine-needle aspiration biopsy (FNAB) can detect malignant cells but can offer no information on invasion or histologic grade. Insufficient specimens (particularly in benign lesions), lack of adequate training in aspiration techniques, and a paucity of dedicated breast cytopathologists pose important problems for FNAB. The implementation of FNAB in the United States has been particularly limited as the result of few highly trained cytopathologists. There is an unacceptably high false-negative rate.

The technique for FNAB of palpable breast lesions has been well described by a National Cancer Institute–sponsored conference in 1996 *(10)*. Arisio et al. *(11)* described a series of 6954 lesions sampled by FNAB (of which 97.3% were palpable lesions). This study excluded 2844 lesions (41%) for which there was no clinical follow-up or

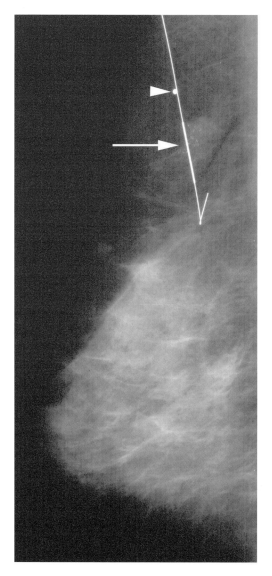

Fig. 5. Mammogram after wire placement shows the skin entry site (arrowhead) and collar (arrow) of the hook wire.

information from subsequent surgical excision. For the 4110 lesions with surgical or 1 yr clinical follow-up, 9% had FNAB findings that were described as inconclusive or inadequate. Of these lesions, 29% were found to be malignant at surgery or clinical follow-up (*in situ* lesions were not included in the malignant category). The authors also reviewed 60 articles published between 1983 and 1996 that reported FNAB of the breast. Sensitivities for the 54 articles limited to palpable lesions ranged from 61 to 98%. Specificities ranged from 56 to 100%. False-positive rates are generally low (0–9.5%), whereas false-negative rates are more variable ranging from 2 to 44%. The rates of inadequate samples ranged from 3.5 to 36%. This study highlights the diffi-culty in interpreting results from different FNAB studies. Direct comparisons are prob-

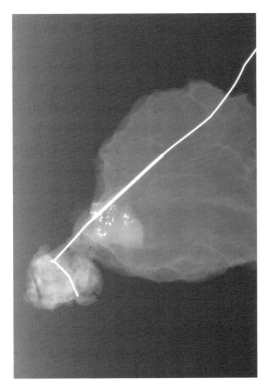

Fig. 6. Specimen radiography shows the distal portion of the hookwire and the excised lesion. Pathology showed invasive ductal carcinoma.

lematic because authors vary on whether or not inadequate and inconclusive specimens are included in the statistical analyses of sensitivity and specificity.

Image-guided FNAB has been reported as a method of diagnosing nonpalpable lesions *(12)*. Stereotactic guidance for FNAB was described in 1989 by Ciatto et al. *(13)*. In this series, positive results were found in 44 cancers, atypia was detected in 13 cancers and five benign lesions, and negative results were obtained in 11 cancers and 109 benign lesions. Inadequate tissue was obtained in six cancers and 30 benign lesions. These authors concluded that "in patients strongly suspected of having cancer at mammography, the decision to perform biopsy must be independent of the cytologic report as false-negative cytologic findings are expected." A more recent series of mammographically guided FNAB of 215 nonpalpable lesions has shown that the likelihood of obtaining samples that are insufficient for diagnosis is as high as 54% *(14)*. Additionally, the radiologist performing FNAB will generally be unable to determine from gross inspection whether the sample is adequate. A cytopathologist is needed on site at the time of the biopsy to evaluate slides for adequacy of cellular material. Such experienced cytopathologists may not be available at all institutions.

A series of 1885 ultrasound-guided FNAB of nonpalpable breast lesions was reported in 1999 *(15)*. This series used FNAB based on guidelines from the National Cancer Institute. Four hundred eighty lesions were shown to be benign cysts. Of the remaining 1405 lesions, 41% were diagnosed as benign and 36% were diagnosed as malignant after FNAB. The remaining 23% of these 1405 lesions were deemed "atypical," "sus-

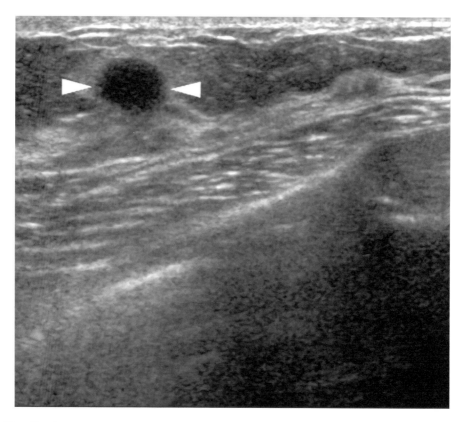

Fig. 7. Right breast ultrasound performed to evaluate a nonpalpable mammographic mass shows an 8-mm hypoechoic mass (arrowheads).

picious," or "nondiagnostic." Follow-up showed a malignancy rate of 3.7% in lesions diagnosed as benign, 99% in lesions diagnosed as malignant, 53% in lesions diagnosed as atypical, 76% in lesions diagnosed as suspicious, and 34% in lesions reported as nondiagnostic.

The disadvantages of FNAB include the absolute requirement for an expert cytopathologist, the inability to yield adequate material in cases of fibrous tumors, the possibility of false-negative and false-positive results, and the inability to differentiate between invasive and noninvasive breast carcinomas.

LARGE-CORE NEEDLE BIOPSY

Large-core needle biopsy (LCNB) is preferred to fine-needle aspiration at most centers because of its ability to better characterize benign and malignant masses. A study by the National Institute of Health's Radiologic Diagnostic Oncology Group designed specifically to compare FNAB and LCNB showed that LCNB has a lower frequency of insufficient samples *(16)*. The frequency of insufficient samples at image-guided FNAB of nonpalpable breast lesions was 34% in this study. Lower insufficient rates were found for malignant lesions sampled using ultrasound guidance in comparison with low suspicion areas of microcalcifications sampled by stereotactic techniques. Regard-

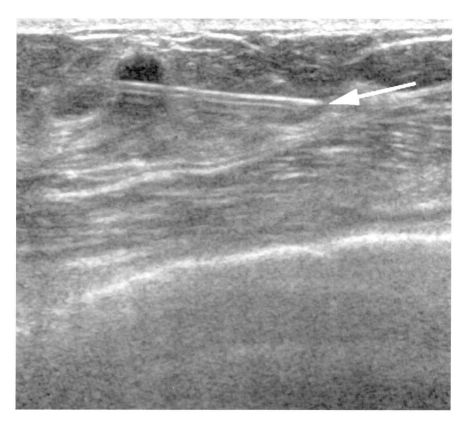

Fig. 8. Image obtained during ultrasound-guided localization shows the needle traversing the lesion. The needle tip (arrow) is seen extending beyond the lesion.

less, the unacceptably high rate of insufficient samples remains as a substantial limitation of FNAB.

Automated Core Needles

Steven Parker initially described stereotactic LCNB with a biopsy gun in 1990 *(17)*. He initially tried 18-gage needles and gradually moved to 16-gage and 14-gage needles to increase sample size. Both "short-throw" (1.15 cm) and "long-throw" (2.3 cm) needles were tried (the "throw" of the needle is equal to the distance it travels during firing). An add-on stereotactic unit to the standard mammography machine was tried and a dedicated prone table (Fig. 10) was developed. In 1991, Parker reported his first series of 102 patients, all of whom had surgical biopsy after stereotactic-guided LCNB *(18)*. There was agreement between pathology at stereotactic LCNB and surgical excision in 96% of the cases. Stereotactic-guided LCNB diagnosed two lesions missed at surgery and surgery diagnosed two lesions missed at LCNB. Subsequently, a multi-institutional study of 6152 lesions was reported in 1994 *(19)*. The cancer miss rate in this series was 1.2%. This compares favorably with failure rates for excisional biopsy after wire localizations, reported to range between 0.2 and 20% *(20–23)*. This multi-institutional study had a very low complication rate (0.2%) (either hematoma or infection). No instance of needle track seeding was reported among patients during surgical or clinical follow-up. A single case

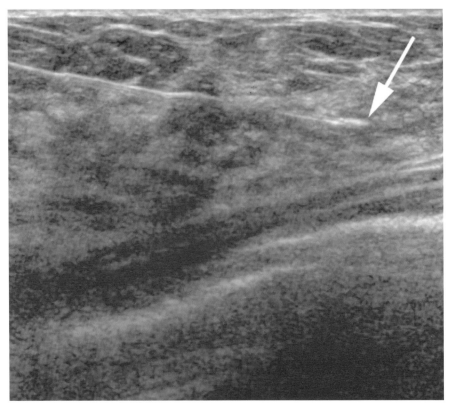

Fig. 9. Image obtained after wire placement shows the distal tip of the hookwire (arrow). Pathology showed fibroadenoma.

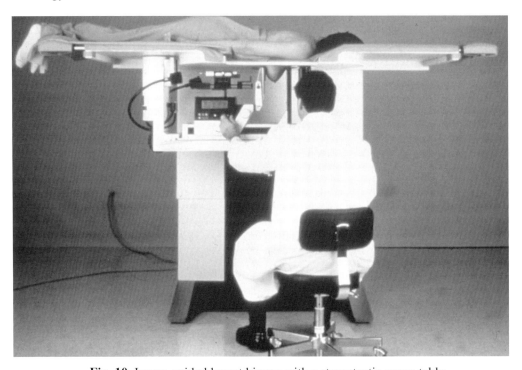

Fig. 10. Image-guided breast biopsy with a stereotactic prone table.

of malignant seeding of the needle track has been reported after stereotactic-guided LCNB of an invasive mucinous carcinoma of the breast *(24)*.

Patients are advised to avoid any medications that could potentially be a blood thinner for 3 d before the biopsy. The patient need not be nothing per oral (NPO) before the procedure.

The patient must be able to remain still for the duration of the procedure (20 min minimum). For the stereotactic table, the patient must be able to be positioned prone (severe cervical spine abnormalities may preclude adequate positioning). The risks of the procedure (infection and bleeding) are discussed and written informed consent obtained. After positioning in the prone position, stereotactic images are obtained at 15° positive and 15° negative to the zero axis. Digital imaging capabilities significantly decrease the amount of time the patient must remain in position. The targeted lesion must be visible in both stereotactic images. X, Y, and Z coordinates are obtained from the stereotactic images (typically these are automatically calculated by the imaging device). After calibration of the device, the needle is moved to the X and Y coordinates. The skin is cleansed with povidone soap and alcohol. The needle is advanced along the Z axis until it touches the skin. This skin entry site is injected with local anesthetic. Additional local anesthetic (often with diluted epinephrine) is administered along the expected needle track. A small skin nick (4–5 mm) is made just large enough to allow easy passage of the biopsy needle through the dermis. The needle is advanced along the Z-axis until the needle is 5 mm shy of the targeted lesion. Prefire stereotactic images are obtained to confirm appropriate targeting (Fig. 11). Adjustments are made as necessary. The needle is fired and post-fire images are obtained to confirm that the needle has traversed the lesion. The automated multipass needle has an inner stylet with a sampling notch that fires forward through the target (Fig. 12). Almost immediately a cutting sleeve fires forward to cover the sampling notch, trapping the core specimen with the needle. The needle is removed from the breast and the core sample retrieved (Fig. 13). The needle is replaced on the stereotactic device and the next sample is obtained. Typically, five passes are made through masses and 8–12 passes through calcification clusters *(25)*. If the targeted lesion is a calcification cluster, a radiograph of the core specimens is obtained to confirm the presence of calcifications (Fig. 14). As described, a separate insertion and removal of the needle is required to obtain each specimen. As increasing numbers of samples are obtained, the later samples are often composed predominantly of blood rather than breast tissue. Adequate sampling of small calcification clusters and small masses is particularly challenging. The technique leaves minimal post biopsy changes at the targeted site. Unfortunately, the automated needle technique does not provide a readily available mechanism for leaving behind a localizing marker if the entire mammographic lesion is removed.

It is estimated that over 90% of mammographic lesions that require biopsy can be sampled by LCNB. Lesions that are too close to the nipple–areolar complex or too close to the chest wall may not be accurately targeted. Calcifications that are too faint to see on stereotactic images should be sampled by wire localization (which can be performed under magnification views). An area of architectural distortion that is highly suggestive of a complex sclerosing lesion (radial scar) is best evaluated by removal en toto. Most prone stereotactic tables have a weight limit of 300 lbs (135 kg). If the patient's breast compresses to less than 2.5 cm, it may not be possible to place the biopsy needle in the breast without puncturing the opposite skin surface.

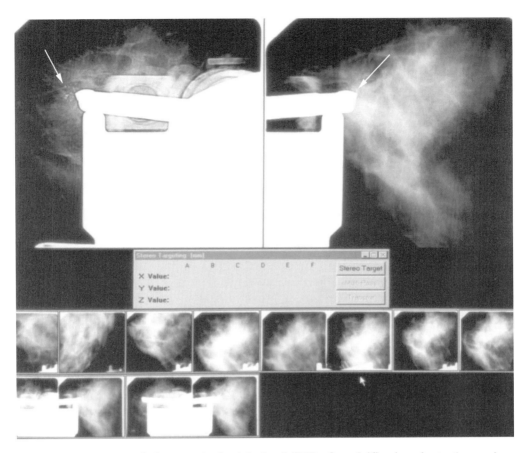

Fig. 11. Stereotactic images obtained during LCNB of a calcification cluster (arrows).

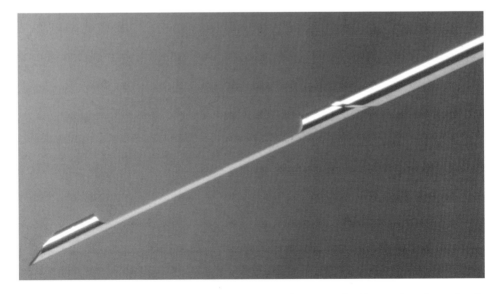

Fig. 12. Distal portion of a 14-gage automated multipass needle (the cutting sleeve has been withdrawn to show the sampling notch).

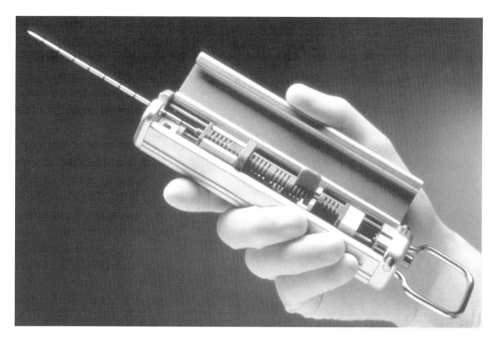

Fig. 13. Reusable automated firing device with 14-gage multipass needle in place.

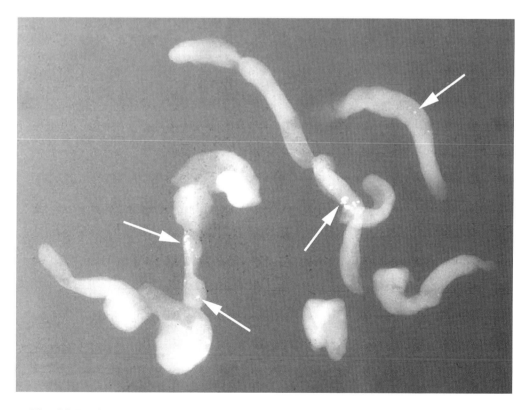

Fig. 14. Radiograph of core samples obtained to confirm excision of targeted calcifications (arrows).

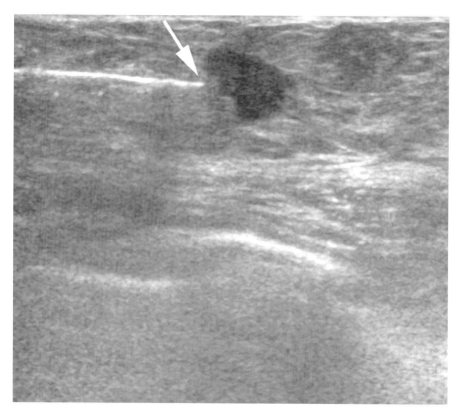

Fig. 15. A 32-yr-old pregnant woman presented with a palpable breast mass. Prefire image during a 14-gage ultrasound-guided LCNB shows the needle tip (arrow) adjacent to the mass.

The percutaneous diagnosis of atypical ductal hyperplasia (ADH) in a lesion that has ductal carcinoma *in situ* (DCIS) has been termed an ADH underestimate; the percutaneous diagnosis of DCIS in a lesion that has infiltrating ductal carcinoma has been termed a DCIS underestimate *(26)*. Under stereotactic guidance with the 14-gage sample size, approx 50% of calcifications clusters that show only atypical ductal hyperplasia at LCNB will underestimate invasive carcinoma or DCIS found at excisional biopsy *(27)*.

Ultrasound-guided 14-gage LCNB was first described in a series of 181 patients by Parker et al. *(28)*. In this report, 49 of these 181 lesions were eventually excised (including 34 malignancies) and showed complete agreement between pathology from the surgical excision and pathology from the LCNB. No cancers were found during follow-up (12–36 mo) of the unexcised benign lesions. This technique is typically easier for patients and faster than LCNB using stereotactic guidance (Figs. 15 and 16). There have been few reports of large series of ultrasound-guided LCNB since Parker et al's original report of 181 ultrasound-guided LCNBs in 1993 *(28)*. Chare et al. *(29)* described a series of 125 lesions sampled by 16-gage ultrasound-guided LCNB. A definite decision regarding patient management could be made in only 88 (70%) lesions in this series. The remaining 37 patients underwent surgical excision, and 12 additional malignancies were found. The lack of adequate tissue sampling in this series may have been related to the smaller (16-gage) needle used. Smith et al. *(30)* reported a series of

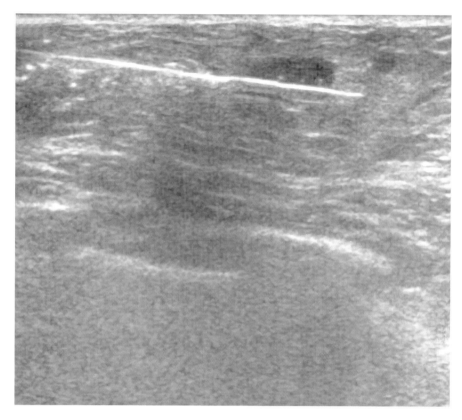

Fig. 16. Post-fire image during a 14-gage ultrasound-guided core biopsy shows the needle traversing the mass. Pathology showed invasive ductal carcinoma.

500 ultrasound-guided LCNBs of solid masses in 446 women *(30)*. Histopathologic results were correlated with imaging findings. Ultrasound-guided LCNB diagnosed a malignancy ($n = 124$) or severe ADH ($n = 4$) in 128 lesions (26%). In the remaining 372 lesions (74%) ultrasound-guided LCNB yielded benign pathology. Follow-up greater than 1 yr ($N = 225$) and/or results of surgical excision ($N = 50$) were obtainable in 275 (74%) of the benign lesions. No malignancies were discovered at surgical excision or during follow-up of this group of benign lesions. There were no complications related to LCNB that required additional treatment. Ultrasound-guided LCNB is a safe and accurate method for evaluating breast lesions that require tissue sampling. Of the malignant lesions in this study, discordance between the histopathology after ultrasound-guided LCNB and the histopathology after surgical excision was rarely seen. Only one of five lesions diagnosed as DCIS by ultrasound-guided LCNB was an underestimation of invasive ductal carcinoma after surgical excision. Two lesions diagnosed as ADH by ultrasound-guided LCNB were an underestimation of DCIS after surgical excision. The remaining two lesions diagnosed as ADH by ultrasound-guided LCNB were an underestimation of invasive ductal carcinoma after surgical excision. As previously stated, ADH diagnosed at LCNB is an indication for surgical biopsy because of the high prevalence of ductal carcinoma *in situ* in these lesions. Rates of underestimation are significantly lower in mass lesions than in sampling of calcification clusters.

Liberman et al. *(31)* have pointed out that cost savings for ultrasound-guided LCNB should exceed those with stereotactic biopsy. The equipment is less expensive and multifunctional ultrasound machines are readily available in most radiology departments. LCNB has a number of advantages over FNAB in the evaluation of breast masses. These include lower inadequacy and equivocal rates and the ability to make a definitive diagnosis of a fibroadenoma. In addition, a core result of normal breast tissue alerts the clinician to the possibility of sampling error and the need for repeat biopsy.

Stereotactic- and ultrasound-guided LCNB use similar biopsy instruments to obtain cores of tissue from breast lesions. Both can be used to sample masses. Although the administration of local anesthesia and even minimal bleeding can obscure the targeted lesion if stereotactic mammographic imaging is used, these factors rarely affect the ability of ultrasound to visualize a solid mass. Microcalcifications are better visualized with stereotactic mammographic imaging than with ultrasound. Most use stereotactic guidance for calcifications and ultrasonographic guidance for mass lesions.

As in any percutaneous sampling procedure, there are potential pitfalls. The radiologist performing the LCNB is generally aware of any technical difficulties that might result in inaccurate sampling. These difficulties include targeting errors, patient movement, and obscuration of the lesion by accumulating blood. If after LCNB, there is concern that the lesion was not accurately targeted, rebiopsy (LCNB or surgical biopsy) is indicated. Similar recommendations exist after surgical biopsy if specimen imaging (mammographic or ultrasonographic) does not clearly show the lesion. If the pathologic findings are nonspecific or indicate only normal breast or fatty tissue and no evidence of a mass-forming lesion, there is a possibility that the lesion has been missed and rebiopsy is recommended *(32)*. A cooperative effort between radiologist, surgeon, and pathologist is required for meticulous radiology–pathology correlation.

Image-guided LCNB is widely available. In a survey of members of the Society of Breast Imaging *(33)*, 71% of respondents reported that both stereotactic and ultrasound-guided LCNBs were available at their institution. In 13% only ultrasound-guided LCNBs were available. However, only 48% of these respondents believe that image-guided LCNB would replace most surgical biopsies.

Directional Vacuum-Assisted (DVA) Biopsy Probes

DVA biopsy probes have several design advantages compared with automated needles. The DVA system consists of a disposable biopsy probe and a reusable drive unit *(34)*. This device can be used with either stereotactic or ultrasonographic imaging guidance. The probes are available in a 14-gage, 11-gage, and an 8-gage size (Fig. 17). For stereotactic biopsy, the probe is typically fired into the breast so that the tip of the probe is just distal to the lesion. However, firing the probe is not necessary for tissue acquisition. Within the biopsy probe is a vacuum channel and a rotating cutting cylinder. Just proximal to the piercing tip of the probe is an aperture through which tissue is drawn by the vacuum. The sample is retrieved by withdrawing only the cutting cylinder that is on the inside of the coaxial pair instead of the outside as in the automated core needle. The sampling notch component of the probe remains in position within the lesion, eliminating the risk of unintentional change in needle position for subsequent sampling. Vacuum can be used to suction blood out of the biopsy cavity during and at the end of the biopsy procedure. Also, because of the vacuum, tissue can be acquired at a

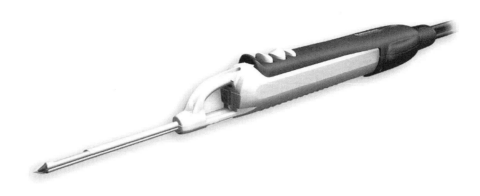

Fig. 17. Eight-gage Mammotome® DVA device.

distance from the probe (up to 5 mm away from the position of the probe), not just within the line of fire. The needle can be rotated 360° around its long axis, resulting in contiguous sampling from a large area of tissue via the eccentrically located sampling notch on the side of the needle. Therefore, multiple specimens may be obtained from a single insertion. Individual specimens are larger than those obtained with the 14-gage automated needle. The larger size of individual specimens and the ease of obtaining multiple specimens allow a substantially larger volume of tissue to be obtained. Berg et al. *(35)* and Burbank et al. *(34)* demonstrated considerable increase in size of the individual specimens obtained with DVA vs automated core needles. A small metallic clip can be deployed at the site of the biopsy to act as a marker should surgical excision be required. This is particularly useful for small lesions in which the mammographic target may be removed at percutaneous biopsy.

Calcifications retrieval rates typically ranges from 95 to 100% by using the DVA biopsy device as compared with the automated LCNB, which had a reported calcifications retrieval rate or 86 to 94% *(36,37)*. It is likely that even this difference is an underestimation of the improvement resulting from the DVA device. As the ease of calcifications retrieval with the DVA biopsy device was discovered, smaller, more challenging calcification clusters that would not have been attempted by automated multipass needles are now routinely sampled by stereotactic DVA biopsy.

The characterization of lesions containing ductal carcinoma *in situ* and atypical ductal hyperplasia has become more accurate with the DVA biopsy probe. The largest series (3873 LCNBs) to examine this issue was reported by Darling et al. in 2000 *(38)*. They showed an ADH underestimate for 14-gage multipass of 44%, for 14-gage DVA of 39%, and for 11-gage DVA of 19%. Similarly, this series shows a DCIS underestimate for 14-gage multipass of 21%, for 14-gage DVA of 17%, and for 11-gage DVA of 10%.

DVA biopsy probes are available for use with ultrasonographic guidance. The operation is similar to that used with stereotactic imaging except that the firing mechanism is not used. The biopsy probe is positioned into or adjacent to the lesion under ultrasonographic guidance and samples are obtained with the vacuum and rotating cutter. This allows for visualization of the cutter as it samples the lesion. Also, any accumulating hematoma can be removed via the vacuum. Marker clips may also be placed at the biopsy site should there be complete removal of the ultrasonographic lesion.

ADVANCED BREAST BIOPSY INSTRUMENTATION (ABBI) DEVICE

The ABBI device is a tissue-sampling instrument that uses stereotactic guidance. It allows the acquisition of tissue volumes larger that those obtained by automated core needles or DVA biopsy. The ABBI system is available in cannula sizes ranging up to 20 mm. The patient is positioned prone on the biopsy table and stereotactic images of the lesion are obtained. Typically, after successfully targeting by a radiologist, a surgeon administers local anesthesia and performs a skin incision for insertion of the needle into the breast. After confirmation of correction position of the needle in the lesion, the surgeon deploys a "T" bar into the breast to mark the lesion. The position of the "T" bar is confirmed by another set of stereotactic images. Additional anesthesia is administered and the skin incision is enlarged to accommodate the ABBI cannula. Cannulas range in size from 5 to 20 mm. The choice of the cannula is based on the size of the lesion. A cylindrical specimen extending from the subcutaneous tissue to distal to area of concern is obtained by activating a knife oscillation motor in the cannula. Electrocautery is applied via an internal snare, which completes the transection of the distal portion of the specimen. The cannula is removed from the breast. The biopsy site is assessed for bleeding and electrocautery used as needed. An image of the breast is obtained to document removal of the area of concern. Packing is inserted into the incision site and later removed for suture of the skin. There are many limitations to this technique. In addition to restrictions on stereotactic biopsy, such as patient weighing more than 300 lbs (135 kg), posterior lesions, and anticoagulation, other limitations exist. The required breast thickness and depth from the skin surface are greater for ABBI biopsy than for DVA biopsy. The ABBI procedure may take longer than core or DVA biopsy such that patients who are unable to lie prone for 30 to 60 min may not be candidates for ABBI. Many lesions (up to 29% in reported series) are not amenable because of strict positioning requirements *(39)*. There is a high failure rate of up to 20% in reported series *(40)*. Failures appear to be related to displacing the lesion rather than piercing the lesion with the localizing needle or "T" bar, fracture of the "T" bar, failure of the snare wire to activate properly, and dislodging the specimen during withdrawal of the blade. Larger tissue samples are obtained with mean specimen volumes of approx 13 cm^3 *(41)*. Smathers et al. *(42)* reported that 90.1% of tissue removed was from normal surrounding tissue only. Although removing such a large volume of tissue may be beneficial for some women (calcifications that represent ADH and DCIS), for most women this procedure is less desirable because it may lead to more deformity and scarring (both on physical examination and on the mammogram). The complication rate of ABBI is significantly higher than that of other percutaneous biopsy methods. Although significant complications (hematoma and infection) from 14-gage automated LCNB and 11-gage DVA biopsy have been reported in 0.2 and 0.1% of cases, respectively, the complication rate in 895 reported ABBI procedures in 1.1% *(40)*.

The theoretic advantage of ABBI is removal of an entire small infiltrating carcinoma in a single procedure in a single specimen. Smathers reported an 85.2% incidence of positive margins whereas other series report tumor present at the margin in 64 to 100% of specimens *(42)*. The ABBI biopsy device is not approved as an excisional device by the Food and Drug Administration. The ABBI biopsy procedure costs 20 times as much as 14-gage automated LCNB and over twice as much as an 11-gage DVA biopsy. It is disturbing to note the low frequency of carcinomas in series of lesions biopsied by the ABBI procedure (11–22%) *(43)*. This may represent a bias towards referring more suspicious lesions for needle localization or LCNB or this may reflect the diminished role of expert breast imagers in ABBI biopsies.

FOLLOW-UP AFTER IMAGE-GUIDED BREAST BIOPSY

Appropriate follow-up is invaluable for the evaluation of any biopsy technique. A study by Goodman et al. *(44)* showed 74% compliance in lesions recommended for surgical excision and 54% known compliance with follow-up recommendations for patients receiving imaging surveillance recommendation. Patient compliance with recommended follow-up is essential to avoid delay in diagnosing missed malignancies. Appropriate follow-up after a benign biopsy result is critical to identify any false-negative image guided breast biopsy results *(45)*.

CONCLUSIONS

Diagnostic breast procedures have been revolutionized by image guidance. Minimally invasive techniques have been developed for obtaining adequate tissue samples from breast lesions. The various techniques have been evaluated and compared. The correlation of findings at percutaneous biopsy with those obtained at surgical excision has proven the reliability of the various percutaneous techniques. This comparison has also identified which percutaneous diagnoses are unreliable and thereby require surgical excision for definitive diagnosis. Minimally invasive image-guided biopsies are less deforming, faster than surgery, and less costly.

REFERENCES

1. Tabar L, Vitak B, Chen HT, Yen M, Duffy SW, Smith RA. Beyond randomized controlled trials: organized mammographic screening substantially reduces breast carcinoma mortality. *Cancer* 2001;91:1724–1731.
2. Jackman RJ, Marzoni FA. Needle localization breast biopsy: why do we fail? *Radiology* 1997;204:677.
3. Kopans DB.: The positive predictive value of mammography. *AJR* 1992;158:521.
4. Kopans DB, Meyer JE. Versatile spring hook-wire breast lesion localizer. *AJR* 1982;138:586–587.
5. Meyer JE, Kopans DB, Stomper PC, Lindfors KK. Occult breast abnormalities: percutaneous preoperative needle localization. *Radiology* 1984;150:335–337.
6. Liberman L, Kaplan J, Van Zee KR, Morris EA, LaTrenta LR, Abramson AF, Dershaw DD. Bracketing wires for preoperative breast needle localization. *AJR* 2001;177:565–572.
7. Stomper PC, Davis SP, Sonnenfeld MR, Meyer JE, Greenes RA, Eberlein TJ. Efficacy of specimen radiography of clinically occult noncalcified lesions. *AJR* 1988;151:43–47.
8. Kopans DB, Meyer, JE, Lindfors KK, Bucchianeri SS. Breast sonography to guide cyst aspiration and wire localization of occult solid lesions. *AJR* 1984;143:489–492.
9. Frenna TH, Meyer JE, Sonnenfeld MD. US of breast biopsy specimens. *Radiology* 1994;190:573.
10. Anonymous. The uniform approach to breast fine-needle aspiration biopsy. NIH Consensus Development Conference. *Am J Surg* 1997;174:371–385.
11. Arisio R, Cuccorese C, Grazia Accinelli, Mano MP, Bordon R, Fessia L. Role of fine-needle aspiration biopsy in breast lesions: analysis of a series of 4,110 cases. *Diagn Cytopathol* 1998;18:462–467.
12. Jackson VP. The status of mammographically guided fine needle aspiration biopsy of nonpalpable breast lesions. *Radiol Clin North Am* 1992;30:155–166.

13. Ciatto S, Rosselli Del Turco M, and Bravetti P. Nonpalpable breast lesions: stereotaxic fine-needle aspiration cytology. *Radiology* 1989;173:57–59.

14. Helvic MA, Baker DE, Adler DD, Andersson I, Naylor B, Buckwalter KA. Radiographically guided fine-needle aspiration of nonpalpable breast lesions. *Radiology* 1990;174:657–661.

15. Boerner S, Fornage BD, Singletary E, Sneige N. Ultrasound-guided fine-needle aspiration (FNA) of nonpalpable breast lesions: a review of 1885 FNA cases using the National Cancer Institute-supported recommendations on the uniform approach to breast FNA. *Cancer* 1999;87:19–24.

16. Pisano ED, Fajardo LL, Tsimikas J, et al. Rate of unsufficient samples for fine-needle aspiration for nonpalpable breast lesions in a multicenter clinical trial: The Radiologic Diagnostic Oncology Group 5 Study. *Cancer* 1998;82:678–688.

17. Parker SH, Lovin JD, Jobe WE, al. Stereotactic breast biopsy with a biopsy gun. *Radiology* 1990;176:741–747.

18. Parker SH, Lovin JD, Jobe WE, Burke BJ, Hopper KD, Yakes WF. Nonpalpable breast lesions: stereotactic automated large-core biopsies. *Radiology* 1991;180:403–407.

19. Parker SH, Burbank F, Jackman RJ, et al. Percutaneous large-core breast biopsy: a multi-institutional study. *Radiology* 1994;193:359–364.

20. Rissanen TJ, Makarainen HP, Matilla SI, et al. Wire localized biopsy of breast lesions: a review of 425 cases found in screening or clinical mammography. *Clin Radiol* 1993;47:14–22.

21. Homer MJ, Smith TJ, Safaii H. Prebiopsy needle localization: methods, problems, and expected result. *Radiol Clin North Am* 1992;30:139–153.

22. Norton LW, Zeligman BE, and Pearlman NW. Accuracy and cost of needle localization breast biopsy. *Arch Surg* 1988;123:947–950.

23. Norton LW, Pearlman NW. Needle localization breast biopsy: accuracy versus cost. *Am J Surg* 1988;156:13B–15B.

24. Harter LP, Curtis JS, Ponto G, Craig PH. Malignant seeding of the needle track during stereotaxic core needle breast biopsy. *Radiology* 1992;185:713–714.

25. Liberman L, Dershaw DD, Rosen PP, Abramson AF, Deutch BM, Hann LE. Stereotactic 14-gage breast biopsy: how many core biopsy specimens are needed: *Radiology* 1994;192;793–795.

26. Burbank F. Stereotactic breast biopsy of atypical ductal hyperplasia and ductal carcinoma in situ lesions: improved accuracy with a directional, vacuum-assisted biopsy instrument. *Radiology* 1997;202:843–847.

27. Meyer JE, Smith DN, Lester SC, et al. Large-core needle biopsy of nonpalpable breast lesions. *JAMA* 1999;281:1638–1641.

28. Parker SH, Jobe WE, Dennis MA, et al . US-guided automated large-core needle biopsy. *Radiology* 1993;187:507–511.

29. Chare MJ. B., Flowers CI, O'Brien CJ, Dawson A. Image-guided core biopsy in patients with breast disease. *Br J Surg* 1996;83:1415–1416.

30. Smith DN, Rosenfield Darling ML, et al. The utility of ultrasonographically guided large-core needle biopsy: results from 500 consecutive breast biopsies. *J Ultrasound Med* 2001;20:43–49.

31. Liberman L, Feng TL, Dershaw DD, Morris EA, Abramson AF. US-guided core breast biopsy: use and cost-effectiveness. *Radiology* 1998;208:717–723.

32. Liberman L, Drotman M, Morris EA, et al. Imaging-histologic discordance at percutaneous breast biopsy: an indicator of missed cancer. *Cancer* 2000;89:2538–2546.

33. March DE, Raslavicus A, Coughlin BF, Klein SV, Makari-Judson G. Use of breast core biopsy in the United States: results of a national survey. *AJR* 1997;169:697–701.

34. Burbank F, Parker SH, Fogarty TJ. Stereotactic breast biopsy: improved harvesting with the Mammotome. *Ann Surg* 1996;62:738–744.

35. Berg WA, Krebs TL, Campassi C, Magder LS, Sun C-CJ. Evaluation of 14- and 11-gauge directional, vacuum-assisted biopsy probes and 14-gauge guns in a breast parenchymal model. *Radiology* 1997;205:203–208.
36. Meyer JE, Smith DN, DiPiro PJ, et al. Stereotactic breast biopsy of clustered microcalcifications with a directional, vacuum-assisted device. *Radiology* ;204:575–576.
37. Liberman L, Smolkin JH, Dershaw DD, Morris EA, Abramson AF, Rosen PP. Calcifications retrieval at stereotactic, 11-gauge, directional, vacuum-assisted breast biopsy. *Radiology* 1998;208:251–260.
38. Darling ML, Smith DN, Lester SC, et al. Atypical ductal hyperplasia and ductal carcinoma in situ as revealed by large-core needle breast biopsy: results of surgical excision. *AJR* 2000;175:1341–1346.
39. Baum JK, Raza S, Keeler B. ABBI breast biopsy: early experience using a combined radiological-surgical approach [abstract]. *AJR* 1998;170:83.
40. Liberman L. Advanced breast biopsy instrumentation (ABBI): analysis of published experience. *AJR* 1999;172:1413–1416.
41. Ferzli GS, Puza T, Van Vorst-Bilotti S, Waters R. Breast biopsies with ABBI: experience with 183 attempted biopsies. *Breast J* 1999;5:26–28.
42. Smathers RL. Advanced breast biopsy instrumentation device: percentages of lesion and surrounding tissue removed. *AJR* 2000:175:801–803.
43. Leibman AJ, Frager D, Cho P. Experience with breast biopsies using the advanced breast biopsy instrumentation system. *AJR* 1999;172:1409–1416.
44. Goodman KA, Birdwell RL, Ikeda DM. Compliance with recommended follow-up after percutaneous breast core biopsy. *AJR* 1998;170:89–92.
45. Lee CH, Philpotts LE, Harvath LJ, Tocino I. Follow-up of breast lesions diagnosed as benign with stereotactic core-needle biopsy: frequency of mammographic change and false-negative rate. *Radiology* 1999;212:189–194.

4

Magnetic Resonance Imaging (MRI) and MRI-Guided Intervention in the Detection and Diagnosis of Breast Cancer

Susan Greenstein Orel, MD

INTRODUCTION

As clinical investigation into the utility of magnetic resonance imaging (MRI) as a breast-imaging tool continues, there is now a large body of evidence demonstrating the increased sensitivity of MRI in the detection of breast cancer compared with conventional imaging methods, with reported sensitivities for the visualization of invasive breast cancer approaching 100% *(1–5)*. The reported sensitivities of MRI for the visualization of ductal carcinoma *in situ* (DCIS) have been more variable, ranging from 40 to 100% *(6–10)*. It has been demonstrated that not only can MRI visualize breast cancer but mammographically, sonographically, and clinically occult breast cancer, both invasive cancer and DCIS, as well. MRI has been shown to be more accurate than mammography and ultrasound in determining the size of the primary breast cancer and in the detection of multifocal, multicentric, and bilateral breast cancer *(11–18)*. In addition to these studies, which have evaluated MRI in the diagnostic setting, there are now reports of MRI-detected breast cancer in the screening setting, specifically in the evaluation of women at high risk for the development of breast cancer *(19–21)*.

Based on the very promising results of these studies, MRI of the breast is rapidly gaining popularity for use in clinical practice, outside of research centers, for the evaluation of patients with breast-related problems that are not felt to be adequately evaluated with the conventional breast imaging methods of mammography and ultrasound. However, as this imaging modality is transferred from a research setting to a clinical setting, there are ongoing technical and image interpretation issues that need to be considered. There are multiple imaging variables that can dramatically alter image quality and, at the present time, there are no clearly defined standards for what would be considered optimal imaging. There are no standard interpretation criteria for evaluating breast MRI examinations. Although the sensitivity of MRI for the detection of breast cancer appears to be very high, the specificity of MRI appears more limited, with an overlap in the appearance of benign and malignant lesions. The majority of MRI studies will demonstrate one or more enhancing lesions. Which, if any, are poten-

From: *Image-Guided Diagnosis and Treatment of Cancer*
Edited by: A. D'Amico, J. S. Loeffler, and J. R. Harris © Humana Press Inc., Totowa, NJ

tially clinically important and warrant tissue diagnosis? Which "lesions" are likely benign and can be followed? Which "lesions" likely represent enhancement of normal tissue during the secretory phase of the menstrual cycle? What should the follow-up interval be: 2 wk, 3 mo, 6 mo, 1 yr? Also, until recently, there has been a lack of commercially available MRI-guided localization and biopsy systems to permit tissue diagnosis of lesions identified only by MRI, which are deemed to be suspicious for malignancy. Finally, clinical indications warranting the use of MRI to image the breast remain to be defined. Technical and interpretation issues, the present status of MRI-guided intervention, potential clinical applications, and pitfalls of contrast-enhanced MR imaging and intervention as a method to detect, diagnose, and stage breast cancer will be described.

THE BREAST MRI EXAMINATION: TECHNICAL CONSIDERATIONS

There is no universally accepted standard or optimal technique for MRI of the breast. There are a multitude of imaging variables, including magnetic field strength (high-field vs mid-field vs low-field), breast surface coil configuration, including unilateral vs bilateral coils, and a wide variety of potential imaging parameters *(22,23)*. Despite the lack of consensus on how contrast-enhanced MRI examination of the breast should best be performed, there are general technical issues, which need to be considered.

Magnetic Field Strength

To date, most clinical investigations of MRI of the breast studies that have been performed on standard high-field MRI systems (1 to 1.5 T). For breast imaging, high-field systems present several obstacles, including high cost, the need for extensive shielding placing these units outside of breast imaging centers, and the potential for relatively long delays in patient scheduling. The lower cost of a dedicated breast MRI system (0.5 T) that can be placed directly within a breast-imaging center and the open-architecture of low-field systems (0.2–0.3 T) are very appealing for breast MRI *(24)*. There are, however, several ongoing limitations of imaging at lower field strength, including longer scan times, suboptimal fat-suppression, and potential limited visualization of small lesions *(23)*. There are no large series comparing the results of imaging at high field with those obtained at lower field strength. Although the issues described above do not preclude performing contrast-enhanced breast MRI at lower field strength, they do raise the concern that breast MRI performed at lower field strength may not simulate the experience at high field.

Breast Coils

Breast MRI is typically performed with the patient in the prone position lying on a platform placed in the MR scanner that allows the breast to extend dependently from the patient *(22,23)*. Prone patient positioning minimizes the effects of respiratory motion and is preferred to supine imaging, which results in lower image quality. A dedicated breast surface coil should be used when performing breast MRI. Many different types of surface coils are available. At the University of Pennsylvania, we have developed a prototype unilateral breast coil using a compression multicoil array with two coils on each of two plates *(25)*. The patient is examined in the prone position with the breast gently compressed between the two plates, which are placed along the medial and lateral sides of the breast. The compression minimizes patient motion and reduces the number of sagittal slices required to image the breast. This configuration also ensures that all of the breast tissue is close to one of the elements of the array, resulting in enhanced signal-to-noise ratio. We are also currently evaluating a bilateral breast coil where both breasts are imaged simultaneously using a bilateral compression array *(26)*. These coils are not, as yet, commercially available.

Intravenous Contrast

The cornerstone of breast MRI is imaging after the intravenous injection of a para-magnetic contrast agent (gadolinium chelate). Most investigators report the use of a dose of 0.1 mmol/kg of body weight. The contrast is injected intravenously, usually as a bolus, followed by a saline flush. To ensure that the postcontrast images can be obtained immediately after the contrast injection, tuning and gain adjustments should be performed before the contrast is injected and should not be readjusted for the remainder of the postcontrast enhanced sequence.

Contrast-Enhanced Sequence: Tradeoff Between Spatial and Temporal Resolution

Investigators evaluating MRI for breast cancer detection have demonstrated the need for rapid acquisition capability (high temporal resolution), where the contrast-enhanced images are obtained ideally in the first 1–4 min after bolus contrast injection *(22,23)*. With rapid imaging, small enhancing lesions can be identified before the enhancement of normal glandular tissue, which usually shows more delayed enhancement. In terms of high spatial resolution, multiple investigators have demonstrated that spatial resolution of approx 1 mm in all three directions is attainable. There are now multiple reports in the literature of MRI-detected breast cancers, both invasive and noninvasive as small as 2–3 mm in size. Unfortunately, high temporal resolution and high spatial resolution are competing strategies. Sensitivity for the detection of small enhancing foci improves with increasing spatial resolution and increasing signal to noise. However, this requires longer imaging times. However, the hightemporal resolution needed for dynamic contrast enhancement is obtained at the cost of a loss of spatial resolution, signal to noise, and/or volume of the breast imaged. With continued developments in MRI software and hardware, it is now becoming possible to image the breast with both high temporal and spatial resolution. In our practice, we currently use a three-dimensional volume, fast spoiled gradient echo sequence. With this sequence, a single breast can be imaged at high resolution in 90 s and a both breasts can be imaged simultaneously in approx 150 s.

Contrast-Enhanced Sequence: Suppression of Fat Signal

In contrast with mammography where lesion detectability is increased in a fatty background, on MRI, an enhancing lesion may not be detected because it becomes so intense to fat after the administration of intravenous contrast. Thus, the signal from fat needs to be eliminated. This can be accomplished with either so-called active or passive fat suppression. We prefer using active fat suppression, using a variation of chemical selective fat suppression *(27)*. There are a variety of other available fat suppression techniques. Alternatively, passive fat suppression can be accomplishing with postprocessing image subtraction (subtracting the precontrast from the postcontrast image. This requires that there be no patient motion between the pre- and the postcontrast sequences. Both methods of fat suppression (chemical fat suppression and image postprocessing image subtraction) can be used together and, in our experience, may aid in the detection of small enhancing lesions.

LESION DIAGNOSIS: MRI-GUIDED
LOCALIZATION/BIOPSY CAPABILITY

Although it has become clear that MRI can be used to detect breast cancers that are mammographically and clinically occult, not all enhancing lesions will prove to be malignant. Reported specificities of MRI have ranged from 37 to 97% *(23)*. With a technique that is highly sensitive but not highly specific, a needle localization or biopsy system is needed to differentiate true positive enhancing malignant lesions from false-positive benign enhancing lesions that are mammographically, sonographically, and clinically occult (Fig. 1). A few prototype MRI-guided localization/biopsy systems have been described, although only recently have breast MRI localization systems become commercially available *(12,28–32)*.

Our current strategy for performing MR-guided breast lesion localization involves scanning the patient in the prone position with mild compression of the breast between medial and lateral plates in the sagittal plane *(12,23)*. We have recently converted from using our prototype biopsy coil to using a commercially available system (USA Instruments). The lateral plate consists of a Lexan plate with a detachable coil, which can be sterilized after each procedure. The plate for needle localization contains a grid of 18-gage holes placed at 2.5-mm intervals. Another plate with 14-gage holes is used for core biopsies. Three-dimensional gradient echo images of the breast are obtained before and after the administration of intravenous gadolinium. Fiducial markers filled with (CuSO4) are placed into holes on the lateral coil to serve as reference markers. The needle position is then calculated relative to the fiducial markers for proper placement of the needle into the lesion. The patient is withdrawn from the MR magnet and an 18-gage MR-compatible needle (EZ-M, Westbury, NY) is inserted horizontally into the appropriate calculated hole while the patient is outside the MR scanner. The patient can then be returned into the MR system for confirmation of needle position. Once needle position is confirmed, either percutaneous sampling or wire placement can then be performed. One limitation of this type of localization system is access only to the lateral breast. For lesions that are in the medial potion of the breast, a lateral approach is clearly not optimal although, in our experience, the lateral approach has not been a clinical problem. Systems with access to the medial breast are being investigated. A second limitation of this type of system is that some lesions located in the axillary tail or near the chest wall may not be amenable to needle localization because the grid-hole platform limits the needle trajectory. In these cases, we position the patient more obliquely to reach the deep posterior and lateral breast tissue.

Even when a lesion can be accurately localized with MRI guidance, a major remaining limitation of MRI-guided needle localization is the inability to verify lesion removal because the MRI-identified lesions are usually not visible with mammographic or noncontrast MRI specimen radiography. Close communication with the surgeon regarding the expected location of the lesion relative to the hookwire is very important. Investigation is ongoing to find a marker that could be placed into the lesion at the time of

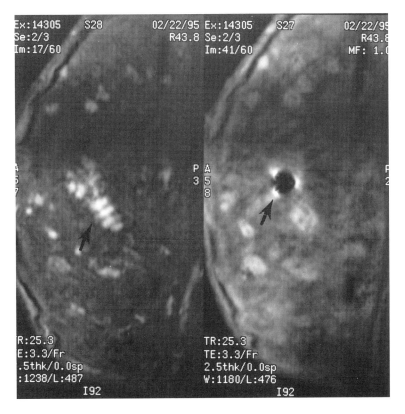

Fig. 1. MRI-guided wire localization. Images of a patient with invasive breast cancer at 6:00. Sagittal, fat-suppressed, contrast-enhanced, three-dimensional, fast spoiled, gradient echo MR image reveals a focal area of ductal enhancement (arrow in left image) in the subareolar breast. The lesion was localized with an MRI-compatible needle (arrow in right image). DCIS was found at excisional biopsy. This represented multifocal breast cancer that was occult to mammography and to physical examination. (Reprinted with permission from ref. *11*.)

localization (i.e., tiny clip similar to that used for stereotactic biopsy) that would be visible on mammographic specimen radiography so that lesion removal could be documented.

An alternative to MR-guided needle localization, which would avoid the problem of specimen radiography, is percutaneous core biopsy, where the lesion could be sampled under direct vision. Although MR-guided fine needle aspiration has been attempted, the problem of insufficient sample material is well known and we do recommend core biopsy instead. MR-compatible needles in the sizes of 18, 16, and 14 gage are available for percutaneous biopsy. Although 14-gage needles are used for routine mammographic or sonographic guidance, smaller needles, particularly 18-gage needles, have been used under direct MR guidance. MR-compatible needles do not cut as sharply as regular steel needles and there is a certain amount of artifact particularly on gradient echo images. The signal void caused by the needle can measure several times the actual needle diameter and does depend on both needle trajectory as well as the construction material. A small lesion can be completely obscured by the needle artifact and the exact location of the needle tip can sometimes not be determined.

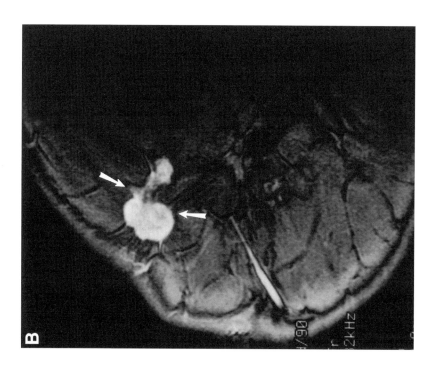

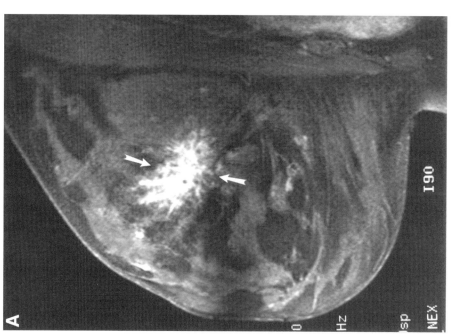

Fig. 2. False-positive enhancement. (**A**) Radial scar. Image of a patient with architectural distortion identified on a screening mammogram. Sagittal, fat-suppressed, contrast-enhanced, three-dimensional, fast spoiled, gradient echo MR image reveals regional enhancement with spiculated borders (arrows). Excisional biopsy revealed a radial scar. (**B**) Fat necrosis. Image of a patient status postlumpectomy and radiation with equivocal changes on a routine follow-up mammogram. Sagittal, fat-suppressed, contrast-enhanced, three-dimensional, fast spoiled, gradient echo MR image reveals a peripherally enhancing mass with irregular borders (arrows). Fat necrosis was found at excisional biopsy. (Reprinted with permission from ref. *41*.)

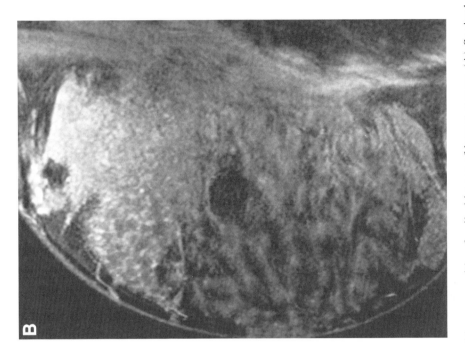

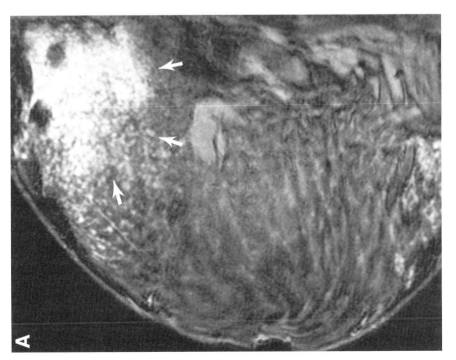

Fig. 3. Hormonal variability of contrast enhancement. Images of a 39-yr-old woman with a family history of breast cancer. (**A**) Sagittal. fat-suppressed, contrast-enhanced, three-dimensional, fast spoiled, gradient echo MR image reveals an area of regional enhancement (arrows) in the superior breast. (**B**) On a follow-up MR study obtained 2 mo later, the area of regional enhancement is no longer present. (Reprinted with permission from ref. *41.*)

We currently perform percutaneous core biopsy with an 18-gage MR-compatible gun to document needle position as well as to obtain several initial samples. Then, we bring the patient outside the MR magnet and perform several additional samples with a 14-gage biopsy gun (BARD, Covington, GA) using the same grid hole. Our experience with MR-guided core biopsy has been limited with several instances of suboptimal specimen adequacy. The use of larger needle sizes, such as the MR-guided vacuum biopsy system developed by Heywang-Kobrunner, is promising *(32)*. This system allows for multiple specimen acquisitions within an area up to 2 cm in size without the needle to withdraw the needle. This results in larger tissue samples as well as less sampling error. This device has been used on more than 120 lesions with successful biopsy in all cases but one.

IMAGE INTERPRETATION: WHAT IS A SIGNIFICANTLY ENHANCING LESION?

After contrast administration, one or more enhancing areas in the breast will often be identified. These enhancing areas must then be further characterized—are any suspicious for breast cancer? Investigators have used differences in enhancement kinetics and morphologic features in attempt to differentiate lesions suspicious for breast cancer from those felt to be benign or likely benign. Early investigation of contrast-enhanced MR imaging of the breast demonstrated that breast cancer consistently enhanced after the administration of intravenous contrast and that cancer could be differentiated from benign lesions with very high specificity *(1,2)*. However, further investigation demonstrated that in addition to breast cancer, many benign lesions demonstrated contrast enhancement *(3,33)*. Reported specificities of MRI have been very variable, ranging from 37 to 97% *(23)*. Contrast enhancement has been seen not only in cancer, but also in fibroadenomas, fibrocystic changes, including sclerosing adenosis, fat necrosis, radial scars, mastitis, atypical hyperplasia, and lobular neoplasia *(3,23,33)* (Fig. 2). In addition, normal breast tissue may enhance after contrast enhancement, and this enhancement has been shown to vary with different phases of the menstrual cycle *(34)* (Fig. 3).

The higher reported specificities have come from studies evaluating the dynamic uptake of contrast. Both quantitative and qualitative methods have been described. It has been suggested, based on the results of these studies, that enhancement kinetics can be used to differentiate malignant from benign lesions where malignant lesions demonstrate a rapid increase in signal intensity after contrast administration often followed by a wash-out of contrast on delayed images whereas benign lesions exhibit a slower, progressive rise in signal intensity without wash-out of contrast *(1,2,4,5,7,35)*. Other investigators, however, have observed an overlap in the enhancement characteristics of benign and malignant lesions, which can probably can be explained, at least in part, by histologic variability of both cancers and benign lesions *(3,33,36,37)*.

Morphologic features have also been described that may be used in selected cases to differentiate malignant from benign lesions. Features that suggest the possibility of malignancy include a mass with irregular or spiculated, borders, a mass with peripheral enhancement, an area of regional enhancement, and ductal enhancement (Figs. 4 and 5). Features suggesting benign disease include a mass with smooth or lobulated borders, a mass demonstrating minimal or no contrast enhancement, a mass with nonenhancing internal septations, and patchy parenchymal enhancement

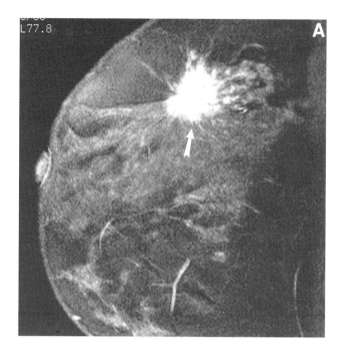

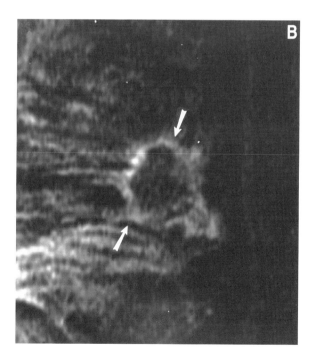

Fig. 4. *(continued on next page)* Lesion morphology: MRI appearances of invasive breast cancer. (**A**) Sagittal, fat-suppressed, contrast-enhanced, three-dimensional, fast spoiled, gradient echo MR image reveals an enhancing spiculated mass (arrow). Invasive ductal carcinoma was found at excisional biopsy. (**B**) Sagittal, fat-suppressed, contrast-enhanced, three-dimensional, fast spoiled, gradient echo MR image reveals a peripherally enhancing spiculated mass (arrows).

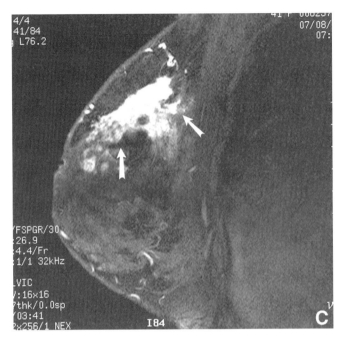

Fig. 4. *(continued)* Invasive ductal carcinoma was found at excisional biopsy. **(C)** Sagittal, fat-suppressed, contrast-enhanced, three-dimensional, fast spoiled, gradient echo MR image reveals an area of regional enhancement (arrows). This area was adjacent to a 1-cm palpable breast cancer but was mammographically, sonographically, and clinically occult. Invasive breast cancer was found at excisional biopsy. (Reprinted with permission from refs. *41* [4B] and *15* [4C].)

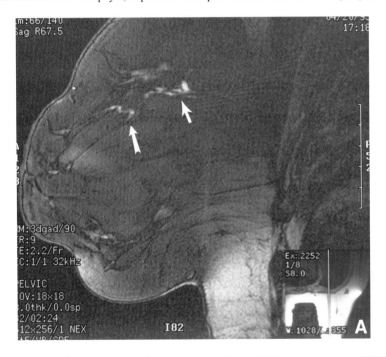

Fig. 5. *(continued on next page)* Lesion morphology: MRI appearances of DCIS. **(A)** Sagittal, fat-suppressed, contrast-enhanced, three-dimensional, fast spoiled, gradient echo MR image

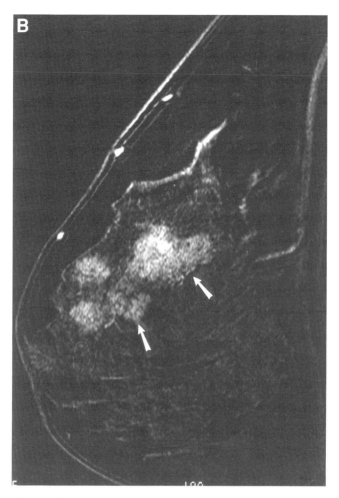

Fig. 5. *(continued)* reveals an area of linear enhancement (arrows). This corresponded to linear calcifications identified at mammography. (**B**) Sagittal, fat-suppressed, contrast-enhanced, three-dimensional, fast spoiled, gradient echo (post-imaging subtraction) MR image reveals an area of regional enhancement (arrows) that was adjacent to a known invasive breast cancer (not illustrated). Extensive DCIS was found at excisional biopsy, which was mammographically, and clinically occult. (Reprinted with permission from refs. *11* [1A] and *23* [4D].)

(3,6,7,11,33,38,39) (Fig. 6). An interpretation model encompassing multiple architectural features has been described, yielding a specificity between 70 and 80% *(40,41)*.

It is becoming increasing clear that although investigators have used either enhancement kinetics or lesion morphology in attempt to differentiate malignant from benign lesions on contrast-enhanced MRI studies, the integration of both kinetic and morphologic information may ultimately be needed to achieve optimal discrimination. The relative significance assigned to enhancement kinetics or lesion morphology will, for now, vary from practice to practice because of differences in experience, available hardware and software, and imaging parameters. Whether high temporal resolution (needed for time intensity curve analysis) should be sacrificed for high spatial resolution (needed for morphologic analysis) or visa versa, or whether both high temporal and spatial

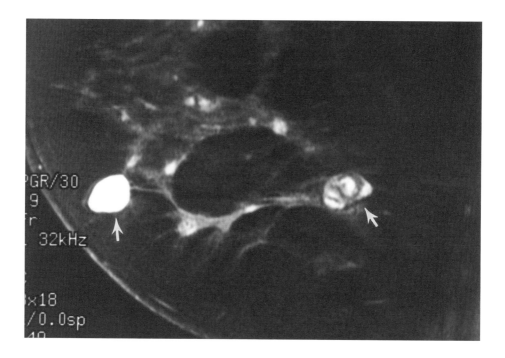

Fig. 6. Lesion morphology: MRI appearances of fibroadenomas. Image of a patient with two developing masses identified at mammography and sonography. Sagittal, fat-suppressed, contrast-enhanced, three-dimensional, fast spoiled, gradient echo MR image reveals two enhancing masses, one homogeneously enhancing with smooth borders (arrow on left side of image) and one with nonenhancing septations (arrow on right side of image). Two fibroadenomas were found at excisional biopsy. (Reprinted with permission from ref. *41*.)

resolution will be obtainable with continuing improvements in MRI technology remains to be defined. A "BI-RADS" type lexicon similar to the one used in mammography, which will encompass lesion descriptors, level of suspicion, and management recommendations is under development *(42)*.

MRI DETECTION, DIAGNOSIS, AND STAGING OF BREAST CANCER: POTENTIAL CLINICAL INDICATIONS

There is a growing demand for the use of MRI to evaluate patients with breast-related problems. Despite the absence of technical standards for optimal imaging and the absence of a unified strategy for image interpretation, these studies are being performed in clinical practice. When breast MRI studies are performed clinically, outside of research protocols, several issues should be kept in mind. In those cases where MRI is being used to further evaluate a questionable mammographic abnormality (i.e., lesion in one view, question of architectural distortion), it is critical that the MRI findings be correlated with the mammographic findings. If no abnormality is identified at MRI, then further patient management must be based on the findings at conventional imaging (mammography and ultrasound). If a lesion is seen on MRI, it must be determined whether this lesion corresponds to the suspected mammographic lesion or, rather, represents an incidental lesion seen only on MRI. If a lesion identified on MRI is indeed incidental and not seen with conventional imaging methods, it must be determined what further, if anything, needs be done about this lesion. Questions that should be raised include: Is the enhancing lesion a "true" lesion or is it just an area of enhancing glandular tissue? Should the lesion undergo biopsy, and if so, how will it be localized if it is seen only on MRI? If there are multiple enhancing lesions, which one(s), if any, are significant, and which, if any, correlate with the mammographic or palpable finding? If the lesion does not undergo biopsy, should a follow-up MRI study be performed, and, if so, at what time interval?

Adjunctive Imaging Test

With the potential for greater sensitivity for the detection of breast cancer than is possible with conventional methods (mammography and ultrasound), MRI may play a role as an adjunctive imaging test when there are equivocal mammographic, sonographic, and/or physical examination findings. There are reports demonstrating that MR imaging can be used as a problem-solving tool in cases where a suspicious lesion is identified only on one mammographic view and in cases where there are equivocal mammographic findings or physical examination findings *(23,43,44)* (Fig. 7). MRI may also play a problem-solving role in the evaluation of patients after breast conservation therapy for breast cancer in which equivocal changes on mammography or physical examination are identified (Fig. 7). For these patients, post-treatment follow-up can sometimes be difficult because post-treatment changes can mimic and obscure recurrent disease (Fig. 8). There are now several studies demonstrating the effectiveness of MRI in identifying recurrent cancer in patients with suspected breast cancer recurrence where the clinical and/or mammographic findings were equivocal. Reported sensitivities have ranged from 93 to 100% with reported specificities ranging from 88 to 100% *(33,45,46)*. False-positive cases have included inflammatory changes and fat necrosis *(47)*. The differentiation of enhancing recurrent cancer from enhancing post-treatment changes can be difficult in the early post-treatment period. Investigators thus far have reported that enhancement secondary to radiation-induced changes can be present for at least 18 mo after treatment. Based on the promising results of clinical investigation thus far, it appears that MRI will play a role in the evaluation of patients after breast conservation. The clinical indication for MRI will most likely be suspected breast cancer recurrence where the physical examination and/or mammographic and sonographic findings are equivocal. At the present time, there are no data on the use of MRI for routine surveillance after breast conservation.

Another potential indication for MRI as an adjunctive imaging test is the evaluation of patients presenting with axillary node malignancy and unknown site of primary tumor (Fig. 9). Reported rates of MRI detected primary breast cancer in patients presenting with axillary node metastases and negative mammogram and physical examination have ranged from 75 to 86% *(23,48,49)*. Based on these initial studies, it appears that MRI will likely be the imaging study of choice in patients presenting with malignant axillary adenopathy and a negative mammogram.

It appears that, as with ultrasound of the breast, MRI can be a very useful clinical tool when breast cancer is suspected but the diagnosis cannot be established by conventional methods. However, there are several caveats to keep in mind if MRI is to be used in this capacity. First, in controlled research settings, it has been demonstrated

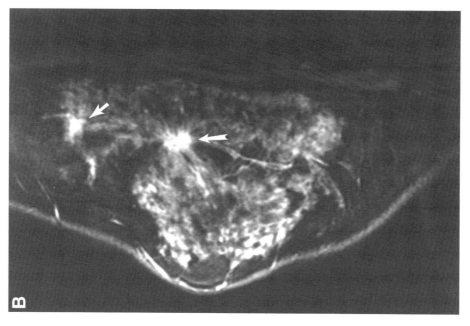

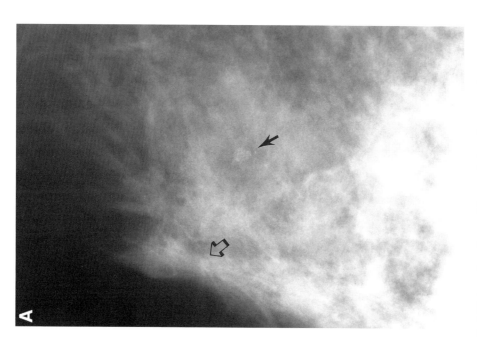

Fig. 7. MR imaging for problem solving. Images of a 50-yr-old patient with two questionable lesions identified at mammography, each seen on only one mammographic view. (**A**) Spot magnification mediolateral oblique view demonstrates a cluster of microcalcifications (solid arrow) and an area of possible architectural distortion (open arrow). Both lesions could not be identified in two views to allow for localization or biopsy. (**B**) Sagittal, fat-suppressed, contrast-enhanced, three-dimensional, fast spoiled, gradient echo MR image reveals two enhancing lesions (arrows).

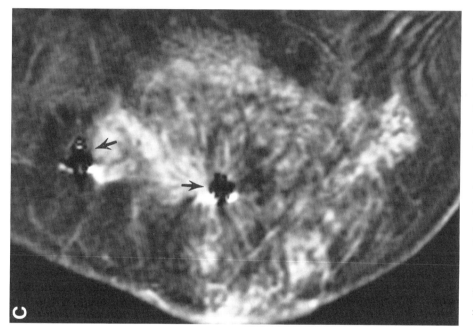

Fig. 7. *(continued)* **(C)** MRI-guided wire localization reveals both lesions to be localized by the MRI needles (arrows). Excisional biopsy revealed two invasive ductal carcinomas (0.8 and 0.5 cm; mammographic specimen radiographs reveals both the cluster of microcalcifications and the area of architectural distortion). (Reprinted with permission from ref. 23.)

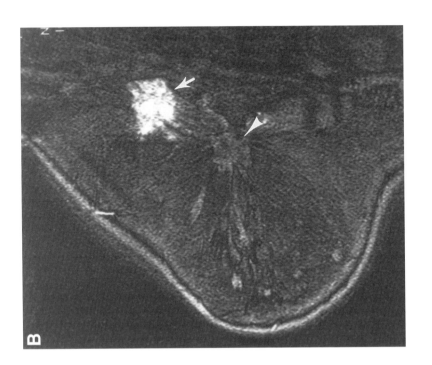

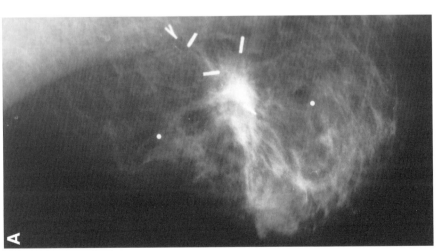

Fig. 8. MR imaging for problem solving after breast conservation therapy. Images of a 41-yr-old patient 3 yr after lumpectomy and radiation for DCIS complaining of discomfort in the axillary tail of her treated breast. (**A**) Mediolateral oblique view mammogram reveals expected post-treatment changes. The standard craniocaudad view and exaggerated craniocaudad view to show the axillary tail (not illustrated) were also unremarkable. Ultrasound examination did not demonstrate any definite abnormalities. (**B**) Sagittal, fat-suppressed, contrast-enhanced, three-dimensional, fast spoiled, gradient echo MR image reveals an enhancing irregular mass (arrow) superior to the biopsy site (arrowhead). MRI-guided wire localization was performed. Invasive breast cancer (1.6 cm) was found at excisional biopsy.

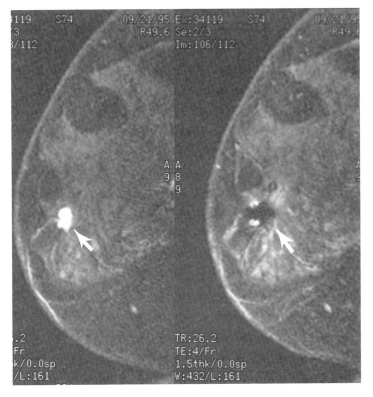

Fig. 9. MR imaging for axillary node malignancy and unknown primary site. Images of a patient presenting with multiple axillary lymph nodes found to contain adenocarcinoma at biopsy. Mammography (not illustrated) reveals dense breast tissue with no suspicious findings. Sagittal, fat-suppressed, contrast enhanced, three-dimensional, fast spoiled, gradient echo MR image reveals a subareolar, 7-mm, peripherally enhancing mass (arrow in left image). MRI-guided wire localization reveals the lesion to be localized by the MRI-compatible needle (arrow in right image). Excisional biopsy revealed a 7-mm invasive ductal carcinoma.

that MRI can reliably identify invasive cancer, and based on several studies, it has been suggested that a negative MRI virtually excludes the presence of invasive cancer. However, the false-negative rate and the negative predictive value of MRI are currently unknown. There have been multiple reports of false-negative MRI studies, including cases of invasive ductal cancer, invasive lobular cancer, and DCIS *(1,3,5,10,11, 15,33,36)*. As is true with a negative mammogram or a negative ultrasound examination in a patient with a suspicious palpable abnormality, a negative MRI examination should not preclude biopsy of a suspicious mammographic, sonographic, or palpable abnormality (Fig. 10).

When MRI is used an adjunctive imaging test to further evaluate an equivocal mammographic or sonographic abnormality, is critically important that the MRI findings be correlated with the mammographic and sonographic findings to ensure that a lesion identified on MRI corresponds to that identified on mammography. If the MRI examination is negative, the recommendation must be based on the mammographic, sonographic, or clinical findings. A single recommendation based on both the conventional work-up and the MRI study should be given.

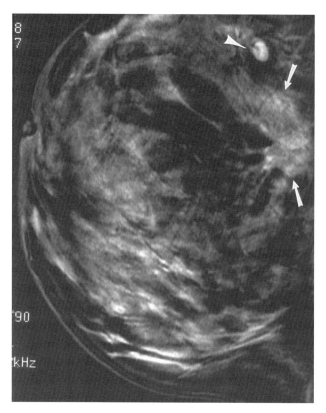

Fig. 10. False-negative MRI study. Image of a 55-yr-old patient presenting with a palpable mass and a negative mammogram. The MRI study was interpreted as showing no abnormality. Excisional biopsy revealed a 5-cm invasive lobular carcinoma. In retrospect, an ill-defined enhancing mass (arrows) was identified (Vitamin E capsule marking the area of palpable concern, [arrowhead]). (Reprinted with permission from ref. *41*.)

MRI for Breast Cancer Staging

In the process of investigating MRI as a means of evaluating mammographic or palpable abnormalities, it became apparent that MRI-enabled detection of mammographically and clinically occult breast cancer. This discovery has lead to the investigation of MRI for breast cancer staging. There are now several reports in the literature demonstrating the ability of MRI to determine the extent of cancer within the breast more accurately than conventional methods *(3,23,50–53)*. Reported rates of MRI detected, mammographically, and clinically occult multifocal or multicentric cancer have ranged from 16 to 37% *(3,23,50–53)*.

Potential clinical indications for the use of MRI in the setting of suspected or newly diagnosed breast cancer include staging patients following a positive fine needle aspiration biopsy or core biopsy before excisional biopsy and identifying the extent of residual disease after excisional biopsy where tumor is identified at the margins of resection (Fig. 11). Preliminary studies have shown that residual or multifocal cancer can be detected on MRI after excisional biopsy and can usually be differentiated from postsurgical changes *(54,55)*. It does appear that MRI could play a role in the evaluation of patients who have undergone excisional biopsy for breast cancer (Fig. 12). The identification of clinically and mammographically unsuspected multifocal or diffuse

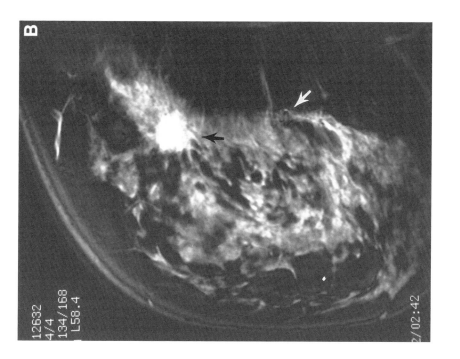

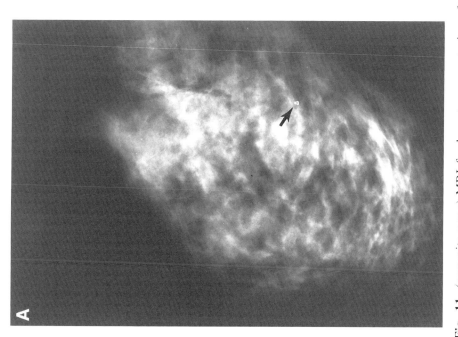

Fig. 11. (*opposite page*) MRI for breast cancer staging after core biopsy. Images of a patient after stereotactic core needle biopsy for mammographically identified microcalcifications. Histopathologic examination revealed DCIS. (**A**) Mediolateral view mammogram demonstrates a core biopsy clip (arrow) in the central breast. No residual microcalcifications were identified. (**B**) Sagittal, fat suppressed, contrast enhanced, three-dimensional, fast spoiled, gradient echo image (9.2/2.1) reveals a 1.5-cm enhancing spiculated mass (black arrow) in the superior breast several centimeters superior to the core biopsy clip (white arrow). The mass was identified on subsequent directed ultrasound examination, and ultrasound-guided wire localization and excisional biopsy revealed invasive ductal carcinoma. Mammographic-guided wire localization and excisional biopsy of the core biopsy clip revealed residual DCIS. The patient subsequently underwent mastectomy. (Reprinted with permission from ref. 23.)

cancer could be used to avoid multiple surgical procedures for patients who will ultimately require mastectomy. There are limitations to MRI after excisional biopsy. Postsurgical alterations can both mimic and obscure residual tumor. In one study, the
false-negative rate was 27% (7 of 26 patients) and the false-positive rate was 19% (4 of
21 patients) *(54)*.

Despite the promising results showing that MRI can be used to stage patients with
newly diagnosed breast cancer with greater accuracy that is possible with conventional
methods, there are pitfalls that must be considered *(15)*. As discussed earlier, in addition to cancer, many benign lesions as well as presumably normal breast tissue may
enhance after contrast administration. The identification of one or more additional
enhancing lesions at a distance from the primary tumor may require an increase in the
amount of tissue excised and/or a second incision; patients may be advised to undergo
mastectomy based on the MRI findings despite the absence of histologic confirmation
that the enhancing lesion(s) represents multifocal breast cancer (Fig. 13). As noted
above, an MRI compatible needle localization system is needed in order to differentiate true-positive from false-positive enhancing lesions. However, with currently available localization systems (none are commercially available), there is no "specimen
radiograph" to document lesion removal. An MRI compatible core biopsy system could
obviate both a potentially unnecessary surgical procedure for a benign enhancing lesion as well as the problems related to documenting lesion removal. Such systems
remain in development.

It is clear that MRI can detect unsuspected additional foci of breast cancer in patients
with newly diagnosed breast cancer. However, there are many unanswered questions
concerning MRI staging of breast cancer. The clinical significance of MRI only detected
additional foci of carcinoma, especially foci of DCIS, in patients with newly diagnosed
breast cancer is not known. Should these lesions be excised or would they be effectively
treated with radiation therapy? Should mastectomy be recommended for patients with
multifocal cancer detected only on MRI, or if the multiple lesions can be successfully
excised, is the patient eligible for breast conservation therapy? What should be done
when multiple enhancing lesions are identified; how many, if any, should be localized?
Which patients are at risk for multifocal or extensive carcinoma and would benefit most
from MRI, that is, patients with a palpable cancer or patients with dense breasts? Continued clinical investigation is needed to address these questions.

Breast Cancer Screening

There is a growing clinical demand for screening breast MRI based on the promising
results of diagnostic MRI. Unfortunately, screening MRI is being performed, outside
of clinical trials, in the absence of data demonstrating the efficacy of MRI as a screening modality. In addition, at the present time, there is no standardized method for performing breast MRI studies and there are no guidelines for interpreting breast MRI
studies. Furthermore, and perhaps most important, MRI-guided breast localization/bi-
opsy systems needed to permit tissue diagnosis of suspicious lesions detected only on
MRI are only, now, just becoming commercially available. The reports of MRI detected,
mammographically, and clinically occult breast cancer have come from diagnostic series
(19–21). Little is know about the efficacy of MRI as a method to screen for breast
cancer. There are recent preliminary reports demonstrating that MRI can detect

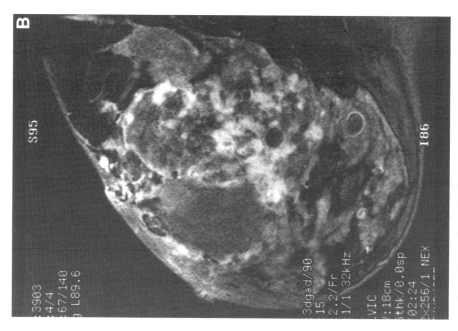

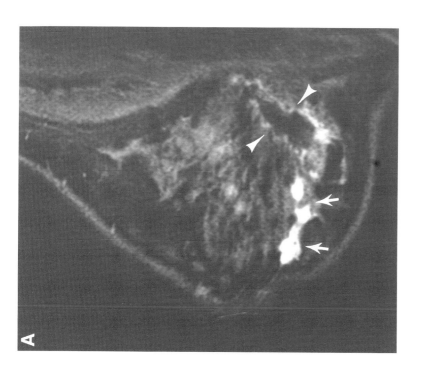

Fig. 12. MRI for breast cancer staging after excisional biopsy with positive margins of resection. (**A**) Sagittal, fat suppressed, contrast-enhanced, three-dimensional, fast spoiled, gradient echo MR image, in a patient status postexcisional biopsy showing invasive ductal carcinoma with positive margins of resection, reveals enhancing lesions (arrows) anterior to the biopsy site (arrowheads). At mastectomy, residual invasive ductal carcinoma was found. (**B**) Sagittal, fat suppressed, contrast-enhanced, three-dimensional, fast spoiled gradient echo MR image, in a patient status postexcisional biopsy showing invasive lobular carcinoma with positive margins of resection, reveals multifocal enhancement (which was seen throughout the breast on additional sections). At mastectomy, diffuse infiltrative lobular carcinoma was found.

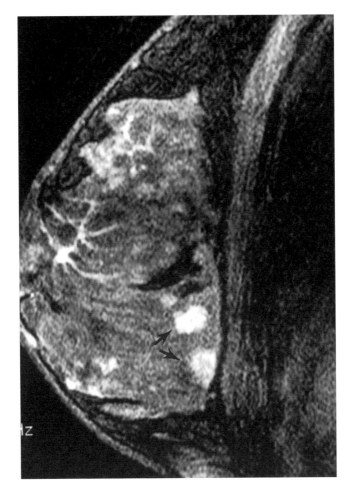

Fig. 13. False-positive enhancement aftrer excisional biopsy for cancer. Sagittal, fat suppressed, contrast-enhanced, three-dimensional, fast spoiled, gradient echo MR image reveals two enhancing lesions (arrows) that were distant from the lumpectomy site. Based on lower inner quadrant location of the masses with respect to the biopsy site (upper outer quadrant), wire localization and excisional biopsy was not deemed to be feasible. Mastectomy was recommended, and the enhancing lesions proved to be fibroadenomas. (Reprinted with permission from ref. *41.)*

mammographically and clinically occult breast cancer in high-risk women, including contralateral breast cancer in women with a history of breast cancer, and breast cancer in known or suspected carriers of BRCA 1 and BRCA 2 mutations *(19–21)* (Fig. 14). There is general agreement among breast MRI researchers that MRI should not be used for routine breast cancer screening at the present time. In terms of high-risk screening, MRI screening should be performed as part of a clinical trial. Patients being considered for MRI should first be evaluated in a cancer risk evaluation before being enrolled in a clinical MRI screening trial. There are now several ongoing MRI high-risk screening trials, including a National Cancer Institute-funded pilot study, and international clini-

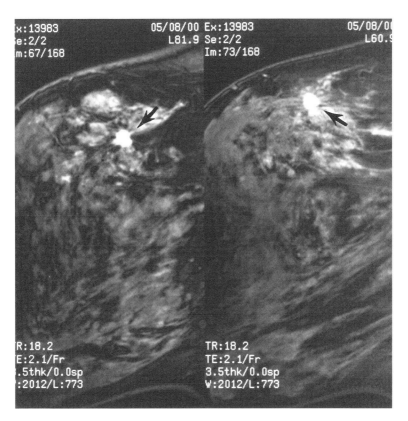

Fig. 14. MRI for breast cancer screening in high-risk patients. Images of a 46-yr-old patient with a family history of breast cancer. Mammogram (not shown) revealed heterogeneously dense breast tissue with no suspicious findings. Sagittal, computer subtracted, fat suppressed, contrast enhanced, three-dimensional, fast spoiled, gradient echo images reveal two 7-mm enhancing lesions (arrows) in the superior lateral aspect of the left breast. Follow-up ultrasound examination demonstrated two hypoechoic lesions (not shown) in the upper outer quadrant corresponding in size and location to the MRI-detected lesions. Ultrasound-guided fine needle aspiration biopsy revealed adenocarcinoma from one lesion and atypia from the second lesion. The patient underwent bilateral mastectomies, and two invasive carcinomas (1.1-cm invasive ductal carcinoma and 3-mm invasive tubular carcinoma) were identified in the left breast. No cancer was found in the right breast. (Reprinted with permission from ref. *23*.)

cal trials in Canada, England, Germany, France, Italy, and the Netherlands. Entrance criteria vary among these trials *(33)*. In general, patients are enrolled from cancer risk evaluation centers. Entrance criteria include: 1) a known carrier of a BRCA 1 or BRCA 2 mutation, 2) a member of family known to carry a BRCA 1 or 2 mutation where the individual status is not known, 3) a personal or family history highly suggestive of BRCA 1 or BRCA 2 involvement (guidelines vary), or 4) an individual with at least a 25 to 30% estimated lifetime risk for developing breast cancer based on the Claus or Gail model. Although MRI has demonstrated tremendous potential as a diagnostic breast imaging modality, the utility of MRI as screening method to detect mammographically and clinically occult breast cancer remains to be determined.

CONCLUSIONS

The results of clinical investigation have demonstrated that MRI can offer clinically important information that cannot be obtained with conventional imaging methods, and that this modality is rapidly becoming an invaluable adjunctive breast imaging tool. MRI appears to be very sensitive for the visualization of both invasive carcinoma and DCIS. Perhaps, most importantly, MRI can detect invasive and noninvasive breast carcinoma that is mammographically, sonographically, and clinically occult, offering the potential for more accurate breast cancer staging and optimized treatment planning. Preliminary investigation into MRI for breast cancer screening of women at increased risk for the development of breast cancer suggests that MRI will play an important role in the imaging evaluation of these patients. Clinical trials are now underway.

MRI is emerging as perhaps the most promising imaging modality for breast cancer detection to date. However, published results are from studies with relatively small numbers of patients. There are ongoing efforts to validate these results in larger-scale clinical trials. This type of clinical investigation is needed to define the technical requirements for optimal imaging, to define interpretation criteria, to develop accurate MRI-guided localization and biopsy systems, to define the clinical indications for which MRI should be used as an adjunct to conventional imaging methods, and to address the issue of cost-effectiveness.

REFERENCES

1. Heywang SH, Wolf A, Pruss E, et al. MR imaging of the breast with Gd-DTPA: use and limitations. *Radiology* 1989;171:95–103.
2. Kaiser WA, Zeitler E. MR imaging of the breast: fast imaging sequences with and without Gd-DTPA. Preliminary observations. *Radiology* 1989;170:681–686.
3. Harms SE, Flamig DP, Hensley KL, et al. MR imaging of the breast with rotating delivery of excitation off resonance: clinical experience with pathologic correlation. *Radiology* 1993;187:493–5.01.
4. Boetes C, Barentsz JO, Mus RD, et al. MR characterization of suspicious breast lesions with a gadolinium-enhanced turboflash subtraction technique. *Radiology* 1994;193:777–781.
5. Gilles R, Guinebretiere JM, Lucidarme O, et al. Nonpalpable breast tumors: diagnosis with contrast-enhanced subtraction dynamic MR imaging. *Radiology* 1994;191:625–631.
6. Soderstrom CE, Harms SE, Copit DS, et al. Three-dimensional RODEO breast MR imaging of lesions containing ductal carcinoma in situ. *Radiology* 1996;201:427–432.
7. Gilles R, Zafrani B, Guinebretiere JM, et al. Ductal carcinoma in situ: MR imaging-histo-pathologic correlation. *Radiology* 1995;196:415–419.
8. Piccoli CW, Matteucci T, Outwater EK, Siegelman ES, Mitchell DG. Breast cancer diagnosis with MR imaging: effect of clinical and mammographic findings on recommendations for biopsy. *Radiology* 1995;196:415–419.
9. Westerhof JP, Fischer U, Moritz JD, Oestmann JW. MR imaging of mammographically detected clustered microcalcifications: is there any value? *Radiology* 1998;207:675–681.
10. Gilles R, Zafrani B, Guinebretiere JM, et al. Ductal carcinoma *in situ*: MR imaging-histo-pathologic correlation. *Radiology* 1995;196:415–419.
11. Orel SG, Mendonca MH, Reynolds C, Schnall MD, Solin LJ, et al. MR imaging of ductal carcinoma in situ. *Radiology* 1997;202:413–420.
12. Orel SG, Schnall MD, Newman RW, et al. MR imaging-guided localization and biopsy of breast lesions: Initial experience. *Radiology* 1994;193:97–102.
13. Rodenko GN, Harms SE, Pruneda JM, et al. MR imaging in the management before sur-

gery of lobular carcinoma of the breast: correlation with pathology. *Am J Roentgenol* 1996;167:1415–1419.

14. Boetes C, Mus RD, Holland R, et al. Breast tumors: comparative accuracy of MR imaging relative to mammography and US for demonstrating extent. *Radiology* 1995;197:43–47.

15. Orel SG, Schnall MD, Powell CM, et al. Staging of suspected breast cancer: effect of MR imaging and MR-guided biopsy. *Radiology* 1995;196:115–122.

16. Essermann L, Hylton N, Yassa L, Barclay J, Frankel S, et al. Utility of magnetic resonance imaging in the management of breast cancer: evidence for improved preoperative staging. *J Clin Oncol* 1999;17:110–119.

17. Fischer U, Kopka L, Grabbe E. Breast carcinoma: effect of preoperative contrast-enhanced MR imaging on the therapeutic approach. *Radiology* 1999;213:881–888.

18. Mumtaz H, Hall-Craggs MA, Davidson T, et al. Staging of symptomatic primary breast cancer with MR imaging. *Am J Roentgenol* 1997;169:417–424.

19. Slantez PJ, Edmister WB, Yeh ED, et al. Occult contralateral breast carcinoma incidentally detected by breast magnetic resonance imaging. *Breast J* 2003;8(3):145–148.

20. Lee S, Orel SG, Woo IJ, et al. MR imaging screening of the contralateral breast in patients with newly diagnosed breast cancer: preliminary results. *Radiology* 2003;226:773–778.

21. Kuhl CK, Schmutzer RK, Leutner CC, et al. Breast MR imaging screening in 192 women proved or suspected to be carriers of a breast cancer susceptibility gene: preliminary results. *Radiology* 2000;215:267–279.

22. Hylton N. M. , Kinkel K. Technical aspects of breast magnetic resonance imaging, in *Topics in Magnetic Resonance Imaging*, Vol. 9 (Brant Zawadzki M, Edelman RR, and Mitchell DG, eds.) Lippincott-Raven, Philadelphia, 1998; pp. 3–16.

23. Orel SG, Schnall MD. MR imaging of the breast for the detection, diagnosis, and staging of breast cancer: state of the Art. *Radiology* 2001;220:13–30.

24. Daniel BL, Butts K, Glover GH, Cooper C, Herfkens FJ. Breast cancer: gadolinium-enhanced MR imaging with a 0.5-T open imager and three-point dixon technique. *Radiology* 1998;207:183–190.

25. Insko EK, Connick TJ, Schnall MD, Orel SG. Multicoil array for high resonance imaging of the breast. *Magn Reson Med* 1997;37:778–784.

26. Greenman RL, Lenkinski RE, Schnall MD. Bilateral imaging using separate interleaved 3D volumes and dynamically switched multiple receive coil arrays. *Magn Reson Med* 1998;39:108–115.

27. Foo T. K. F., Sawyer AM, Faulkner WH, et al. Inversion in the steady state: contrast optimization and reduced imaging time with fast three-dimensional inversion-recovery-prepared GRE pulse sequences. *Radiology* 1994;191:85–90.

28. Fischer U, Vosshenrich R, Doler W, et al. MR imaging-guided breast intervention: experience with two systems. *Radiology* 1995;195:533–538.

29. Heywang-Koebrunner SH, Halle MD, et al. Optimal procedure and coil design for MR imaging-guided transcutaneous needle localization and biopsy. *Radiology* 1994;193:267.

30. Kuhl CK, Elevelt A, Leutner CC, et al. Interventional breast MR imaging: clinical use of stereotactic localization and biopsy device. *Radiology* 1997;204:667–675.

31. Daniel BL, Birdwell RL, Ikeda DM, et al. Breast lesion localization: a free-hand interactive MR imaging technique. *Radiology* 1998;207:455–463.

32. Heywang-Koebrunner SH, Heinig A, Schauloeffel-Schulz U, et al. MR-percutaneous vacuum breast biopsy of breast lesions: initial experience with 100 lesions. *Radiology* (RSNA) 1999; 289.

33. Orel SG, Schnall MD, LiVolsi VA, Troupin RH. Suspicious breast lesions: MR imaging with radiologic-pathologic correlation. *Radiology* 1994;190:485–493.

34. Kuhl CK, Bieling HB, Gieseke J, et al. Healthy premenopausal breast parenchyma in dynamic contrast-enhanced MR imaging of the breast: normal contrast medium enhancement and cyclical-phase dependency. *Radiology* 1997;203:137–144.

35. Kuhl CK, Mielcareck P, Klaschik S, et al. Dynamic breast MR Imaging: are signal intensity time course data useful for differential diagnosis of enhancing lesions? *Radiology* 1999;211:101–110.

36. Stomper PC, Herman S, Klippenstein DL, et al. Suspect breast lesions: findings at dynamic gadolinium-enhanced MR imaging correlated with mammographic and pathologic features. *Radiology* 1995;197:387–395.

37. Orel S. G. Differentiating benign from malignant enhancing lesions identified at MR imaging of the breast: are time-signal intensity curves an accurate predictor. *Radiology* 1999;211:5–7.

38. Buadu LD, Murakami J, Murayama S, et al. Patterns of peripheral enhancement in breast masses: correlation of findings on contrast medium enhanced MRI with histologic features and tumor angiogenesis. *J Comp Assist Tomogr* 1997;21:421–430.

39. Sherif H, Mahfouz AE, Oellinger H, et al. Peripheral washout sign on contrast-enhanced MR images of the breast. *Radiology* 1997;205:209–2.13.

40. Nunes LW, Schnall MD, Orel SG, et al. Breast MR imaging: interpretation model. *Radiology* 1997;202:833–841.

41. Nunes LW, Schnall MD, Siegelman ES, et al. Diagnostic performance characteristics of architectural features revealed by high spatial-resolution MR imaging of the breast. *Am J Roentgenol* 1997;169:409–415.

42. Harms SE, ed. Technical report of the international working group on breast MRI. *J Magn Reson Imaging* 1999;10:978–1015.

43. Lee CH, Smith RC, Levine JA, Troiano RN, Tocino I. Clinical usefulness of MR imaging of the breast in the evaluation of the problematic mammogram. *Am J Roentgenol* 1999;173:1323–1329.

44. Orel S. G. High-resolution MR imaging for the detection, diagnosis, and staging of breast cancer. *RadioGraphics* 1998;18:903–912.

45. Mumatz H, Davidson T, Hall-Craggs MA, et al. Comparison of magnetic resonance imaging and conventional triple assessment in locally recurrent breast cancer. *Br J Surg* 1997;84:1147–1151.

46. Muuller RD, Barkhausen J, Sauerwein W, Langer R. Assessment of local recurrence after breast-conserving therapy with MRI. *J Comput Assist Tomogr* 1998;22:408–412

47. Solomon B, Orel SG, Reynolds C, Schnall MD. Delayed development of enhancement in fat necrosis after breast conservation therapy: a potential pitfall of MR imaging of the breast. *Am J Roentgenol* 1998;170:966–968.

48. Morris EA, Schwartz LH, Dershaw DD, et al. MR imaging of the breast in patients with occult primary breast carcinoma. *Radiology* 1997;205:437–440.

49. Orel SG, Weinstein SP, Schnall MD, et al. Breast MR imaging in patients with axillary node metastases and unknown primary malignancy. *Radiology* 1999;212:543–549.

50. Orel SG, Schnall MD, Powell CM, et al. Staging of suspected breast cancer: effect of MR imaging and MR-guided biopsy. *Radiology* 1995;196:115–122.

51. Essermann L, Hylton N, Yassa L, et al. Utility of magnetic resonance imaging in the management of breast cancer: evidence for improved preoperative staging. *J Clin Oncol* 1999;17:110–119.

52. Fischer U, Kopka L, Grabbe E. Breast carcinoma: effect of preoperative contrast-enhanced MR imaging on the therapeutic approach. *Radiology* 1999;213:881–888.

53. Mumtaz H, Hall-Craggs MA, Davidson T, et al. Staging of symptomatic primary breast cancer with MR imaging. *AJR Am J Roentgenol* 1997;169:417–424.

54. Orel SG, Reynolds C, Schnall MD. Breast carcinoma: MR imaging before re-excisional biopsy. *Radiology* 1997;205:429–436.

55. Soderstrom CE, Harms SE, Farrell RS, Pruneda JM, Flamig DP. Detection with MR imaging of residual tumor in the breast soon after surgery. *Am J Roentgenol* 1997;168:485–488.

5

Magnetic Resonance Imaging-Guided Stereotactic Biopsy in the Central Nervous System

Ion-Florin Talos, MD and Peter M. Black, MD, PhD

INTRODUCTION

Neurobiopsy allows for sampling of central nervous system (CNS) lesions with high accuracy and represents one of the most common neurosurgical procedures. The rapid development of new imaging modalities (computed tomography [CT] and magnetic resonance imaging [MRI]) and surgical navigation techniques over the past three decades have significantly impacted brain biopsy techniques. Moreover, they have altered the indications spectrum for biopsies of CNS lesions. Tumors previously considered inoperable because of their deep location and/or involvement of functionally critical structures gradually became more accessible for radical surgical therapy.

In the early 1970s, CT imaging was used for targeting intracranial lesions in a freehand manner. The introduction of stereotactic frames followed. This has allowed for translating the image data into the patient's coordinate system and has led to an increased targeting precision *(1,2)*.

Frame-based stereotactic systems next evolved into so called "frameless" devices, wherein the bulky metal frame was replaced by a set of external fiducial markers attached to the patient's head. This apparatus is, in effect, an "ultra" miniaturized version of the stereotactic frame.

The subsequent introduction of intraoperative MRI (iMRI), powered by high-performance computing and surgical navigation, represented a watershed in the evolution of stereotaxy. iMRI offers multiple advantages to the surgeon: multiplanar image acquisitions; high anatomic accuracy and high sensitivity; accurate localization and targeting of intracranial lesions; excellent compensation for changes in brain morphology and position with subsequent displacement of the lesion; and immediate detection of complications, such as hemorrhage, edema, and ischemia *(3–7)*.

MRI FOR CNS TUMORS

Low-grade gliomas (astrocytomas, oligodendrogliomas, oligoastrocytomas) as well as low-grade glioneural tumors (gangliogliomas, dysembryoplastic neuroepithelial tumors) appear as hypointense masses on T1- and T2-weighted images. In most cases, there is no contrast enhancement because the blood–brain barrier is usually intact. The mass effect, if any, is generally mild and there is no or minimal surrounding edema (Fig. 1).

From: *Image-Guided Diagnosis and Treatment of Cancer*
Edited by: A. D'Amico, J. S. Loeffler, and J. R. Harris © Humana Press Inc., Totowa, NJ

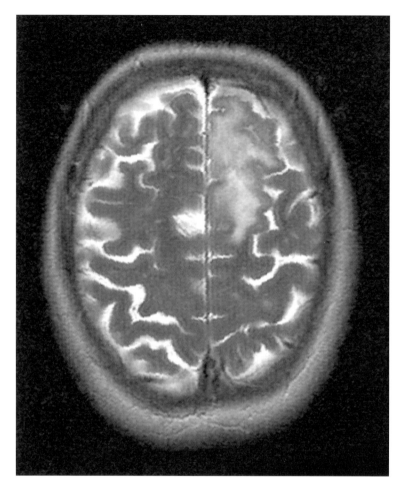

Fig. 1. Left frontal oligodendroglioma WHO II/IV (axial T2-weighted fast spin echo MRI).

Unlike their low-grade counterparts, high-grade gliomas (anaplastic astrocytomas, glioblastomas) appear on MRI as heterogenous enhancing mass lesions with surrounding edema (Fig. 2). The enhancement pattern suggests recruitment of abnormal vessels (i.e., angiogenesis resulting in neovascularity). The neoplastic tissue doesn't possess an effective blood–brain barrier, which is a useful diagnostic feature. Additionally, glioblastomas show areas of necrosis. However, contrast enhancement is not specific for tumor growth, it simply points out areas of disrupted blood–brain barrier, irrespective of etiology.

It is a widely accepted fact that tumor cells tend to migrate along white matter fibers and vascular structures *(8)*. Thin-section pathological analysis has demonstrated the presence of tumor cells beyond the peritumoral edema zone into apparently normal tissue. Hence, there is currently no available imaging method capable to show the entire extent of a high-grade glioma.

Radiotherapy is commonly used in high-grade glioma cases as an adjuvant after surgical debulking. Radiation induces complex changes in the tumor bed and surrounding tissue (gliosis, necrosis, increased vascular permeability with attendant edema,

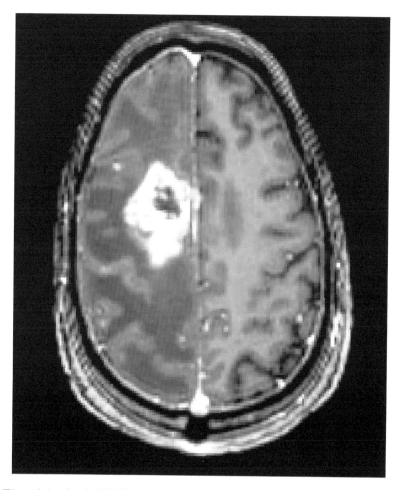

Fig. 2. T1-weighted axial SPGR in a case of right frontal recurrent glioblastoma multiforme after intravenous administration of 20 cc gadolinium.

microthrombosis followed by microinfarctions). The radiographic correlate of radiation induced changes are zones of necrosis surrounded by enhancing margins and edema, frequently indistinguishable from residual or recurrent tumor *(9)*. However, this distinction is imperative for choosing the appropriate biopsy target.

Help can be provided by using MR spectroscopy *(10)*, dynamic contrast imaging *(11)*, or nuclear medicine scans, such as single-photon emission computed tomography (SPECT) and positron emission tomography (PET).

MR spectroscopy can detect zones of increased metabolic turnover, suspicious for tumor tissue. The most commonly used metabolic markers are phosphocholine and NAA (*N*-acetyl aspartate/creatine ratio). Dynamic contrast imaging takes advantage of the presence of neovascularity within high-grade gliomas *(11)*. The abnormal tumor vessels are inherently permeable and thus the rate and degree of enhancement is demonstrably greater at the site of tumor recurrence than in areas of radionecrosis, which are hypovascular. In this technique, a two-dimensional fast spoiled gradient echo (2D FSPGR) sequence is performed whereas gadolinium is injected intravenously (2D FSPGR, echo time [TE] minimum, 45° flip angle, 1 number of excitations [NEX], sequential, multiphase, interleaved, variable bandwidth, extended dynamic range, 10 phases/location, field of view [FOV] 22 cm, matrix 256 × 128, 1.87 s/image). The result is a series of images depicting regional rates of enhancement through the tumor volume.

Schwartz et al. *(11)* have reported a series of 24 patients who underwent dynamic MRI while in the operative magnet. This technique allowed to distinguish recurrent tumor from radiation-induced changes with an accuracy of more than 90%. The authors found that the signal intensity increase at first pass through active tumor was 50% versus 15% in regions of radiation induced changes.

Detecting recurrent tumor with SPECT is based, similarly to dynamic contrast imaging, on the tumor neovascularity *(12–14)*. The PET method *(15–17)* is based, as is MR spectroscopy, on detecting an increased metabolic rate in the area of recurrent tumor.

Metastatic tumors to the CNS present as solitary or multiple contrast-enhancing mass lesions surrounded by edema. Occasionally, central necrosis may be present, making the differential diagnosis to glioblastoma extremely difficult. Further complicating matters, in about one third of metastatic brain tumor cases, the primary tumor is unknown or cannot be identified at the time of diagnosis. Brain abscess often shows a very similar radiologic appearance.

FUNCTIONAL MRI AND ANISOTROPIC DIFFUSION TENSOR IMAGING IN CNS TUMORS

The use of MRI is not limited to localization and improved definition of the lesion. For a surgical procedure to be safe, information regarding the relationship of the target to functionally critical cortical areas and deep white matter structures is imperatively needed.

Functional MRI (fMRI) is of paramount value for surgical planning in lesions located in or around eloquent cortex. The currently used technique is based on variations in local blood oxygenation and regional blood flow changes induced by neuronal activation.

The blood oxygenation level-dependent effect is a result of increased regional blood flow and blood volume in response to regional neuronal activation. Because the increased oxygen supply exceeds the neuronal oxygen consumption, the result is an increased oxy-/deoxyhemoglobin ratio. Oxyhemoglobin's diamagnetic properties lead to decreased local magnetic susceptibility and thus increased MR signal in T2*-weighted sequences *(18)*.

The interpretation of fMRI data is based on statistical analysis of the temporal variations in voxel intensity distribution during rest and activity. The functional maps are obtained by displaying the distribution of the voxels activated by various physiological tasks (i.e., motor, sensory, visual). The resulting data are critical in establishing the optimal entry point of the biopsy probe (Fig. 3).

The importance of fMRI data for brain biopsies must be stressed even more because as a result of the small skull access, electrical cortical mapping is not practicable.

Anisotropic diffusion tensor imaging (DTI) is a noninvasive method of imaging white matter fiber tracts. Information regarding the topographic relationships between lesion and fiber tracts is crucial for surgical planning. DTI takes advantage of the anisotropic material properties of the cerebral white matter, which consists of tightly packed fiber tracts with various orientations. Unlike in the case of isotropic materials, where water proton diffusion is free in all directions, in the cerebral white mater, water diffu-

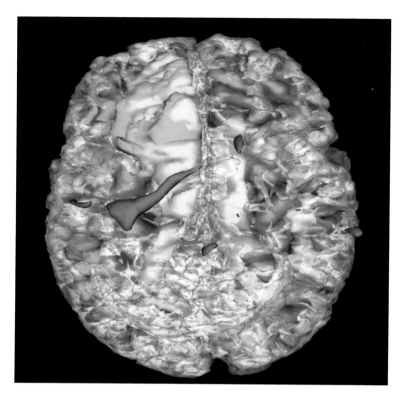

Fig. 3. fMRI (finger-tapping task) in a case of left frontal glioma. Three-dimensional
tumor reconstruction (green), motor activation (red).

sion is facilitated along the fibers and restricted in the direction perpendicular to them
because of the cell membrane and myelin sheath. By imaging the anisotropic water
proton diffusion, one can depict the trajectory and extent of different fiber tracts.

White matter fiber tracts can be depicted by displaying either the eigenvectors of the
diffusion tensor *(19)* (Fig. 4), by color coding of the directional information *(20)*, or,
better, by computer-aided 3D tractography *(21)* (Fig. 5).

Intra-axial tumors are intrinsically linked with white matter tracts. They can be infil-
trate, displace, or destroy these structures. Accurate information in this respect is more
relevant for tumor resection. However, precise knowledge of fiber tracts location in
respect to the lesion enables the surgeon to avoid postoperative neurologic deficit as a
result of fiber tract injury.

MRI FOR INTRAOPERATIVE DETECTION OF COMPLICATIONS

Hyperacute blood collections can be detected by using gradient echo sequences with
long TE (40–60 ms) *(22)*. After an acute hemorrhage, the hematoma compresses the
surrounding brain. This leads to local hypoxia which, in turn, causes an increased oxygen extraction at the hematoma–brain interface *(22)*. The resulting deoxy-hemoglobin
can be visualized on gradient echo sequences with increasing TE. Increasing TE on
gradient echo sequences leads to "blooming" of hyperacute blood (increasing dark signal), whereas air collections will not change their signal characteristics. Conventional
T1-weighted sequences might be also useful in the differential diagnosis.

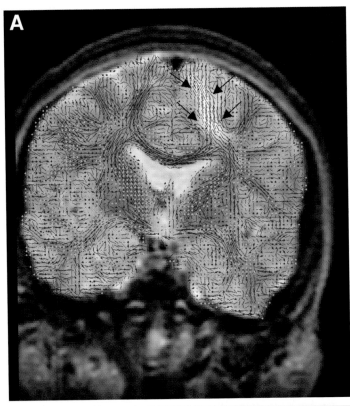

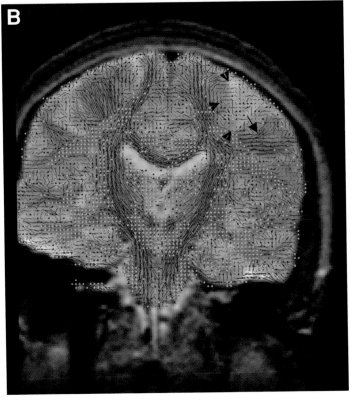

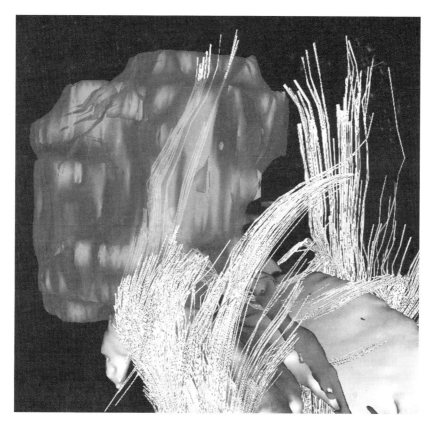

Fig. 5. Same case as in Fig. 4. 3D tractography demonstrating descending fibers passing through the tumor. Left posterior lateral view (transparent gray).

"FRAMELESS" STEREOTAXY AND INTRAOPERATIVE MRI

During the last decade, several so-called "frameless" stereotactic navigation systems have been developed. Basically, using 3D digitizers, stereotactic navigation systems serve the purpose of establishing the correspondence between virtual "image space" (CT, MRI) and physical "patient space" in the operating room, including the lesion to be biopsied/ resected as well as the surgical instruments being used. The instrument's position in the operating field is displayed in one or multiple (reformatted) image planes. The process of aligning image space to patient space is commonly referred to as registration. Registration and instrument tracking for surgical navigation can be based on articulated arms *(23–25)* or acoustic *(26)*, optical *(27)*, or electromagnetic waves *(28–30)*.

Each of the above-mentioned navigation systems has capabilities for "rigid" registration, but none is able to accommodate changes in brain morphology and position, which inherently occur to some extent during surgery *(31,32)*. These changes, com-

Fig. 4. *(opposite page)* Coronal DTI superimposed on T2-weighted coronal images in a case of left frontal oligodendroglioma WHO II/IV. **(A)** Tumor infiltration of descending, as well as corpus callosum fibers (arrows). **(B)** The tumor displaces the surrounding white matter tracts (arrow). No fiber structure can be identified inside the T2 hyperintensity (arrowheads).

monly referred to as brain shift, which typically set on after durotomy, are induced by cerebrospinal fluid drainage consecutive to opening of the subarachnoid and sometimes ventricular system, brain edema, $paCO_2$-dependent changes in the vascular tone, effect of anesthetic and diuretic agents administered during the procedure, drainage of cystic lesions, and effect of the gravitational force.

It is now a widely accepted fact that brain shift occurs according to a nonlinear pattern *(31,32)*. As a result of this phenomenon, in the absence of intraoperative imaging, preoperatively acquired data looses its accuracy and therefore its value for surgical targeting. This fact is even more important for biopsies, where even slight changes in the lesion's position might compromise the results.

Although progress has been made *(33,34)*, the use of ultrasonography (USD) for intraoperative imaging is limited by low sensitivity and specificity as well as low signal-to-noise ratio of this method. CT has a higher sensitivity and higher signal-to-noise ratio compared with USD.

However, its use for intraoperative imaging is limited by factors, such as exposure to radiation for the patient and surgical team, restricted patient access, inferior sensitivity and specificity when compared with MRI, and high artifact susceptibility in the posterior cranial fossa *(35)*.

Because of its noninvasive nature, its capability of providing high definition of soft tissue and vessel anatomy and pathology, fMRI, metabolic (MR spectroscopy, dynamic contrast imaging) and fine structural (anisotropic diffusion tensor imaging) information, its sensitivity to temperature changes (key feature for monitoring LASER or focused ultrasound tumor ablations), MRI is superior to any other imaging method for intracranial tumors *(3,7,36)*. Among the disadvantages of iMRI are the currently high cost, the need for MR-compatible surgical instruments, restricted space for the surgical team, and risk for heating.

Since the introduction of iMRI in 1994, various systems have been implemented *(3,7,36–38)*.

Currently available iMRI systems can be classified as low, middle, and high field, vertically or horizontally open designs, fixed or mobile. It is beyond the scope of this chapter to provide detailed descriptions of the various iMRI systems currently in use around the world.

Several factors limit the use of horizontal scanner designs for intraoperative imaging: it does not allow direct patient access; for each imaging cycle, the patient has to be moved into the magnet's bore, with the actual surgery being performed outside the magnet; and a new registration needs to be performed after each image update to preserve the accuracy of the stereotactic navigation system.

The use of low-field, mobile iMRI units *(38)* (0.1 T field strength) is widely limited by the low-image quality, limited spectrum of available MR sequences, as well as a strongly restricted FOV.

MULTIMODALITY IMAGE FUSION: PUTTING THE PIECES TOGETHER

As previously mentioned, unlike any other imaging method, MRI has the potential of describing cortical function (fMRI), detailed structure (MR angiography, anisotropic diffusion tensor imaging), and metabolism (MR spectroscopy). Because of low magnetic field and relatively weak gradients, as well as the time constraints imposed by the surgical procedure, it is difficult to exploit the full potential of diagnostic MRI during surgery. For sophisticated, preoperative imaging to be of real value for surgery, it has to be incorporated into the patient's frame of reference, as he/she is positioned in the open magnet for surgery.

For this purpose, we developed, in collaboration with the Artificial Intelligence Laboratory at the Massachusetts Institute of Technology, a software application package called the 3D Slicer *(39)*. The software's architecture is modular so that incorporating new software modules can easily expand its functionality.

The main modules enable the 3D Slicer with the following functionality: simultaneous visualization of multimodal volume data (MRI, MR angiography [MRA], anisotropic diffusion, CT, PET, SPECT) through multiplane reformatting, rigid body registration of different scans as well as images/3D models to patient *(40)*, semiautomatic and manual segmentation, generation of 3D anatomical models *(41)*, measurement of angles, distances and volumes, and intraoperative navigation.

Typically, the display is multilayered, consisting of a foreground, background, and label layer. The transparency of the foreground layer can be altered gradually, so that a combination of two different scans of the same volume can be displayed (e.g., CT for the bone structures, structural MRI for the intracranial content).

The raw volumetric data can be resampled and displayed along orthogonal, conventional planes, or along arbitrary oblique planes, parallel to the biopsy probe or perpendicular to it. This feature has proven very useful for simulating biopsy needle trajectories.

To insure the accuracy of the multimodality data throughout the procedure, we have developed a biomechanical simulation method that is able to capture the brain deformation field from the intraoperative image updates and to infer it to preoperative data within a time compatible with the time constraints of the surgery, typically less than 10 min *(42)*.

THE iMRI SYSTEM AT BRIGHAM AND WOMEN'S HOSPITAL

In performing image-guided neurosurgery at our institution, we typically use a vertically open, "double-donut"-shaped interventional MR scanner (SignaSP, General Electric, Milwaukee, MN) with 0.5-T field strength. The MR scanner incorporates an optical instrument tracking system that consists of three high-resolution infrared cameras mounted in the magnet's bore above the surgical field; a star-shaped hand piece ("locator") equipped with light-emitting diodes on each of the three arms; a centrally located hole in which a biopsy needle or other instrument of predetermined length can be inserted; and a computer unit. The patient can be positioned supine, prone, or lateral decubitus; the operating table can be docked along the scanner's longitudinal ("front dock") or transversal axis ("side dock"). When the table is front-docked, two surgeons can access the patient simultaneously. The head is positioned in the scanner's field of view (FOV) and immobilized using a MR-compatible, carbon-fiber Mayfield clamp. A flexible RF coil is then wrapped around the region of interest and left in place for the duration of the procedure. The operative field is prepped and draped in the usual manner and lastly, drapes are applied to the inner surface of each "donut" of the scanner.

Before skin incision, a set of axial, coronal, and sagittal T1-weighted spin-echo (TR/ TE 700/29, FOV 22, matrix 256 × 128, NEX 1, 3-mm thickness, 0.5-mm gap) and T2-weighted fast spin echo images (TR/TE 5000/99, FOV 22, matrix 256 × 128, NEX 2, 3-

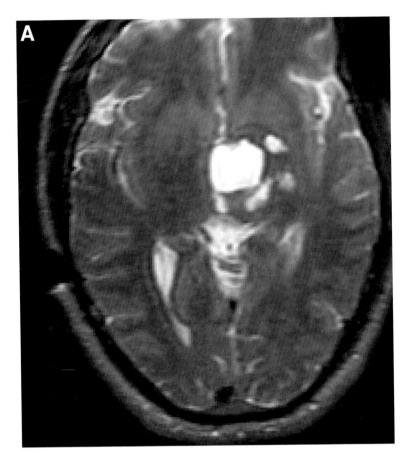

Fig. 6. Polycystic lesion of the left thalamus. (**A**) Preoperative T2-weighted axial fast spin echo. (**B**) Coronal. (**C**) Sagittal SPGR displayed along with a 3D reconstruction of the ventricles (blue) and cyst (red). Yellow: simulated biopsy needle.

mm thickness, gap 0.5-mm, echo train 8) is acquired. The imaging is completed with a T1-weighted, 3D SPGR sequence (TR/TE 28/12.5, FOV 22, matrix 256 × 128, NEX 1, 2.5-mm thickness, gap 0). The initial imaging requires 10–15 min on average.

We have modified the original hardware design by adding a visualization workstation, which runs the navigation software (3D Slicer). The visualization workstation receives data on the locator's position and orientation, which is updated at a rate of 10 Hz. The pre- and intraoperative images, as well as the 3D models, can be displayed simultaneously on the workstation's 20-inch monitor as well as on the two LCD monitors mounted in the bore of the magnet.

Head localization in the scanner space is achieved by the imaging process itself. Instrument localization is achieved using the optical tracking system. The FOV of the optical tracking system is aligned precisely to the scanner's FOV; though the dimensions of the latter slightly exceed those of the former, a feature that enables accurate tracking of instruments even in situations where the light-emitting diode locator lies beyond the scanner's FOV.

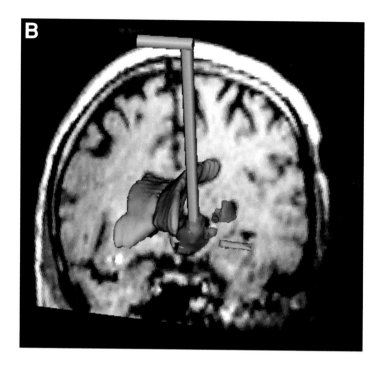

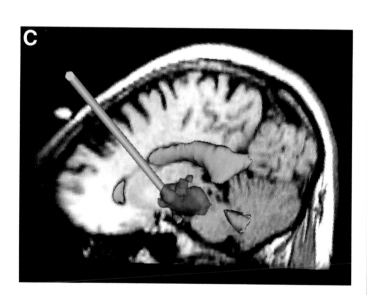

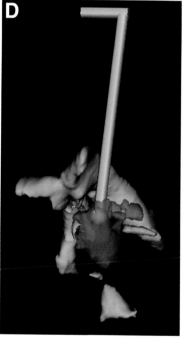

Fig 6. *(continued)* (**D**) 3D models viewed from left anterior inferior. One of the challenges of this procedure was taqrgetting the lesion from a secure entry point, without penetrating the left lateral ventricle.

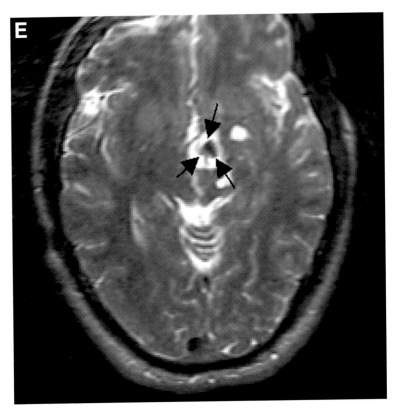

Fig. 6. *(continued)* (**E**) Intraoperative axial T2 fast spin echo showing the needle tip (arrows) in the center of the cyst.

Rigid registration of preoperative data (i.e., MR slices, 3D models) to the patient's head (as it is positioned for surgery) is readily accomplished by either manual or fully automatic means in the 3D Slicer environment. The initial intraoperative SPGR serves as a frame of reference for this purpose. The average time required for registration is between 60 and 90 s.

We can then simulate different surgical approaches by moving the locator without the attached instruments in the FOV (Fig. 6).

After selecting the optimal trajectory, the targeting device is immobilized using a Bookwalter arm or a trajectory guide screwed to the patient's skull (Daum GmbH, Germany). After drilling a burr hole and durotomy, real-time imaging is used to monitor the needle progression towards the lesion. After the target is reached, a new high-resolution scan is acquired to verify the correct needle position. In phantom tests, we have shown that the targeting accuracy of this method falls well within the range established for frame-based systems (1–2 mm) *(4)*.

Since 1995, we have performed a total of 154 brain biopsies using intraoperative MRI. For determining the optimal target region, we use dynamic contrast images, MR spectroscopy, or 201Tl-SPECT coregistered with the structural MRI scan. According to the literature, the diagnostic yield for brain biopsies ranges from 80 to 100% *(10,43)*.

Reasons for diagnostic failure in brain biopsy include small sample size, inaccurate tissue targeting resulting in sampling error, very small target size, lesions that are difficult to penetrate, as well as pediculated (mobile) intraventricular lesions.

In our series, we were able to localize the target and confirm the correct biopsy needle position within the MR abnormality in 100% of cases. Four biopsies yielded normal brain tissue, resulting in a 97.4% diagnostic yield. The literature also indicates that the rate of postoperative hemorrhage after brain biopsy ranges from 0 to 11.5% *(10)*.

In our series, we encountered two cases of immediate postoperative bleeding (1.2%), both of which were immediately detected using heme-sensitive imaging (*see* MRI for Introperative Detection of Complications). In both cases, hematomas were evacuated during the same session and an excellent postoperative outcome was achieved. There was no case of permanent neurologic deficit in this series.

CONCLUSION

iMRI and frameless stereotaxy have radically changed the way biopsies of the CNS are performed. iMRI, combined with multimodality image fusion, provides a more complete picture not only of the intracranial pathology, but also of the surrounding functional anatomy that has to be preserved by all possible means. Unlike in the case of frame-based systems, confirmation of the correct probe position can be achieved immediately and the "brain shift" issue can be easily overcome. Postoperative complications, such as hemorrhage, can be detected with ease and counter-measures immediately taken. Overall, iMRI is an extremely helpful tool for increasing both accuracy and safety of brain biopsies.

REFERENCES

1. Landi AMR, DeGrandi C, Crespi A, Montanari G, Sganzerla EP, Gaini SM. Accuracy of stereotactic localisation with magnetic resonance compared to CT scan: experimental findings. *Acta Neurochir* 2001;143:59:1–601.
2. Schulder MFP, Lavenhar MA, Carmel PW. The relationship of imaging techniques to the accuracy of frameless stereotaxy. *Stereotact Funct Neurosurg* 1999;72:131–141.
3. Black PM, Alexander E III, Martin C, et al. Craniotomy for tumor treatment in an intraoperative magnetic resonance imaging unit. *Neurosurgery* 1999;45:42:1–433.
4. Moriarty TM, Quinones-Hinojosa A, Larson PS, et al. Frameless stereotactic neurosurgery using intraoperative magnetic resonance imaging: stereotactic brain biopsy. *Neurosurgery* 2000;47:113:1–1146.
5. Dietrich J, et al. [Brain tumor resections in an open 0.5-T MRT. 2 years' experiences from the neuroradiological viewpoint]. *Radiology* 1999;39:98:1–94.
6. Schneider JP, et al. Gross-total surgery of supratentorial low-grade gliomas under intraoperative MR guidance. *Am J Neuroradiol* 2001;22:81–98.
7. Liu H, Hall WA, Martin AJ, Maxwell RE, Truwit CL. (2000) MR-guided and MR-monitored neurosurgical procedures at 1.5 T. *J Computer Assist Tomogr* 2000;24:90:1–918.
8. Giese A, Westphal M. Glioma invasion in the central nervous system. *Neurosurgery* 1996;39:23:1–50; discussion 25:1–2.
9. Kumar, AJ, Leeds NE, Fuller GN, et al. Malignant gliomas: MR imaging spectrum of radiation therapy-and chemotherapy-induced necrosis of the brain after treatment. *Radiology* 2000;217:37:1–384.
10. Hall WA, Martin A, Liu H, Truwit CL. Improving diagnostic yield in brain biopsy: Coupling spectroscopic targeting with real-time needle placement. *J Magn Reson Imaging* 2001;13:11–15.

11. Schwartz RB, Hsu L, Kacher DF, et al. Intraoperative dynamic MR imaging: localization of sites of brain tumor recurrence after high-dose radiotherapy. *J Magn Reson Imaging* 1998;8:108:1–1089.

12. Cipri S, et al. Clinical evaluation of thallium-201 single photon emission computed tomography in equivocal neuroradiological supratentorial lesions. *J Neurosurg Sci* 2001;45: 71–82.

13. Kinuya K, et al. Differential diagnosis in patients with ring-like thallium-201 uptake in brain SPECT. *Ann Nucl Med* 2002;16: 411–421.

14. Lam WW, et al. Pre-operative grading of intracranial glioma. *Acta Radiol* 2001;42: 541–554.

15. Schlemmer HP, et al. Differentiation of radiation necrosis from tumor progression using proton magnetic resonance spectroscopy. *Neuroradiology* 2002;44 211–222.

16. Chao ST, et al. The sensitivity and specificity of FDG PET in distinguishing recurrent brain tumor from radionecrosis in patients treated with stereotactic radiosurgery. *Int J Cancer* 2001;96:191–197.

17. De Witte O, et al. Positron emission tomography with injection of methionine as a prognostic factor in glioma. *J Neurosurg* 2001;95:741–750.

18. Logothetis NK, Pauls J, Augath M, Trinath T, Oeltermann A. Neurophysiological investigation of the basis of the fMRI signal. *Nature* 2001;412:151–157.

19. Mamata H, Mamata Y, Westin C-F, Shenton ME, Kikinis R, Jolesz FA, Maier SE. High-resolution line-scan diffusion-tensor MRI of white matter fiber tract anatomy. *AJNR Am J Neuroradiol* 2002;23:61–75.

20. Pajevic S, Pierpaoli C. Color schemes to represent the orientation of anisotropic tissues from diffusion tensor data: application to white matter fiber tract mapping in the human brain. *Magn Reson Med* 1999;42:521–540.

21. Catani M, Howard RJ, Pajevic S, Jones DK. Virtulal in vivo dissection of white matter fasciculi in the human brain. *Neuroimage* 2002;17:71–94.

22. Atlas SW, Thulborn KR. MR detection of hyperacute parenchymal hemorrhage of the brain. *Am J Neuroradiol* 1998;19: 1471–1507.

23. Golfinos JG, et al. Clinical use of a frameless stereotactic arm: results of 325 cases. *J Neurosurg* 1995;83:191–205.

24. Guthrie BL, Adler JR Jr. Computer-assisted preoperative planning, interactive surgery, and frameless stereotaxy. *Clin Neurosurg* 1992;38:111–131.

25. Olivier A et al. Frameless stereotaxy for surgery of the epilepsies: preliminary experience. Technical note. *J Neurosurg* 1994;81:621–33.

26. Barnett GH, et al. Use of a frameless, armless stereotactic wand for brain tumor localization with two-dimensional and three-dimensional neuroimaging. *Neurosurgery* 1993;33:671–678.

27. Pattisapu JV, Walker ML, Heilbrun MP. Stereotactic surgery in children. *Pediatr Neurosci* 1989;15:61–65.

28. Walker DG, Ohaegbulam C, Black PM. Frameless stereotaxy as an alternative to fluoroscopy for transsphenoidal surgery: use of the InstaTrak-3000 and a novel headset. *J Clin Neurosci* 2002;9:291–297.

29. Zaaroor M, Bejerano Y, Weinfeld Z, Ben-Haim S. Novel magnetic technology for intraoperative intracranial frameless navigation: in vivo and in vitro results. *Neurosurgery* 2001;48:1101–1108.

30. Manwaring, KHMM, Moss SD. Magnetic field guided endoscopic dissection through a burr hole may avoid more invasive craniotomies. A preliminary report. *Acta Neurochir Suppl (Wien)*1994;61:31–39.

31. Nabavi A, Black PM, Gering DT, et al. Serial intraoperative magnetic resonance imaging of brain shift. *Neurosurgery* 2001;48:781–798.

32. Nimsky C, Ganslandt O, Cerny S, Hastreiter P, Greiner G, Fahlbusch G. Quantification of, visualization of, and compensation for brain shift using intraoperative magnetic resonance imaging. *Neurosurgery* 2000;47:1071–1080.

33. Bonsanto MM, et al. Initial experience with an ultrasound-integrated single-RACK neuronavigation system. *Acta Neurochir (Wien)* 2001;143:1121–1132.
34. Trantakis C, et al. Iterative neuronavigation using 3D ultrasound. A feasibility study. *Neurol Res* 2002;24:661–670.
35. Lee JY, et al. Brain surgery with image guidance: current recommendations based on a 20-year assessment. *Stereotact Funct Neurosurg* 2000;75:31–48.
36. Sutherland GR, Kaibara T, Louw D, Hoult DI, Tomanek B, Saunders J. A mobile high-field magnetic resonance system for neurosurgery. *J Neurosurg* 1999;91:804–813.
37. Fahlbusch R, Ganslandt O, Nimsky C. Intraoperative imaging with open magnetic resonance imaging and neuronavigation. *Childs Nerv Syst* 2000;16:821–831.
38. Hadani M, Feldman Z, Berkenstadt H, Ram Z. Novel, compact, intraoperative magnetic resonance imaging-guided system for conventional neurosurgical operating rooms. *Neurosurgery* 2001;48 791–808.
39. Gering DT, et al. An integrated visualization system for surgical planning and guidance using image fusion and an open MR. *J Magn Reson Imaging* 2001;13:961–975.
40. Wells WM III, Kikinis R, Jolesz FA. Adaptive segmentation of MRI Data. *IEEE Trans Med Imaging* 1996;15:421–443.
41. Lorensen W, Marching cubes: a high resolution 3D surface construction algorithm. *Computer Graphics* 1987;21:161–189.
42. Warfield SK, Talos F, Tei A, et al. Real-time registration of volumetric brain MRI by biomechanical simulation of deformation during image guided neurosurgery. *Comput Visual Sci* 2002;5:1–11.
43. Truwit CL, Liu H. Prospective stereotaxy: a novel method of trajectory alignment using real-time image guidance. *J Magn Reson Imaging* 2001;13: 451–457.

II
IMAGE-GUIDED THERAPY

6

Transrectal Ultrasound-Guided Prostate Brachytherapy

John Sylvester, MD, **John Blasko,** MD, and **Peter Grimm,** DO

INTRODUCTION

The most common solid malignancy in men, prostate cancer is now being diagnosed, in most men, in the very earliest stages, in the United States (1). This surge in earlier-stage diagnosis is the result, in large part, of the introduction and increased use of the prostate-specific antigen (PSA) blood test (2). Traditional therapeutic options of radical prostatectomy and external beam radiation therapy have come under more scrutiny because PSA tests in follow-up reveal disease control rates have been found to be lower than previously thought (3–6). Neither radical prostatectomy nor external beam radiation therapy (EBRT) appear to result in superior cancer control, vs each other, when major pretreatment prognostic variables are taken into consideration (7–11). Moreover, patient-reported toxicity rates have been found to be considerably higher than the previous physician-reported rates (12).

Ultrasound-guided transperineal interstitial permanent prostate brachytherapy (TIPPB) is a form of radiation therapy, wherein radioactive 125-I or 103-Pd sources are permanently inserted into the prostate. These isotopes deliver very high doses to the prostate and 2 to 5 mm of surrounding tissue, but because of their low energy deliver low doses to the adjacent rectum and bladder.

The demand for TIPPB has recently soared. The oncology roundtable a Washington DC think tank has estimated that up to 50% of patients with early-stage prostate cancer are now receiving ultrasound-guided TIPPB (13) The rise in popularity is most likely the result of 5- and 10-yr disease control rates that rival that of the top surgical centers, perceived lower toxicity, and the single-treatment, outpatient nature of the therapy (14).

HISTORICAL BACKROUND

Brachytherapy has long been postulated to be a possible option for the treatment of localized prostate cancer. Alexander Graham Bell suggested it might be a possible treatment as far back as 1903. In 1911 Pasteur suggested the insertion of radium into the prostate to eradicate malignancy (15). In 1922, Denning published a study of 100 patients treated with transurethral radium insertion for prostate cancer (16). The cancer control rates were reasonable compared with the other options of the day; however, complication rates were high, as it was not possible to measure the dose of radiation

From: *Image-Guided Diagnosis and Treatment of Cancer*
Edited by: A. D'Amico, J. S. Loeffler, and J. R. Harris © Humana Press Inc., Totowa, NJ

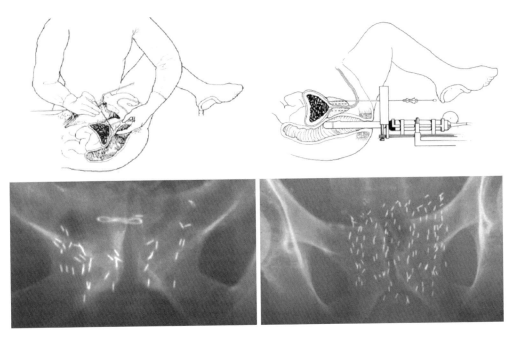

Fig. 1. Graphic illustration of retropubic and transperineal brachytherapy techniques and pelvic X-rays showing typical seed distribution patterns.

delivered. This form of treatment fell out of favor as surgical and anesthetic technique improved. The advent of megavoltage radiation therapy, the ability to measure radiation dose, and the lower side effect profile (compared to surgery) all combined to make externalbeam radiation therapy popular in the 1960s to 1990s.

Scardino and Carlton *(17)* reintroduced permanent prostate brachytherapy in the late 1960s using 198-Au interstitial implantation combined with external beam radiation therapy. The use of permanent interstitial 125-I seed implantation was pioneered at Memorial Sloan Kettering Cancer Center (MSKCC) by Dr. Whitmore and colleagues. They used an open laparotomy retropubic approach. They attempted to place the seeds evenly throughout the gland using a nomogram to calculate the number of seeds of a particular activity to use *(18)*. This therapy gained wide popularity in the 1970s and early 1980s, but with follow-up it became apparent that disease control rates were inferior to those of surgery and EBRT of that era. The technical innovations in that era did not allow for clear visualization of the seeds as they were inserted into the prostate and as a result relatively poor coverage of the gland frequently occurred even in the hands of experts. Quality of implantation was evaluated with postoperative orthogonal X-rays. All too frequently, inadequate coverage was obtained (Fig. 1).

The end points used to evaluate treatment outcomes in this pre-PSA era were local control and survival *(7,8,20)*. In those centers that performed both EBRT and brachytherapy, similar survival rates were seen in stage A and B prostate cancer *(20–24)*. Either both modalities performed equally well or both were equally ineffective. Either theory is reasonable. In these older men with early stage disease (a disease that has a slow natural progression), they could be expected to die of other causes thinking their prostate cancer was "cured," but still harboring subclinical disease. Thus, survival end points could be misleading.

Local control became the primary end point in many series. This too was problematic because local failure was only crudely diagnosed by a worsening palpable abnormality on serial digital rectal examination (DRE) or increasing obstructive urinary symptoms. Post-treatment prostate biopsies were rarely performed and modern actuarial statistical analysis was not available. Comparing local control rates between surgery, EBRT, and brachytherapy was difficult. Those institutions that performed both brachytherapy and EBRT did not see any significant difference in local control in their early stage A and B1 cancers, but as grade and stage of disease increased, brachytherapy produced worse results *(22,24,25)*.

Excellent local control was achieved in patients that received (by orthogonal X-ray) high-quality implants and had low-grade and early-stage cancer *(20,21,26)*. The group from MSKCC published a 60% local control rate in those patients received a matched peripheral dose of >140 Gy vs 20% if the matched peripheral dose was less than 140 Gy. In another report by Hilaris and colleagues *(27)* the 15-yr survival was 70% in patients with stage B1 prostate cancer treated with 125-I seed brachytherapy. These data indicate that disease outcomes were more dependent on proper patient selection and quality seed implantation than on disease resistance to permanent interstitial brachytherapy. Unfortunately, it was not possible to consistently perform high-quality implants with the technology of that era, thus brachytherapy once again fell out of favor.

MODERN-ERA TECHNICAL IMPROVEMENTS

The decade of the 1980s brought with it a myriad of advances that would be applied to the diagnosis and treatment of prostate cancer *(28)*. Martinez et al. *(29)* treated patients with a combination of a brachytherapy transperineal applicator and EBRT. At Long Beach Memorial Hospital in Southern California, Syed and Puthawala pioneered temporary low-dose rate transperineal brachytherapy placed at open laparotomy after staging lymph node dissection *(30)*. In Denmark, Holm et al. *(31)* took advantage of advances in transrectal ultrasound imaging to guide the placement of 125-I seeds under ultrasonic visualization, by a transperineal approach, directly into the prostate. This resulted in relatively even distribution of seeds throughout the prostate as viewed on orthogonal X-ray films. In 1983, they published this pioneering technique. This major advance in ultrasound imaging combined with improved radiation therapy treatment planning systems now allowed the brachytherapist to take a preoperative series of transverse images of the prostate, calculate the number, mCi strength, and three-dimensional position of each radioactive seed before the implantation procedure and then in the operating room perform the insertion of the 125-I seeds into the prostate using a template-guided transperineal approach while visualizing the placement of the seeds under real-time transrectal ultrasonography. These advances significantly increased the chance that the prostate being treated would receive the proper number, strength, and positioning of radioactive sources, thus a consistently higher-quality implant.

Blasko et al. *(32)* performed the first transrectal ultrasound (TRUS)-guided, template-guided closed 125-I TIPPB procedure in the United States, at a small community hospital in north Seattle, in late 1985. The Seattle approach involved dosimetric preplanning. First the patient underwent a TRUS volume study, which involved an outpatient scan of the prostate from base to apex in 5-mm steps. Onto these films the radiation oncologist drew the target volume, which include the entire prostate with a few millimeters of surrounding tissue a an extra margin. A customized three-dimensional conformal pre-plan was the developed that denoted each needle's position within the prostate and the number and strength and position (in X, Y, and Z coordinates) of the 125-I seeds within each needle. For any particular patient, the seed strength remained consent. A week or two later, the patient radiation oncologist, referring urologist, ultrasound apparatus, and seeds met up in the operating room. The seeds were preloaded into the needles (2–7 seeds per needle with 5.5 mm spacing absorbable sutures between each seed) just before the start of the case. Under spinal anesthesia, the patient and TRUS probe was positioned to match the positioning obtained at the time of the TRUS volume study. The TIPPB then was accomplished under direct transrectal ultrasound guidance *(32)* (Fig. 1).

Postoperative dosimetry was performed by way of orthogonal X-rays the first 6 yr, qualitative computerized tomography scan dosimetry was used once it became available in the early 1990s, and quantitative dose volume histograms in the mid- to late-1990s. In the 1990s more advanced computerized radiation therapy treatment planning systems tailored for prostate brachytherapy became available, training programs in TIPPB run by the leaders in the field, and dramatic improvements in template, stepper, stabilization, and needle design along with improvements in procedure techniques led to improved accuracy and speed of implantation. Encouraging toxicity reports, 5-yr biochemical relapse–free survival (BRFS) data and the addition of another radioactive isotope (103-Pd) helped to spread the availability of this procedure to large and small hospitals throughout the United States and internationally. It is now performed as an outpatient 45-min procedure at many institutions.

With the spread of this procedure has come a variety of minor technical differences from one facility to the next. Several centers have published improved precision and consistency resulting from technical advances that have occurred over the past decade *(31,33–35)*. There are centers that exclusively use 103-Pd seeds because of its lower energy and higher dose rate and those that use 125-I, those that use 103-Pd for higher Gleason score cancers and those that use 125-I for lower Gleason score cancers *(28)*. Most centers use loose seeds, but some prefer seeds encased in absorbable vicryl suture material (RAPID Strand™) because of the lower seed embolization rate associated with RAPID Stand™ (0.7%) vs loose seeds (11%) *(36)*. Although most centers have dropped computed tomography (CT)-planed TIPPB, D'Amico and colleagues are actively exploring magnetic resonance imaging (MRI)-guided TIPPB *(33,37,38)*. There are centers that publish on the use of the Mick™ applicator system and those that report on the preloaded needle approach *(39–42)*. Differences in technique are expected to grow as more and more physicians perform this procedure and as more technical advances are made. It is common to find centers and individual physicians attaching a name or "brand" to the technique they prefer, such as "real-time interactive" or "The Seattle Technique." Despite these technical differences, the vast majority of active institutions currently use real-time TRUS guidance via a closed template-guided transperineal technique, using preplaning in the operating room at the start of the procedure or a few weeks before the procedure in the clinic. Most use a modified uniform seed dispersal pattern and evaluate implant quality quantitatively with postoperative CT scan-based dosimetry. Virtually all are in agreement that the key to successful outcomes lies in appropriate patient selection and high-quality postimplant CT-based dosimetry, orthogonal film dosimetry is no longer sufficient *(43–47)*.

Current TIPPBs involve proper patient selection, conformal computerized planning, implantation procedure, and postoperative dosimetric evaluation and continued patient follow-up.

PATIENT SELECTION

There are three key elements involved in the selection of patients for ultrasound-guided TIPPB: cancer elements, technical elements, and toxicity elements. The patient should be a good candidate in all three areas before TIPPB becomes a reasonable management option. If a patients does not meet all three major patient selection criteria, he should be counseled to look into a different treatment option because no one therapy or strategy has been proven to be superior.

Cancer elements deal with the extent of disease: local, regional and distant. Patients with proven lymph node involvement or distant metastatic disease are not going to benefit from TIPPB and they are not candidates for TIPPB because they will suffer acute toxicity without any legitimate chance for cure. Palliation of the local symptoms of disease progression are more easily treated (with less toxicity) by surgical approaches, such as transurethral resection of the prostate (TURP) or transurethral microwave therapy, androgen ablation or external beam radiation therapy, or a combination of these approaches.

Patients with clinically apparent T3 disease are usually not considered ideal candidates for TIPPB because the number of patients treated with this approach is too small to adequately analyze. Theoretically, one would be concerned that TIPPB plus EBRT would underdose the peripheral extent of disease. These patients are probably better managed by three-dimensional conformal EBRT + androgen ablation or high dose-rate (HDR) brachytherapy plus EBRT with or without androgen ablation.

The ideal candidate for 125-I or 103-Pd TIPPB monotherapy should have a low risk of microscopic extension of disease much beyond 1–3 mm. The risk of microscopic disease extension outside the prostate has been reported by Partin and colleagues *(48,49)*. They correlated the risk of extra-capsular penetration (ECP), seminal vesicle (SV) involvement, and lymph node (LN) involvement based on the pretreatment biopsy Gleason score, clinical stage by DRE, and pretreatment PSA level to disease extent as seen at pathologic examination of over 4000 radical prostatectomy specimens. This has recently been updated and the risk of disease extension has fallen, probably the result of era-specific earlier disease detection *(50)*.

Some patients with documented ECP at radical prostatectomy have a low BRFS rate and others a high BRFS. Davis et al. *(51)* and by Sohayda and colleagues *(52)* have separately published the actual radial extension of disease outside of the prostate capsule, as measured in millimeters on postoperative radical prostatectomy specimens. They independently demonstrated that the risk of extension much beyond 1–3 mm is low in the low-intermediate risk cohorts. The margin modern TIPPB covers is frequently over 5 mm.

Epstein et al. *(53)* showed that some radical prostatectomy patients with pathologically documented ECP had low BRFS and others relatively high BRFS. They correlated the risk of failure to the pathologic Gleason score, LN, and SV status. Those with negative SV, negative LN, and a Gleason score <7 enjoyed a 75% BRFS, whereas those with Gleason score 7 had only a 50% BRFS. Thus, even patients with ECP can observe a low risk of biochemical failure with the tight margins surgery provides, if the Gleason score is <7.

The Seattle Prostate Institute and the American Brachytherapy Society (ABS), D'Amico and others have defined low-risk patients as those with Gleason score <7, PSA 10 ng/ml, and stage cT2c or lower *(43,54,55)*. These patients have a low risk of significant ECP based on data from Epstein, Partin, and Davis above and have experienced excellent BFRS with seed implantation monotherapy with either 103-Pd or 125-I *(56–61)*. Some surgeons perform combined EBRT + TIPPB on all patients, even low-risk group patients, but the BRFS in these studies do not appear to be superior to those using TIPPB alone *(62,63)*. An exception to TIPPB monotherapy in low-risk patients may involve patients with a high percentage of positive biopsies. D'Amico et al. *(64)* demonstrated that patients undergoing radical prostatectomy who had a high percentage of positive biopsy cores suffered a significantly higher biochemical failure rate than those with a low percentage of positive biopsy cores *(64)*. Whether this is an independent risk factor in TIPPB patients has yet to be analyzed.

The Seattle Prostate Institute defines intermediate-risk patients as those with one unfavorable risk factor: PSA >10 ng/ml or Gleason score >7, or cT2c disease or higher by DRE. High-risk patients have two or three of the above poorer prognostic factors *(55)*.

Few studies have many patients in the high-risk group treated by monotherapy. The initial TIPPB experience at Hospital of the University of Pennsylvania showed poor BRFS with the high-risk patients treated with monotherapy, but the quality of these initial implants is in question because of learning-curve issues and the relative lack of postoperative CT dosimetry *(54)*. Data from the Seattle Prostate institute with 103-Pd monotherapy showed better results than that published with three-dimensional conformal therapy or surgery, but it was a small number of patients and has not yet been duplicated by others *(55)*. Thus, high-risk patients that undergo ultrasound-guided TIPPB receive combined therapy consisting of 45 Gy EBRT followed a few weeks later by a 100 Gy 103-Pd boost or 110 Gy 125-I boost.

The challenge comes with the intermediate-risk cohorts. In these patients some studies show excellent 5- and 10-yr BRFS with TIPPB monotherapy, whereas others (usually during their learning curve) have not *(14,54,55,60,65–69)*. The Seattle group recently reported the outcomes of their intermediate-risk patients treated with TIPPB with or without EBRT. The data did not show any statistically significant difference, but the patients treated with combined therapy had worse pretreatment risk factors and longer follow-up, yet enjoyed a 4% better BRFS (not statistically significant) *(70)*. Most likely, some of the more favorable intermediate-risk patients, that is, those with cT1c and Gleason <7, a low percentage of positive biopsies, and a PSA between 10–15 ng/mL, will do well with TIPPB monotherapy. Other intermediate-risk patients with worse prognostic factors are probably served best by EBRT plus TIPPB, but the data are not yet conclusive for this patient risk cohort. Table 1 shows the current treatment

Table 1
Treatment Selection Guidelines
Recommended by the Seattle Prostate Institute

Risk group	Tx guideline
Low	TIPPB Monotherapy
Intermediate	TIPPB ± EBRT
High	TIPPB + EBRT

guidelines recommended by the Seattle Prostate Institute, which are consistent with those advocated by the American Brachytherapy Society *(43)*.

Technical issues and patient tolerance issues need to be accessed before a patient becomes a candidate for TRUS-guided TIPPB. Gland size is evaluated before beginning any therapy. If the prostate is much greater than 60 cc, the implant becomes technically more challenging. Large prostates require more needles and seeds to achieve adequate coverage of the gland dosimetrically. The more needles used during an implant, the more bleeding within and around the gland occur. This can interfere with prostate visualization, making it difficult to accurately place the needles and seeds. Prostate swelling occurs also. This, combined with bleeding into the perineum, will move the base of the prostate further away from the template, and when combined with worsening visualization of the gland, can make it difficult to adequately track the base position of the prostate. This, in turn, can lead to under dosage of the base. Thus, ideally the prostate should be less than 60 cc or reducible to less than 60 cc with androgen ablation.

A history of a previous TURP can be a relative contraindication to TIPPB. Centers have noted higher rates of incontinence when TURP patients are treated with TIPPB *(44,71)*. This is especially true in patients treated with a pure uniform loading dosimetric approach, which delivers a significantly higher dose to the urethra *(72)*. Those studies that report low incontinence rates in patients with a history of a previous TURP suffer from short follow-up *(73,74)*. It took several years for incontinence to develop in patients in the Seattle series *(44)*. Therefore, patients with a history of a small TURP years ago should be counseled that their risk of incontinence may be higher than non-TURP patients. They should also have a dosimetric plan that is more heavily peripherally weighted. A large TURP defect is an absolute contraindication to TRUS TIPPB because there is not enough tissue to hold the radioactive sources for adequate dosimetry.

Patients with severe obstructive voiding symptoms are at higher risk for experiencing acute urinary retention postimplantation and may require a TURP at a later date because of continued retention or obstructive symptoms. A TURP postimplantation would also increase their risk for incontinence. Some patients can become candidates for implantation if their urinary symptoms respond well to alpha-blockers. There are no data suggesting that a response to androgen ablation will decrease their risk of postimplant urinary complaints. To the contrary, unpublished data from Seattle and other centers suggest that pretreatment with androgen ablation may increase the risk of acute urinary retention.

There are insufficient data on pretreatment transurethral microwave therapy. Challenging patients (such as those with a history of a small previous TURP, prior low-dose pelvic radiation therapy, large prostate volume, large median lobe, unusual pelvic anatomy, or poor quality implant as noted at time of postimplantation dosimetry) may benefit from a consultation with a radiation oncologist that is an expert at prostate brachytherapy.

TREATMENT PLANNING

The advantage of TIPPB is the ability to deliver doses of radiation significantly higher than that achievable with any form of external beam radiation, low-dose, or high-dose rate temporary implantation, all in a single outpatient treatment. Several studies support the assumption that higher doses of radiation delivered accurately to the prostate will result in superior BRFS *(28,46,47,75–79)*. Despite the expected dose inhomogeneity seen with TRUS TIPPB, the radiobiologic effective dose delivered by TIPPB is significantly higher than that delivered by three-dimensional conformal intensity modulated radiation therapy (IMRT) *(28,43,80–82)*.

Dose inhomogeneity is intrinsic to any temporary or permanent brachytherapy procedure, such as TIPPB, because the radiation emanates from individuals radioactive sources (seeds). Thus the dose immediately adjacent the seed will be higher than that a few millimeters away. Standardization of the prescription dose has been described, as previously noted, as the matched peripheral dose. The definition is the dose delivered to a volume equal to an ellipsoid volume with the same average dimension as the prostate gland. As this definition can be confusing, most radiation oncologists consider the prescription dose to be the minimum dose that encompasses the target volume. The target volume is usually the entire prostate plus 1–5 mm of surrounding normal tissue. This is frequently referred to as the minimum peripheral dose (MPD).

In the past, standard dose nomograms were used to direct the number of seeds needed for implantation, this is a reasonable approach if the prostate is a smooth ellipsoid shape. Modern dosimetry develops a target volume based on an individual patient's prostate as determined through radiographic or ultrasonic imaging. MRI and ultrasound scans are relatively accurate in estimating the size and shape of the prostate gland, whereas CT scans typically overestimate the prostate volume vs radical prostatectomy specimens *(83)*.

Most centers currently prescribe an MPD of 145 Gy for 125-I monotherapy implants and 125 Gy for 103-Pd implants. However, the internal dosimetry and the margin of normal tissue included in the MPD can vary widely from center to center. This is the result of differences in seed loading patterns, strength, and dosimetric philosophy.

A pure uniform-loaded implant will drive up the dose to the center (periurethral) region of the prostate to greater than 200–300 Gy for 125-I implants. These were the type of implants initially used in Seattle. In uniform dosimetry implants each seed is 1 cm apart (from seed center to seed center). This type of implant typically uses a relatively high number of seeds of low activity. These implants will be more expensive because of the higher number of seeds. It has the theoretical advantage of requiring less precision in the placement of each individual seed (as each seed contributes less than 1% of the total dose, and thus perhaps a lower risk of local failure). But the patient, especially a TURP patient, may be expected to experience more urinary side effects *(72)*.

A peripherally weighted implant is one in which the sources are place just within the peripheral edge of the implant. These use a relatively low number of high-activity seeds. Theoretically, these implants have the advantage of delivering a lower dose to the urethra (than uniform implants) and thus less urinary toxicity (especially in TURP patients). However, even slight misplacement or migration of a few seeds can result in hot spots by the rectum, neurovascular bundle or urethra, and along with this a cold area within the peripheral zone of the prostate and thus a higher risk of local failure and biochemical failure. These implants are less expensive because of the low number of seeds but are intuitively more challenging technically and should probably not be done by beginners. Modified uniform-peripheral loading or modified peripheral-uniform loading incorporates the best of both of these philosophies and minimizes the potential drawbacks. The vast majority of centers in the United States currently use a modified uniform-peripheral approach. This approach uses relatively fewer seeds in the center of the gland and more in the periphery. This decreases the importance of the precise placement of an individual seed, as a moderately high number of seeds are typically used, thus cold spots within the prostate are less likely than with a peripherally loaded implant. The dose to the center of the gland is less than with a uniform loaded implant. This approach would be expected to result in less urethral toxicity and less local and biochemical failures.

It will be difficult to perform clinical studies to evaluate which dosimetric philosophy is "best" because of differences in skill from one brachytherapist to another and differences in patient selection and use of EBRT combined with TIPPB.

It is important to keep in mind the anatomy of the prostate and periprostatic structures and any predisposing conditions the individual patient may have when planning an implant. For example, a TURP patient with intermediate-risk disease for which a combination of EBRT and TIPPB may be planned, a peripherally weighted implant may be most reasonable. The EBRT will probably work as radiation spackle, filling in potential cold areas, and the peripheral loading will probably decrease the urethral dose, thus decreasing the risk of urethral and urinary complications.

However, for most patients most centers use TRUS ultrasound preplanning (in the clinic or the operating room [OR]) and a fusion of the Manchester (peripheral loading) and Quimby (uniform loading) systems to develop a modified uniform-peripheral loaded implant plan, (Fig. 2) and then reproduce that in the OR under real-time ultrasound guidance *(28,84,85)*. This is consistent with the ABS recommendations *(43)*.

TRUS VOLUME STUDY

The TRUS volume study is a critical step in both patient selection and treatment planning. It is used to evaluate prostate size and possible prostate defects (TURP), which is part of the patient selection process. It is also used to plan out the precise seed distribution pattern to be used in the OR at time of implantation *(28)*.

The TRUS volume study can be performed in the OR immediately prior to the actual implant itself; in this case, it is not as helpful for patient selection issues. The Seattle method involves performing the TRUS in the clinic immediately before the initial consultation for those patients that on prescreening paper work appear to be good implant

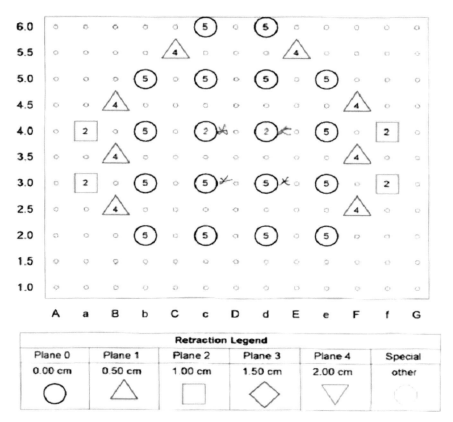

Fig. 2. Example of needle loading plan for TIPPB.

candidates. This allows a more thorough consultation because all the important data needed for decision making will be available at time of consultation.

The procedure uses a TRUS probe that has brachytherapy treatment-planning software and sagittal and transverse imaging capability. The patient performs his bowel prep, including Fleets' Enema™ before the procedure, to improve prostate visualization.

He is positioned in an extended lithotomy position, legs in the same type leg holder used in the OR. The exam table has been modified by adding OR-style metal side bars on to it to hold the leg stirrups, stepper unit, ultrasound probe itself, and stabilization apparatus. The ultrasound technologist inserts the probe into the patients rectum and attaches it to the stepper unit with itself attached to the stabilization apparatus that should have fine-tune adjustments for small vertical, horizontal, and depth changes. The ultrasonographer uses a 5.0, 6.0, or 6.5 MHz frequency if using a machine with frequency options. The lower frequencies penetrate the gland better and will allow for better visualization of the anterior aspects of the prostate and adequate visualization of the posterior portions of the gland (for volume study and implantation purposes). The ultrasonographer then verifies that the patient/prostate/probe positioning is symmetric. Then, while in midgland, the ultrasonographer adjusts the probe so that the posterior row used at time of implantation lines up 1 mm within the prostate (at the midgland position). Next, the prostate is centered on the D row so that the same volume of prostate is present to the left of the D row as to the right of the D row. The ultrasound technologist then takes a sagittal picture measuring the length of the prostate and on this picture, marks are made delineating the apex and the base. Next, he or she identifies the base and takes pictures in the transverse position from 5 mm cranial to the base to 5 mm caudal to the apex. At each 5-mm step, the technologist freezes the picture, traces the outline of the prostate at that particular transverse image record, and prints the picture. This is repeated in 5-mm intervals from base to apex. By convention, we identify the base transverse image (slice) as the 0.0 cm image or "the top." The next transverse image is 0.5 cm into the prostate (caudal of the bladder) and is called the 0.5-cm image. Each subsequent image is taken 0.5-cm caudal to the previous image and identified as the 1.0-, 1.5-, 2.0-cm images, and so on until the final (apical) image is reached. The number of transverse slices needed equals two times the length of the prostate plus 1. A 3.5 cm–long gland requires eight transverse slices (not including the extra slice above the base and below the apex), per the formula below:

$$\text{The number of transverse slices needed} = 2 \times \text{length} + 1 \tag{1}$$

The normal prostate does not wrap around the rectum and form dog ears on either side of the ultrasound probe. If this occurs during the TRUS, it indicates the ultrasound probe is compressing the prostate. One should not do a TRUS or implant on a significantly compressed prostate. Although it is true that the image quality will be better because of a tighter probe rectal wall interface, the quality of the implant will suffer as the gland resumes its normal uncompressed state after the TRUS or implant.

To avoid or eliminate this compression, the probe angle should be changed or a different posterior row used (e.g., row 2 instead of row 1.5 for Siemens™ or row 1.5 instead of row 1.0 for B&K™). At the end of the procedure, the pubic arch can be identified. The narrowest portion of the pubic arch is printed and overlaid on the largest transverse image of the prostate to evaluate for possible pubic arch interference. Special pubic arch identification software is used at the Seattle Prostate Institute. Another option is simply to draw the narrowest portion of the pubic arch directly on the ultrasound monitor with an erasable marker and scan up to the largest transverse image of the prostate to see if there is significant overlap. If less than 10% of the prostate is "blocked" by the arch, the patient is still a candidate for TIPPB. In these cases, simply use a smaller (more horizontal) probe angle in the OR. This will allow the needle to more readily pass up under the arch (Fig. 3). The films of the TRUS then go to the radiation oncologist for target volume determination. The target volume is larger than the prostate volume, particularly at the base and apex.

TARGET VOLUME DETERMINATION

Either directly on the treatment-planning computer or on the films from the TRUS volume study, the radiation oncologist outlines transverse slice by transverse slice the target volume. The goal is to produce a treatment plan that will adequately encompass the prostate and several millimeters of surrounding tissue to the 100% MPD and avoid underdosing the base and apex of the prostate. At the same time overdosing the urethra, rectum, and bulb of the penis needs to be avoided.

The sagittal image and above formula will allow one to chose the proper number of transverse images to outline the target volume. In Seattle, the basic format followed involves using the adjacent transverse image prostate volume as a template for the

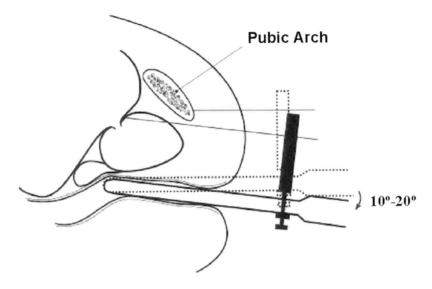

Fig. 3. Angulation technique used to overcome minor pubic arch interference.

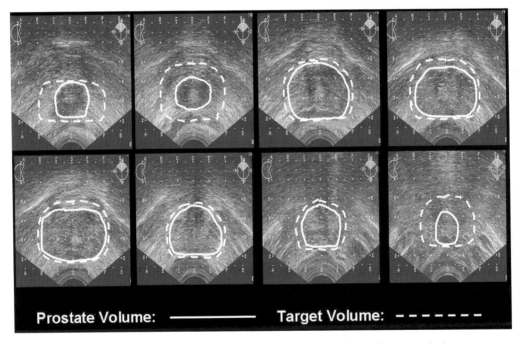

Fig. 4. Prostate volume and target volumes designated on volume study images.

target volume that one is drawing. Thus, the base target volume equals the prostate volume of the 0.5-cm image. The target volume for the 0.5-cm image equals the prostate volume of the 1.0-cm image, and so on. After the largest prostate image is passed, the process is reversed. If the 2.0-cm image is the largest prostate volume it will be the template used for the 1.5-, 2.0-, and 2.5-cm image. The 3.0-cm image will use the 2.5-cm prostate volume as its target volume template, and so on until the apical slice is reached (Fig. 4). An extra margin anterior to the most anterior extent of the prostate should not be drawn because this area is made up of large periprostatic blood vessels. To limit the dose to the bulb of the penis, no more than 0.5- to 1.0-cm margin caudal to the apex should be given. A larger margin is drawn laterally at the base and apex to improve the dose to these areas. The dosimetrist then runs the plan to be used in the OR at a later date, or, right then and there in the OR if intraoperative treatment planning is preferred.

DOSES/ISOTOPES

Debate continues as to the best dose to deliver to the prostate to sterilize all malignant cells. External beam dose escalation studies seem to indicate that higher doses result in higher BRFS rates. Data from MSKCC, M.D. Anderson, Fox Chase Cancer Center, The Cleveland Clinic, and elsewhere all support use of higher doses *(76,86–88)*. However, there are no controlled dose escalation studies involving TIPPB.

The doses used in modern TIPPB were derived from the old retropubic era. The Seattle team chose a prescription MPD of 160 Gy (144 TG-43) in an attempt to achieve a MPD >140 Gy on postoperative dosimetry. MSKCC reported that local control rates by DRE were superior when the MPD achieved on postoperative orthogonal film dosimetry was 140 Gy vs <140 Gy (60% vs 20% local control, respectively) *(21)*. Grimm and colleagues *(60,91)* recently reported a local control rate of 97% by DRE and postimplant serial biopsies on patients treated with 125-I monotherapy from 1988 to 1990. Stock et al. *(46)* reported superior BRFS rates with implants that achieved a CT scan postoperative dosimetry D90 of >140 Gy (TG-43) on 125-I monotherapy implants. Potters and colleagues *(47)* reported superior BRFS in those monotherapy patients that achieved a postoperative CT scan D90 of >90% *(47)*. These studies involve relatively small numbers of patients treated at single institutions and are retrospective reviews. Thus, the final answer in terms of the ideal postoperative dosimetric benchmark is not yet know, but a D90 of >90% in TIPPB monotherapy patients appears to be a reasonable goal at this time.

The dose prescribed depends on which isotope is to be used at time of implantation. The ABS and most experienced prostate brachytherapists recommend a prescribed MPD of 125 Gy for 103-Pd monotherapy implants and 144Gy for 125-I implants *(35,82,89,90)*. 103-Pd uses a lower prescribed MPD because it dose rate is higher than 125-I. 103-Pd has a dose rate of 18–20 cGy per hour and a half-life of 17 d whereas 125-I has a dose rate of 7 cGy per hour and a half-life of 59.4 d. By using different prescribed MPDs for 125-I and 103-Pd one would be expected to achieve the same biologic effect *(92)*.

103-Pd, which was first introduced into clinical practice in 1986, has a photon energy of 21 Kev. 125-I, which has a photon energy of 28 Kev, was introduced in 1965. The differences in energy and dose rate have led to discussions regarding which isotope is more appropriate to use in various clinical situations. Ling et al. has developed mathematical models that indicate that 125-I may be more effective for slow growing tumors and 103-Pd for faster growing tumors *(81,92)*. It has been assumed by many clinicians that high Gleason score cancers grow faster and thus should be treated with 103-Pd and low Gleason score tumors should be treated by 125-I *(85)*. Interestingly, Haustermans and colleagues *(93)* showed no correlation between cell kinetics and histology in human prostate biopsies. Moreover, retrospective reviews do not show any superiority of one isotope over the other in practice *(94)*. A randomized trial at the University of Washington-VA Medical Center in Seattle and Schiffler Cancer Center in West Virginia looking at 125-I vs 103-Pd is almost completed *(95,96)*. The ABS does not recommend one isotope over the other *(43)*.

Task Group 43 (TG-43) reported on interstitial brachytherapy dosimetry in 1995. TG-43 recommended a new single-source dose calculation that predicted a 10 to 18% lower dose rate than before. To achieve the same biologic effect as before TG-43, while using the new TG-43 dosimetric formula, brachytherapists now prescribe 144-145 Gy instead of 160 Gy for 125-I implants *(97)*.

Brachytherapists typically prescribe an MPD of 144 to 145 Gy, The preplanned V100 is the volume of the target volume that receives 100% of the prescribed dose. The V100 is usually planned to be 99 to 100%. The V150 (volume receiving 150% of planned dose) is planned to be approx 35–50%. The V200 should be less than 20% *(85)*.

Clearly, the doses delivered by TIPPB are significantly higher than that achievable by three-dimensional conformal/IMRT external beam radiation therapy. Ling et al. have attempted to run these calculations and noted that a 144 Gy MPD 125-I implant delivers approx 120 Gy external beam equivalent dose *(81,92)*.

With modified peripheral loading the prostate plus several millimeter margin beyond the prostate typically receives 145 Gy with a TIPPB 125-I implant, but the majority of the peripheral zone of the gland is in the 150% isodose curve and receives 145 to 217Gy. It is difficult to compare radiobiologic equivalent doses with TIPPB vs external beam vs HDR brachytherapy. Modified uniform peripheral loading brachytherapists typically use a relatively high number of low-moderate strength seeds (i.e., 0.297–0.326 mCi for 125-I monotherapy or 1.6–1.8 mCi for 103 Pd monotherapy implants). The use of significantly different strength seeds will require different loading distributions and can result in different doses to the interior of the gland. These differences may affect the final postoperative dosimetry and thus the BRFS rates. Thus, the loading philosophy used and the quality of the postoperative implant dosimetry should be kept in mind when comparing results (BRFS and toxicity) achieved at one institution vs another.

IMPLANT PROCEDURE

The implant procedure itself is a 30- to 60-min outpatient procedure that can be performed under spinal or general anesthesia. Most centers prophylactically treat with intravenous antibiotics at time of the implant procedure. The equipment required in the OR include the ultrasound machine, transrectal probe, stepper unit to hold the probe, and a needle guidance template that inserts into the stabilization apparatus that holds the stepper unit and probe. The template needs to undergo needle path verification adjustments before the first case. This verification procedure should be repeated periodically.

Physicians can use either preloaded needles or a MICK™ apparatus to deposit the seeds.

If preloaded needles are to be used, one needs to purchase needle-holding boxes, preferably with needles held in a horizontal position and the ultrasound grid positions

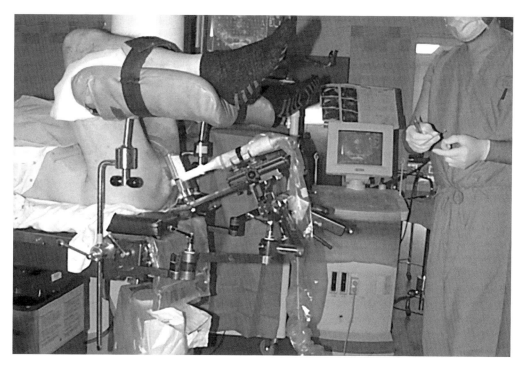

Fig. 5. Patient positioned for TIPPB procedure.

clearly marked on the needle holding box. The stabilization apparatus should have fine tuning adjustments for minor shifts in the *x*, *y*, and *z* axes. Fluoroscopy is helpful to have on hand, especially when the MICK™ apparatus is used.

The patient is positioned in the dorsal lithotomy position. The physician needs to verify that the patient is centered on the table symmetrically. The patient's femurs should be perpendicular to the floor, or even slightly beyond perpendicular in extended lithotomy position to rock to pelvis and help avoid pubic arch interference (Fig. 5). After a standard perineal prep, an aerated KY Jelly™ urethrogram is started. This allows visualization of the urethra and sulci adjacent to the verumontanum, without distortion of the gland *(98)*. Some use a Foley catheter to visualize the urethra, but this can lead to prostate gland distortion and does not visualize the sulci on either side of the verumontanum.

Next the stabilization apparatus is connected to the OR table and the stepper unit and transrectal-ultrasound probe attached. The probe is inserted into the rectum visualizing the prostate. It is important to apply enough pressure with the probe onto the anterior wall of the rectum to adequately visualize the prostate, but not to distort it. When the probe is properly positioned the prostate will be centered about the central axis of the ultrasound grid on the monitor. At the midgland transverse image plane, the posterior row of the implant should be 1 to 2 mm within the prostate (Fig. 6). The base should be identified next and marked on the stepper unit. At the base of the gland one sees bladder, prostate, loose connective tissue, and seminal vesicles. This is sometimes referred to as a head and bow tie appearance (Fig. 7). This plane is the 0.0 imaging plane. The

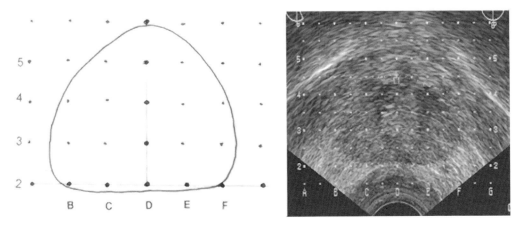

Fig. 6. Proper positioning of the template grid relative to the prostate midgland.

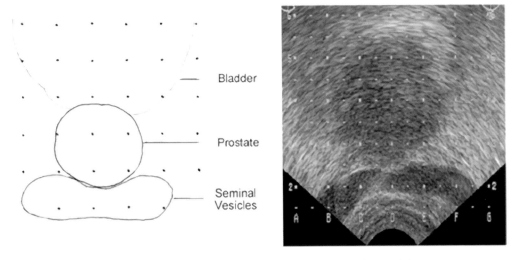

Fig. 7. Proper positioning of the template relative to the base of the prostate.

other planes are referenced in 0.5-cm increments from this 0.0 prostate/bladder inter-face plane. The physicians then double-checks that the type of seed (125-I or 103-Pd), strength, and needle arrangement matches the preplan for that particular patient.

The procedure of seed insertion into the prostate then begins. There are differences in technique at various centers. There is no one correct way of performing the proce-dure itself. Some prefer to use preloaded needles, others the MICK™ system, some prefer 125-I others 103-Pd, some peripheral loading, others modified uniform-periph-eral, some loose seeds, and others seeds stranded in absorbable vicryl suture (RAPID Strand™). Some prefer preplans, others prefer to do the planing in the operating room. Many have published on these differences in technique *(35,40,56,66,99)*.

There are certain principles that are observed regardless of the differences in tech-nique used. Physicians need to constantly monitor the prostate positioning throughout the implant procedure and correct for gland position changes as they occur. The needles distort the gland shape and cause bleeding and gland swelling. This moves the gland away from the perineum during the case and average of 1.5 cm *(65)*. Prostate movement may have contributed to the relatively poor BRFS attained in patients with pretreatment PSAs of greater than 10 ng/mL treated with CT planned but not CT or ultrasound-guided TIPPB monotherapy *(33,57)*. To avoid underdosing the base of the gland during the implant procedure, the brachytherapist overinserts the needle then retracts it to the proper depth and doublechecks that needle's final position on transverse and sagittal imaging before depositing the seeds (Figs. 8 and 9). The prostate also moves medially when inserting peripheral needles, anteriorly when inserting posterior needles, and posteriorly when inserting anterior needles. Thus aiming the needle 1 to 3 mm in the direction of the expected gland movement will usually compensate for that movement so that the radioactive sources end up in the proper position after the needle is withdrawn. Some use stabilization needles to help reduce gland movement, but others do not because the presence of the needles inhibits rapid needle insertion and rapid needle insertion itself will decrease gland distortion and movement.

Once a needle is in the proper x–y coordinate, one can verify the depth (z axis) by various maneuvers including ruler measurements vs the template and, most importantly, sagittal imaging. The sources (seeds) are then deposited and the next needle inserted if one needle at a time is the technique used, or the next needle is withdrawn depositing seeds along its track if the technique used involves having several needles in the gland at once. Those needles near the center of the prostate may drop seeds too close to the urethra. In order to avoid overdosing the urethra, inject a few cc's of aerated KY Jelly™ when addressing the peri-urethral needles. These seeds should usually be at least 5 mm away from the urethra, so it is usually necessary to place the needles containing these seeds a few mm lateral to their planned target coordinates.

Particular attention needs to be taken regarding the posterior row of needles (and their seeds). The needle should be at least 1 mm within the prostate in the midgland in monotherapy implants and 2 to 3 mm within the prostate in boost implants.

The pubic arch can interfere with needle insertion into the prostate, particularly in patients with larger (>50 cc) prostates. If this interference occurs it usually is involves the anterior lateral needle positions. Positioning the patient in a more extended lithotomy position will rotate the pubic arch anteriorly and frequently move the arch out of the way. Using a flatter probe angle can help one avoid the pubic arch as well. However, a flatter probe angle will bring the posterior needles closer to the rectum at the apex of the prostate. This needs to be compensated for when inserting the posterior needles (i.e., a higher template needle position should be used or the probe angle again changed). If the above fails to eliminate the pubic arch blockage, insert the needle into the needle guidance template 0.5 cm posterior and 0.5 cm medial to the target position, then angle the needle bevel anterior lateral and insert. This maneuver usually works. If it fails, save that needle for the end of the case, then change the probe angle so it is negative 5 to 20 degrees and then insert the needle. This last maneuver will virtually always allow the needle to reach a position very close to its planned position, and as the needle involved is usually intended for an anterior position within the prostate (and usually only 2–3 seeds) the rectum is not usually a problem. At the end of the proce-

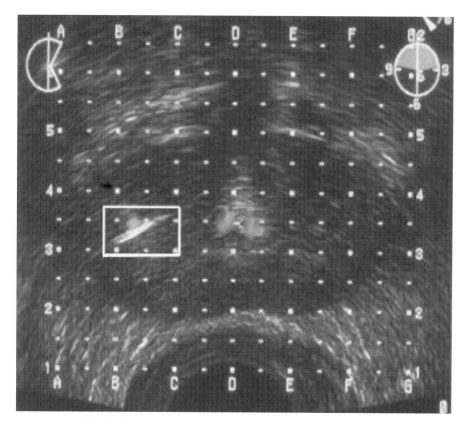

Fig. 8. Needle tip visualization on transverse TRUS image.

dure, a fluoroscopic evaluation is performed. This qualitative evaluation allows the brachytherapist to address any obvious "cold spots." Such areas can be implanted under simultaneous fluoroscopic and ultrasound guidance (Fig. 10).

Cystoscopy is often performed at the end of the procedure to remove any blood clots or seeds from the bladder, but it is optional. Seeds and blood clots can be easily removed by placing a catheter and using a syringe to evacuate material from inside the bladder, this may be less traumatic to a gland already swollen by multiple needle insertions.

Immediately postimplantation radiation exposure measurements are taken in the OR or recovery room of the patient. These measurements are of the radiation exposure at the surface and at 50 or 100 cm from the patient's surface. OR and Foley catheter and drainage bag surveys are also performed to verify that no seeds have been left behind. Typical postoperative orders include an ice pack to the perineum for 20 min and discharge to home with an alpha-blocker (i.e., Flomax™), an antibiotic, a nonsteroidal anti-inflammatory drug, and appointment for CT scan for postoperative dosimetry purposes.

In terms of radiation safety precautions, the energy of the 125-I and 103-Pd are so low that minimal exposure will occur to friends and relatives of the patient. Michalski noted that the average dose a spouse (of a TIPPB patient) received during the year after the implant was 10 mRem. This is approximately equal to living in Denver for 3 to 4 mo or taking one round trip airplane flight from New York to Tokyo *(100)*.

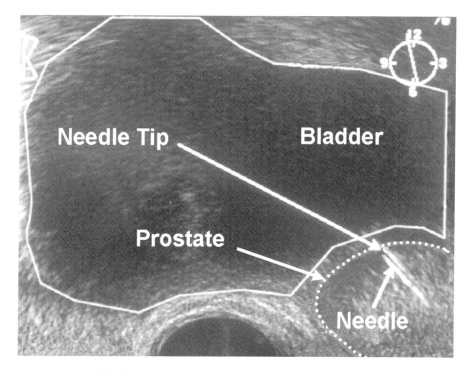

Fig. 9. Needle tip visualization on sagital TRUS image.

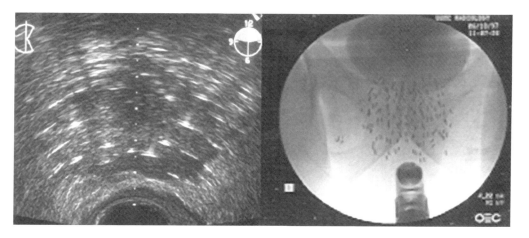

Fig. 10. Combined TRUS and fluoroscopic imaging used at close of TIPPB procedure to identify and correct unintended gaps in seed distribution.

POSTOPERATIVE DOSIMETRIC EVALUATION

Orthogonal film dosimetry was used in the past for postoperative implant quality evaluation. Unfortunately orthogonal film dosimetry does not evaluate source position vs prostate position. Thus, studies that report high-quality implants based on postoperative orthogonal film dosimetry may not truly have achieved high-quality implants.

Modern postoperative implant quality evaluation uses CT-based dosimetry. Although not without problems, CT dosimetry will show the radioactive sources in cross-sectional images where they lie within the prostate (Fig. 11). Dose volume histograms (DVHs) and isodose curves can then be derived with the aid of computer treatment-planning software (Fig. 12). Problems with CT scan-based dosimetry involve artifact caused by the seeds, by artificial hips, difficulty in identifying the apex of the gland, and difficulty in distinguishing the prostate capsule from the periprostatic vascular structures. These latter factors can result in the CT scan overestimating the size of the prostate vs ultrasound, MRI, or operative measurements *(83,101,102)*. The preceding can make it challenging to outline the prostate margin accurately on the postoperative CT scan. To help overcome inconsistencies and physician bias in prostate contouring some centers use the preoperative TRUS to outline the prostate contour on the CT (after correct magnification done) *(97)*. Prestidge and colleagues and others have documented that prostate swelling after implantation can be as high as 41% (vs the pretreatment volume). Serial CT scans show continual shrinkage of the gland over time. As the prostate swells the seeds move further apart and as the prostate shrinks the seeds move back together. This can affect the postoperative dosimetry isodose curves. If a tight margin or no margin is given in the preplan, this prostate swelling and later shrinkage can impact the postoperative DVHs. Therefore, even if one accurately outlines the prostate contour on the postoperative CT scan, the DVHs from one center to another may vary depending on how many days or weeks postoperatively the CT scan was performed. This complicates comparisons of implant quality from one center to the next *(104,105)*

By 4 wk postoperation, most the prostate swelling has resolved and therefore performing postoperative dosimetry at this time is reasonable if the logistics work out with the patient population *(105)*. At centers where some of the patients travel large distances, postoperative dosimetry performed on d 0 or d 1 may be more practical.

Qualitative evaluation with orthogonal films or CT scans without DVH analysis has indicated superior quality implants with modern TIPPB techniques as compared with retropubic techniques of the 1970s *(19,31–33,40,99,106–109)*. Modern CT scan DVH analysis further documents the superiority of the modern TIPPB technique *(46,47)*.

Stock et al. *(46)* documented better BRFS in the patients treated with 125-I monotherapy that achieved a D90 of greater than 140 Gy than those with a D90 less than 140 Gy. Potters et al. *(47)* reported significantly better BRFS in monotherapy TIPPB (125-I or 103-Pd) patients with a postoperative D90 of greater than 90%. Grimm and colleagues *(60)* have shown that monotherapy patients treated from 1986 to 1987 (the first 2 yr TIPPB implants were performed in the United States) achieved significantly worse BRFS than monotherapy patients treated at the same Seattle institution, by the same physicians, from 1988 to 1990. It should be noted that these two cohorts of 125-I monotherapy patients had equivalent follow-up and were treated in the same era. These implants were performed before the availability of DVH analysis, but it is likely that the patients treated from 1988 to 1990 received higher-quality implants than the initial discovery-curve patients treated from 1986 to 1987. These studies all support the hypothesis that higher-quality implants result in better BRFS in monotherapy TIPPB patients. Postoperative dosimetry provides important immediate feedback on the individual patient's implant. If there is a significant region of underdosing, it can be

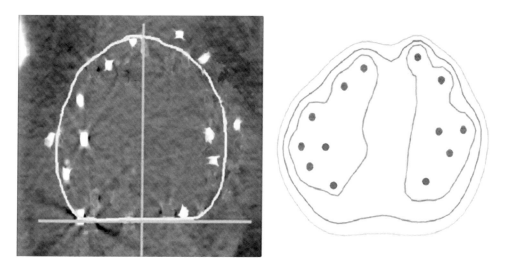

Fig. 11. Postoperative CT image with superimposed prostate outline and corresponding dose volume histogram.

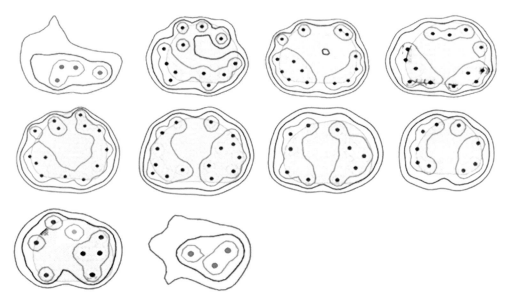

Fig. 12. Complete series of dose volume histograms for a TIPPB procedure.

addressed with supplemental EBRT, HDR, or further strategically placed seeds at a second TIPPB procedure.

Postoperative dosimetry also shows the individual brachytherapist his or her own dosimetry trends. If consistent underdosing of the base or over dosing of the anterior wall of the rectum is seen, the brachytherapist can alter his or her implant technique or preplan to correct for the problem.

Currently, the ABS recommends CT scan-based postoperative dosimetry and that it be reported when TIPPB results are published *(43)*. Postoperative DVH analysis should be performed on each patient, and it should be performed on approx the same postoperative day within a single institution, within 30 d of the procedure. It should include isodose curves overlaid on the prostate, D90, V100, and V150 determinations. Many centers also include V200 and rectal and urethral doses. Some centers are looking at doses to the bulb of the penis as well *(110)*.

TOXICITY OF MODERN TIPPB

Major acute operative morbidity is extremely rare. Severe bleeding requiring transfusions or admission to intensive care for any postoperative acute events and or death have not been noted in the literature *(30,111)*. The Seattle Prostate Institute physicians have performed over 7000 TIPPB procedures and have noted no serious intraoperative or postoperative morbidity.

Acute postoperative side effects are common and are primarily RTOG grade I–II irritative and obstructive lower urinary symptoms, including increased urinary frequency, urgency, dysuria, and weakening of the urinary stream *(38,44,55,112)*. The symptoms are at their worst wk 2 to 6 postoperative but typically are bothersome for 2 to 6 mo. During this time it is standard practice to treat with alpha-blockers. Acute urinary retention occurs in approx 10% of patients. Several factors have been implicated in single institution univariate analysis, including large gland size, high pretreatment urinary symptom score, and pretreatment with androgen ablation. On multivariate analysis most of these risk factors drop out or are not reproducible between various institutions *(38,41,42,66,71,112,113)*.

A recent patient self-administered questionnaire of Seattle patients revealed a 12% risk of acute urinary retention. The average duration of retention was 13 d, and 2% required a Foley, suprapubic, or intermittent self-catheterization for more than 6 mo. The only identifiable risk factor on multivariate analysis was pretreatment with androgen ablation *(115)*. In the small percentage of patients that experience retention of more than a few weeks duration, self catheterization is taught or a suprapubic catheter is placed until the swelling and retention resolves. If retention does not resolve, surgical intervention with a transurethral incision of the prostate or small TURP is usually indicated. It must be emphasized that these procedures should not be performed until at least 6 mo (preferably >9 mo) after TIPPB *(112,115)*. Patients that undergo TURP before or shortly after a uniformly loaded (high urethral doses) TIPPB have a significant risk of developing urinary incontinence *(19,71)*. Patients that undergo a peripheral-loaded TIPPB implant may be at lower risk for incontinence, but published reports with this technique have relatively short follow up, and small patient numbers.

Increased bowel frequency and urgency is uncommon and when it occurs responds to diet and medications, such as Imodium™. Hematuria and hematospermia is to be expected for a few days, occasionally a few weeks after TIPPB. Perhaps half the sexually active patients will experience some level of pain with orgasm; this can persist for weeks to months. The prostatic fluid component (majority) of the ejaculate will decrease dramatically following TIPPB, but sperm will still be present. Whether or not the sperm is significantly damaged by the radiation exposure is unknown, but to be safe birth control measures are recommended for those couples that are still fertile. Ejaculation of a seed is rarely reported. The Seattle team is aware of less than five patients that have noted this event over the past 15 yr *(116)*.

Recently several quality-of-life (QOL) studies have looked at TIPPB vs EBRT vs radical prostatectomy. Lee et al. *(117)* prospectively evaluated the acute toxicity of therapy on 90 patients treated with TIPPB, EBRT, or radical prostatectomy. Using a patient self-reported questionnaire, Functional Assessment of Cancer Therapy—Prostate, filled out at time 0 (before treatment) and, 1, 3, and 12 mo after treatment, the impact on patients' QOL was evaluated. This analysis showed a decrease in QOL with radical prostatectomy and TIPPB at 1 mo postoperation but the QOL returned to near baseline by the 1-yr mark *(117)*. Davis and colleagues *(118)* compared the QOL of patients they treated with radical prostatectomy, EBRT, or TIPPB using five validated QOL instruments. This is also patient self-reported data. They noted the patients treated with radical prostatectomy reported significantly worse QOL in terms of urinary functioning and sexual function and bother (Figs. 13 and 14). The patients treated with EBRT reported significantly worse QOL in regards to bowel function and fear of cancer recurrence (Fig. 15) *(118)*.

Late toxicity after TIPPB is much less common. Patients frequently chose TIPPB in the belief that the risk of cancer recurrence is low, but also in the belief that the risk of permanent bowel, urinary and sexual impairment is low.

Radiation proctitis occurs in approx 2 to 5% of monotherapy patients and 10% of combination EBRT plus TIPPB patients. It is not usually apparent until 1 and 2 yr postimplant and rarely manifests after 3 yr *(38,42,57,67,68,71)*. Postoperative dosimetry/ DVH analysis has shown a direct correlation between the volume of rectum receiving 100% of the prescription dose and the rate of radiation proctitis. Snyder and colleagues noted the percentage of patients developing radiation proctitis was 0% if less than 0.8 cc of rectum received the prescription dose, 8% if >1.3 to 1.8 cc, 24% if >1.8 to 2.3, and 25.5% if > 2.3 cc of rectum received the prescription dose *(119)*. This is usually RTOG grade I–II and treatment consists of conservative measures, low roughage diet, Metamucil™, suppositories. Rectal fistula is rare in patients not undergoing electrocaughtery *(19,111)*. Electrocaughtery is to be avoided. Biopsies to diagnosis radiation proctitis should be avoided also, as this is a clinical diagnosis. Biopsies and electrocaughtery may increase the risk of a nonhealing ulcer or fistula.

Most reports in the literature note that long-term urinary morbidity and/or incontinence is rare after TIPPB. In patients without severe obstructive urinary symptoms, significant benign prostatic hypertrophy and without previous TURP the risk of chronic cystitis or incontinence after TIPPB is less than 3% *(19,111)*. The risk of incontinence is dependent on many factors. These include patient age at treatment, history of TURP, length of follow-up, uniform loading vs peripheral or modified uniform-peripheral loading techniques, definition of incontinence, and patient vs physician reports. The Seattle team reported a rate of incontinence (stress or gravity) of 17% in TURP patients with 2.5 yr follow-up. The rate increased to 32% in TURP patients when 6 yr of follow-up was reached. However, even with long follow-up, they noted incontinence in only 0.4% of non-TURP patients *(44,60,111,120)*. Beyer et al.'s *(66)* series and Kaye's *(68)* series both treated patients with relatively uniform loaded implants like Seattle and report a rate of incontinence of only 0 to 1% in their non-TURP patients as well.

The Seattle team used a uniform technique early on then later switched to a modified uniform-peripheral loading philosophy. Talcott et al. *(72)* reported a higher rate of incontinence in Seattle patients, than noted above. He reported that 10% of non-TURP

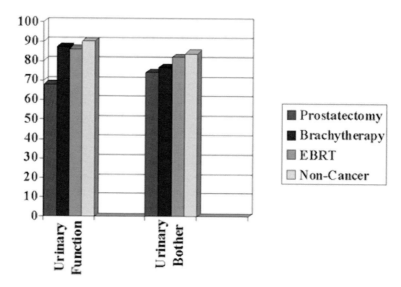

Fig. 13. Patient-reported assessment of urinary function and bother by treatment type.

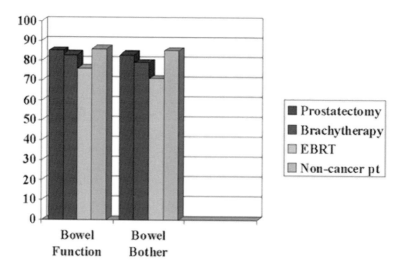

Fig. 14. Patient-reported assessment of bowel function and bother by treatment type.

men reported leakage of "more than a few drops." It should be noted that some of the non-TURP men may have indeed had some sort of urethral surgical procedures, that some had pure uniform-loaded implants, and that they were an average age of 75 yr old at time of the report *(72)*. Uniform loading dramatically increases the urethral dose and 5% of men age 70 will leak more than a few drops, with a higher percentage at age 75, without any treatment. Peripheral loading may decrease the risk of incontinence in TURP patients. A 6% incidence was reported at MSKCC *(38,57)*. This lower incidence of incontinence in TURP patients may be the result of the peripheral loading used or short follow-up or a combination of both.

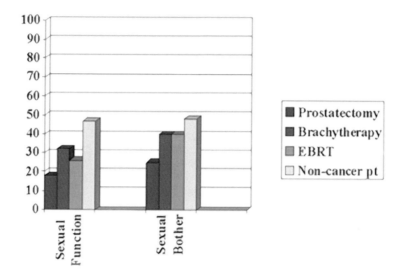

Fig. 15. Patient-reported assessment of sexual function and bother by treatment type.

The bulk of available reports seem to indicate a low rate of incontinence in men treated with TIPPB with either a peripheral or modified uniform-peripheral loading technique, in non-TURP patients. At this time it may be reasonable to avoid TIPPB in TURP patients or to discuss the controversy with the patient and use a more peripheral-loaded technique if the patients decides on TIPPB.

Sexual functioning and impotency are more challenging to evaluate because of differences in definition of potency, age differences in baseline functioning, co-morbid diseases, and the sexual functioning and interest of the patient's partner. The Seattle team has reported the results of a patient self-reported questionnaire. Those patients that noted full normal erection ability before implantation maintained the ability to obtain an erection "adequate for intercourse" in 80% of seed monotherapy patients and in 69% of patients treated with EBRT plus a brachytherapy boost *(65,97,121)*. Wallner *(57)* reported that at 3 yr status postimplantation 81% maintained erection ability. Kaye and colleagues *(68)* reported that 75% of their TIPPB patients maintained erection function at 1 yr postimplant.

Merrick et al. *(110)* have correlated dose to the bulb of the penis to erectile dysfunction. In a small series of retrospectively reviewed patients he noted that 19 of 23 patients lost erectile function when the D50 to the bulb of the penis was greater than 40% of the minimal peripheral dose while 19 of 23 maintained erectile function if the D50 was less than 40% of the minimal peripheral dose.

RESULTS

There remains considerable debate as to how to best define BRFS after EBRT or TIPPB, particularly in the urological literature *(122)*. The American Society of Therapeutic Radiology and Oncology (ASTRO) definition of biochemical failure used in most EBRT and many TIPPB reports, is criticized for underestimating biochemical failure because it requires three increases in PSA postimplant before a failure is called.

After TIPPB, the PSA falls slowly. The half-life of PSA fall after TIPPB with 103-Pd is over 90 d but only 3.8 d after radial prostatectomy (RP) *(120,123)*.

Each year 5 to 10% of patients die of other diseases with no biochemical or clinical evidence of prostate cancer recurrence *(124)*. If TIPPB cures 100% of patients treated, the 5 and 10 yr BFRS would be less than 100% if a definition of PSA less than 1.0 ng/mL or 0.5 mg/mL were used. This is because patients will die of other disease before PSA nadir is reached, whereas their PSA levels are still falling but not yet below 1.0 ng/mL or 0.5 ng/mL, and thus be marked a biochemical failure. Thus, it is inappropriate to define BRFS based on a fixed PSA value such as 1.0 or 0.5 ng/mL. An ASTRO-like BRFS PSA progression free definition; using two or three PSA increases as a cut point for biochemical failure is more reasonable. Nevertheless, these different definitions in BFRS will continue to spark debate between the radiation oncology and urology communities.

Another difficulty is the elimination of many patients in the RP series based on pathologic findings, such as seminal vesicle invasion, positive margins or positive lymph nodes. The EBRT and TIPPB literature cannot eliminate these patients from their series. More recently some RP series have reported BRFS based on pretreatment biopsy Gleason score, DRE, and PSA *(64,125,126)*. However, even when comparing results based on pretreatment risk factors comparisons between different institutions still is problematic due to differences in pathologic Gleason scoring, and other potential selection biases *(47,127,128)*.

D'Amico and Kupellian have reported 5-yr radical prostatectomy BRFS results from three centers and Zelefsky recently reported the MSKCC 5-yr high-dose three-dimensional conformal EBRT BRFS results, by low intermediate and high-risk group cohorts. These are noted in Table 2.

Table 3 displays the 5-yr BRFS for patients treated with TIPPB monotherapy or TIPPB plus EBRT. The 5-yr BRFS is 88 to 95% for the low-risk patient cohort. Intermediate-risk patients treated with TIPPB ± EBRT have a reported 58 to 96% BRFS. High-risk patient cohorts a 54 to 79% *(14,61,63,120,129)*. Nonrandomized data from the Seattle Prostate Institute show no significant difference in 5-yr BRFS between patients treated with TIPPB monotherapy and TIPPB plus EBRT *(130)*. It should be noted that the patients that received the additional EBRT in the Seattle series received it for a reason (multiple positive biopsies, perineural invasion) and thus are not entirely comparable to the TIPPB monotherapy cohort.

Long-term BRFS reports have be published out of Seattle. Blasko and colleagues *(130)* documented the results of 230 patients treated with 103-Pd monotherapy. This article included many patients with unfavorable (community hospital pathologist assigned) Gleason scores. They reported an 83.5% 9-yr BRFS for the patient group as a whole. The half-life of PSA fall status post implantation was 96.2 d. Because 5 to 10% of patients died of nonprostate-related disease each year during follow-up, with falling PSA and no evidence of clinical failure, an absolute PSA level of less than 0.5 ng/mL was considered an inappropriate biochemical endpoint for these low dose–rate brachytherapy patients. The Seattle group uses a modified ASTRO definition whereby two PSA increases (not three) are required before a patient is noted to be a biochemical failure. By risk group, the 5-yr BRFS was 94, 82, and 65% for low-, intermediate-, and

Table 2
5-Yr Biochemical PSA NED

Risk group	RP D'Amico (HUP) *(64)*	RP D'Amico (B&W) *(64)*	RP Kupelian (Cleveland) *(125)*	3D-CRT Zelefsky (5-yr FU) *(86)*[a]
Low	85%	83%	81%	90%
Intermediate	65%	50%	40%	70%
High	32%	28%	–	47%

[a]39% with NHT, three-increase PSA failure definition.

Table 3
TIPPB: 4- to 6-Yr BRFS

	Blasko (*n*=230) 5 yr *(120)*	Lederman (*n*=339) 6 yr *(63)*	Merrick (*n*=262) 5 yr *(61)*	Stone (*n*=182) 4 yr *(129)*	Sylvester (*n*=634) 5 yr *(134)*
Low	94%	88%	96%	91%	92%
Intermediate	82%	75%	96%	58%	84%
High	65%	51%	79%	—	62%
Percent EBRT	0%	100%	57%	0%	36%

high-risk groups, respectively. There were a small number of patients in the high-risk group *(120)*.

Grimm published the 10-yr BRFS outcomes on patients treated by the Seattle Prostate Institute physicians from 1988 to 1990. With an average follow-up of 94.5 mo in the living patients, the 10-yr BRFS in the low-risk cohort was 87%. The local control rate was 97%, the metastatic disease free survival rate was 97%, and the cause specific survival was 100%. Polascik has criticized the Seattle data because of the high number of needle biopsy Gleason score 2–4 cancers contained in the series *(131)*. These patients were probably undergraded. It is interesting to note that reports by Steinberg and colleagues *(127)* from the same institution (The John Hopkins Hospital) demonstrate that undergrading was the rule at outside hospitals during that era. They noted that only 4 of 87 outside biopsy Gleason score 2–4 cancers were called Gleason score 2–4 by the Hopkins pathologists, and those 4 were all upgraded at surgery. Of the outside Gleason score cancers they reviewed, they upgraded 78% to Gleason score 5–6 and 17.5% to Gleason score 7 or higher. Epstien has gone on to propose that Gleason score 2–4 should not be made on the basis of needle biopsies *(128)*. In separate reports Iczkowski et al. *(132)* and Allsbrook and colleagues *(133)* have published on the tendency for community pathologists to undergrade prostate biopsies. It is important to realize that the Gleason grading in all the Seattle reports was performed by pathologists at a small community hospital in north Seattle in the late 1980s and early 1990s. Thus, the vast majority of the Gleason score 2–4 cancers in the Seattle series would have been upgraded to Gleason 5–7 or higher if reviewed by expert prostate pathologists.

The 10-yr BRFS rates of the 634 consecutively treated patients treated in Seattle with I-125/Pd-103 ± EBRT from 1987 to 1993 were reported at the 2001 annual

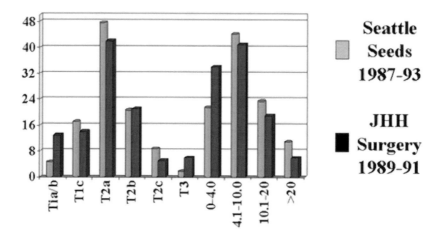

Fig. 16. Pretreatment PSA and stage: Johns Hopkins and Seattle series.

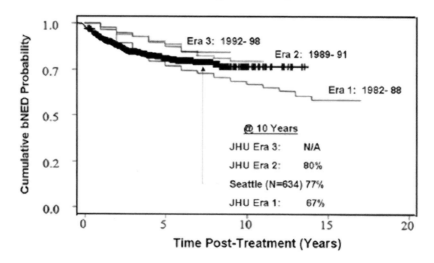

Fig. 17. Long-term BRFS results: Johns Hopkins and Seattle series.

Table 4
Seattle Series: TIPPB 9- to 10-Yr BRFS

	Blasko[a] (n=230) 9 yr (120)	Grimm[b] (n=125) 10 yr (60)	Sylvester[c] (n=232) 10 yr (114)	Seattle[d] (n=402) 10 yr (114)
Low	—	87%	85%	87%
Intermediate	—	76%	77%	73%
High	—	—	47%	45%
Total	84%	85%	70%	77%
Percent EBRT	0%	0%	100%	36%

[a]Pd^{103} monotherapy.
[b]I^{125} monotherapy.
[c]EBRT + Pd^{103}/I^{125}.
[d]Pd^{103} or I^{125} monotherapy.

ASTRO meeting. The low-, intermediate-, and high-risk group rates are presented in Table 4. The 9- to 10-yr Seattle data are presented in Table 4. The long-term Seattle results are similar to those achieved with radical prostatectomy as reported by Han, Walsh, and colleagues from the Johns Hopkins series (Fig. 17). Both patient cohorts had comparable stage and PSA characteristics (Fig. 16).

CONCLUSION

Modern TRUS-guided interstitial permanent brachytherapy is a 45-min single outpatient treatment for the majority of men with early-stage prostate cancer. It has documented 5- and 10-yr biochemical, overall, and disease-specific relapse-free survival rates that equal the best that radical prostatectomy has thus far achieved. These favorable findings should firmly establish permanent prostate brachytherapy as a primary treatment option for early stage prostate cancer.

Current disadvantages include the learning curve that practitioners typically experience before they can perform high-quality implants on a consistent basis. Fortunately, postimplant CT dosimetry can identify any underdosed areas or cold spots that may exist. This allows inadequate implants performed during the learning period to acted upon and corrected in a timely manner. In this regard, developments in the field of implant dosimetry are underway that should bring significant progress in the future.

At present, pretreatment dosimetry planning is the norm at the great majority of centers where permanent prostate brachytherapy is available. Real-time, intraoperative dosimetry based on needle position is in use at several institutions, but it is a matter of some concern that needle position does not always correlate with final seed position. Efforts to improve the real-time technique are under way, the major obstacle being the current inability of ultrasound to reliably identify each seed as it is deposited into the prostate.

Future advances in ultrasound technology that allow the simultaneous recognition of seeds and exporting of location coordinates into dosimetry software modules will give clinicians the ability to produce instantaneous isodose distributions in real time in the OR. With these advances, practitioners should be able to perform virtually perfect implants on every patient and shorten, or altogether eliminate, the learning curve. They should also allow for significant reduction in dose to sensitive normal structures such as the urethra, rectum, and the bulb of the penis.

REFERENCES

1. Mettlin C, Jones GW, Murphy GP. Trends in prostate cancer care in the United States, 1974–1990: observations from the patient care evaluation studies of the American College of Surgeons Commission on Cancer. *CA Cancer J Clin* 1993;4:83–91.
2. Garfinkel L , Mushinski M. Cancer incidence, mortality and survival: trends in four leading sites. *Stat Bull Metrop Insur Co* 1994;75:19–27.
3. Fleming C, Wasson JH, Albertsen PC, Barry MJ, Wennberg JE. A decision analysis of alternative treatment strategies for clinically localized prostate cancer. Prostate Patient Outcomes Research Team [see comments]. *JAMA* 1993;269:2650–2658.
4. Talcott JA, Rieker P, Propert K, et. al. Complications of treatment for early prostate cancer: a prospective, multi-insitutional outcomes study [asbtr]. *Proc Am Soc Clin Oncol* 1994;13:A711.

5. Litwin MS. Health-related quality of life after treatment for localized prostate cancer. _Cancer_1995;75(Suppl):2000–2003.
6. Johansson JE, Adami HO, Andersson SO, Bergstrom R, Holmberg L, Krusemo UB. High 10-year survival rate in patients with early, untreated prostatic cancer [see comments]. _JAMA_1992;267:2191–2196.
7. Blasko JC, Wallner K, Grimm PD, Ragde H. Prostate specific antigen based disease control following ultrasound guided 125iodine implantation for stage T1/T2 prostatic carcinoma. _J Urol_ 1995;154:1096–1099.
8. Zietman AL, Coen JJ, Shipley WU, Willett CG, Efird JT. Radical radiation therapy in the management of prostatic adenocarcinoma: the initial prostate specific antigen value as a predictor of treatment outcome. _J Urol_ 1994;151:640–645.
9. Trapasso JG, deKernion JB, Smith RB, Dorey F. The incidence and significance of detectable levels of serum prostate specific antigen after radical prostatectomy. _J Urol_ 1994;152:1821–1825.
10. Zagars GK, Pollack A, Kavadi VS, von Eschenbach AC. Prostate-specific antigen and radiation therapy for clinically localized prostate cancer. _Int J Radiat Oncol Biol Phys_ 1995;32;293–306.
11. Zagars GK. Prostate-specific antigen as a prognostic factor for prostate cancer treated by external beam radiotherapy. _Int J Radiat Oncol Biol Phys_ 1992;23;47–53.
12. Talcott JA, Rieker P, Clark JA, et al. Patient-reported symptoms after primary therapy for early prostate cancer: results of a prospective cohort study. _J Clin Oncol_ 1998;16;275–283.
13. Prostate Canvcer Brachytherapy: Clinical and Financial Imperatives for Permanent Implantation, in Oncology Roundtable Annual Meeting. Washington, DC, The Advisory Board Co., 2000;15.
14. Sylvester JE, Blasko J, Grimm P. Brachytherapy as Monotherapy, in _Prostate Cancer: Principles and Practice_ (Kantoff P, Carroll PC, D'Amico AV, eds). Philadelphia, Lippincot Williams & Wilkins, 2001; pp. 336–357.
15. Porter AT, Blasko JC, Grimm PD, Reddy SM, Ragde H. Brachytherapy for prostate cancer [see comments]. _CA Cancer J Clin_ 1995;45:165–178.
16. Denning CL. Carcinoma of the prostate seminal vesicles treated with radium. _Surg Gynecol Obstet_ 1922;34:99–118.
17. Scardino P, Carlton C. Combined interstitial and external irradiation for prostatic cancer, in _Principles and Management of Urologic Cancer_ (Javadpour N, ed.). Baltimore, Williams & Wilkins, 983; 392–408.
18. Whitmore WF Jr, Hilaris B, Grabstald H. Retropubic implantation to iodine 125 in the treatment of prostatic cancer. _J Urol_ 1972;108:918–920.
19. Blasko JC, Grimm PD, Ragde H. Brachytherapy and organ preservation in the management of carcinoma of the prostate. _Semin Radiat Oncol_ 1993;3:240–249
20. DeLaney TF, Shipley WU, O'Leary MP, Biggs PJ, Prout GR Jr. Preoperative irradiation, lymphadenectomy, and 125iodine implantation for patients with localized carcinoma of the prostate. _Int J Radiat Oncol Biol Phys_ 1986;12:1779–1785.
21. Fuks Z, Leibel SA, Wallner KE, Begg CB, Fair WR, Anderson LL, Hilaris BS, Whitmore WF. The effect of local control on metastatic dissemination in carcinoma of the prostate: long-term results in patients treated with 125I implantation. _Int J Radiat Oncol Biol Phys_ 1991;21:537–547.
22. Giles GM, Brady LW. 125-Iodine implantation after lymphadenectomy in early carcinoma of the prostate. _Int J Radiat Oncol Biol Phys_1986;12:2117–2125.
23. Kuban DA, el-Mahdi AM, Schellhammer PF. I-125 interstitial implantation for prostate cancer. What have we learned 10 years later? _Cancer_ 1989;63:2415–2420.
24. Schellhammer PF, Whitmore WF, Kuban DA, El-Mahdi AM, Ladaga LE. Morbidity and mortality of local failure after definitive therapy for prostate cancer. _J Urol_ 1989;141:567–571.

25. Morton JD, Harrison LB, Peschel RE. Prostatic cancer therapy: comparison of external-beam radiation and I-125 seed implantation treatment of stages B and C neoplasms. *Radiology* 1986;159:249–252.

26. Kovacs G, Galalae R, Loch T, Bertermann H, Kohr P, Schneider R, Kimming B. Prostate preservation by combined external beam and HDR brachytherapy in nodal negative prostate cancer. *Strahlenther Onkol* 1999;175(Suppl 2):87–88.

27. Hilaris B, Fuks Z, Nori D, et al.Interstitial irradiation in prostatic cancer: report of 10-year results, in *Interventional Radiation Therapy Techniques/Brachytherapy* (Rolf, ed) Berlin, Springer-Verlag, 1991; p 235.

28. Sylvester J, Blasko JC, Grimm P, Ragde H. Interstitial implantation techniques in prostate cancer. *J Surg Oncol* 1997;66:65–75.

29. Martinez A, Edmundson GK, Cox RS, Gunderson LL, Howes AE. Combination of external beam irradiation and multiple-site perineal applicator (MUPIT) for treatment of locally advanced or recurrent prostatic, anorectal, and gynecologic malignancies. *Int J Radiat Oncol Biol Phys* 1985;11:391–398.

30. Puthawala A, Syed A, Tansey L. Temporary iridium implant in the management of carcinoma of the prostate. *Endocurie Hyper Oncol* 1985;1:25–33.

31. Holm HH, Juul N, Pedersen JF, Hansen H, Stroyer I. Transperineal 125-iodine seed implantation in prostatic cancer guided by transrectal ultrasonography. *J Urol* 1983;130:283–286.

32. Blasko JC, Radge H, Schumacher D. Transperineal percutaneous iodine-125 implantation for prostatic carcinoma using transrectal ultrasound and template guidance. *Endocuriether Hyperthermia Oncol* 1987;3:131–139.

33. Wallner K, Chiu-Tsao ST, Roy J, et al. An improved method for computerized tomography-planned transperineal 125iodine prostate implants. *J Urol* 1991;146:90–95.

34. Beyer DC, Priestley JB Jr. Biochemical disease-free survival following 125I prostate implantation. *Int J Radiat Oncol Biol Phys* 1997;37:559–563.

35. Grimm PD, Blasko JC, Ragde H. Ultrasound-guided transperineal implantation of Iodine-125 and Palladium-103 for the treatment of early-stage prostate cancer: technical concepts in planning, operative technique, and evaluation, in *New Techniques in Prostate Surgery*, vol 2 (Schellhammer PF,ed). Philadelphia W.B. Saunders Co., 1994; pp. 113–126.

36. Tapen EM, Blasko JC, Grimm PD, Ragde H, Luse R, Clifford S, et al. Reduction of radioactive seed embolization to the lung following prostate brachytherapy. *Int J Radiat Oncol Biol Phys* 1998;42:1063–1067.

37. Willins J, Wallner K. CT-based dosimetry for transperineal I-125 prostate brachytherapy. *Int J Radiat Oncol Biol Phys* 1997;39:347–353.

38. Arterbery VE, Wallner K, Roy J, Fuks Z. Short-term morbidity from CT-planned transperineal I-125 prostate implants. *Int J Radiat Oncol Biol Phys* 1993;25:661–667.

39. Priestly JB Jr, Beyer DC. Guided brachytherapy for treatment of confined prostate cancer. *Urology* 1992;40:27–32.

40. Stock RG, Stone NN, Wesson MF, DeWyngaert JK. A modified technique allowing interactive ultrasound-guided three- dimensional transperineal prostate implantation. *Int J Radiat Oncol Biol Phys* 1995;32:219–225.

41. D'Amico AV, Coleman CN. Role of interstitial radiotherapy in the management of clinically organ-confined prostate cancer: the jury is still out [see comments]. *J Clin Oncol* 1996;14:304–315.

42. Dattoli MJ, Wasserman SG, Koval JM, Sorace RA, Cash J, Wallner KE. Conformal brachytherapy boost to external beam irradiation for localized high risk prostate cancer [abstr]. *Int J Radiat Oncol Biol Phys* 1995;32(Suppl):251.

43. Nag S, Beyer D, Friedland J, Grimm P, Nath R. American Brachytherapy Society (ABS) recommendations for transperineal permanent brachytherapy of prostate cancer. *Int J Radiat Oncol Biol Phys* 1999;44:789–799.

44. Blasko JC, Ragde H, Luse RW, Sylvester JE, Cavanagh W, Grimm PD. Should brachytherapy be considered a therapeutic option in localized prostate cancer? *Urol Clin North Am* 1996;23:633–649.

45. Wallner K, Blasko J, Dattoli M. *Prostate Brachytherapy Made Complicated*. Seattle, Smart Medicine Press, 1997.

46. Stock RG, Stone NN, Tabert A, Iannuzzi C, DeWyngaert JK. A dose-response study for I-125 prostate implants. *Int J Radiat Oncol Biol Phys* 1998;41:101–108.

47. Potters L, Cao Y, Calugaru E, Torre T, Fearn P, Wang XH. A comprehensive review of CT-based dosimetry parameters and biochemical control in patients treated with permanent prostate brachytherapy. *Int J Radiat Oncol Biol Phys* 2001;50:605–614.

48. Partin AW, Yoo J, Carter HBet al. The use of prostate specific antigen, clinical stage and Gleason score to predict pathological stage in men with localized prostate cancer [see comments]. *J Urol* 1993;150110–114.

49 Partin AW, Kattan MW, Subong EN, et al. Combination of prostate-specific antigen, clinical stage, and Gleason score to predict pathological stage of localized prostate cancer. A multi-institutional update [see comments] [published erratum appears in *JAMA* 1997;9;278:118]. *JAMA* 1997;277:1445–1451.

50. Partin AW, Mangold LA, Lamm DM, Walsh PC, Epstein JI, Pearson JD. Contemporary update of prostate cancer staging nomograms (Partin Tables) for the new millennium. *Urology* 2001;58:843–848.

51. Davis BJ, Pisansky TM, Wilson TM, et al. The radial distance of extraprostatic extension of prostate carcinoma: implications for prostate brachytherapy. *Cancer* 1999;85:2630–2637.

52. Sohayda C, Kupelian PA, Ciezki J, Levin HJ, Klein EA. Extent of extracapsular extension: implications for planning for conformal radiotherapy and brachytherapy [abstr]. *Int J Radiat Oncol Biol Phys*1998;42(Suppl):132.

53. Epstein JI, Carmichael MJ, Pizov G, Walsh PC. Influence of capsular penetration on progression following radical prostatectomy: a study of 196 cases with long-term followup. *J Urol* 1993;150:135–141.

54. D'Amico AV, Whittington R, Malkowicz SB, et al. Biochemical outcome after radical prostatectomy, external beam radiation therapy, or interstitial radiation therapy for clinically localized prostate cancer. *JAMA* 1998;280:969–974.

55. Blasko JC, Grimm PD, Ragde H. External beam irradiation with palladium-103 implantation for prostate carcinoma. *Int J Radiat Oncol Biol Phys* 1994;30(Suppl):219.

56. Wallner K. I-125 brachytherapy for early stage prostate cancer: new techniques may achieve better results. *Oncology* 1991;5:115–126.

57. Wallner K, Roy J, Harrison L. Tumor control and morbidity following transperineal iodine 125 implantation for stage T1/T2 prostatic carcinoma. *J Clin Oncol* 1996;14:449–453.

58. Schellhammer PF, Ladaga LE, El-Mahdi A. Histological characteristics of prostatic biopsies after 125iodine implantation. *J Urol* 1980;123:700–705.

59. Prestidge BR, Hoak DC, Grimm PD, Ragde H, Cavanagh W, Blasko JC. Posttreatment biopsy results following interstitial brachytherapy in early-stage prostate cancer. *Int J Radiat Oncol Biol Phys* 1997;37:31–39.

60. Grimm P, Blasko J, Sylvester JE, Meier RM, Cavanagh W. 10-year biochemical (prostate-specific antigen) control of prostate cancer with 125-I brachytherapy. *Int J Radiat Oncol Biol Phys* 2001;51:31–40.

61. Merrick GS, Butler WM, Galbreath RW, Lief JH. Five-year biochemical outcome following permanent interstitial brachytherapy for clinical T1-T3 prostate cancer. *Int J Radiat Oncol Biol Phys* 2001;51:41–48.

62. Roy JN, Ling CC, Wallner KE, Anderson LL. Determining source strength and source distribution for a transperineal prostate implant. *Endocurie/Hyperthermia Oncol* 1996;1235–41.

63. Lederman GS, Cavanagh W, Albert PS, et al. Retrospective stratification of a consecu-

tive cohort of prostate cancer patients treated with a combined regimen of external-beam radiotherapy and brachytherapy. *Int J Radiat Oncol Biol Phys* 2001;49:1297–3003.

64. D'Amico AV, Whittington R, Malkowicz SB, et al. Clinical utility of the percentage of positive prostate biopsies in defining biochemical outcome after radical prostatectomy for patients with clinically localized prostate cancer [see comments]. *J Clin Oncol* 2000;18:1164–1172.

65. Grimm P. Clinical results of prostate brachytherapy, in Radiological Society of North America Annual Meeting. Chicago, IL, 1998.

66. Beyer DC, Priestley JB. Biochemical disease-free survival following I-125 prostate implantation [abstr]. *Int J Radiat Oncol Biol Phys* 1995;32(Suppl):254.

67. Wallner K, Roy J, Zelefsky M, Fuks Z, Harrison L. Short-term freedom from disease progression after I-125 prostate implantation. *Int J Radiat Oncol Biol Phys* 1994;30:405–409.

68. Kaye KW, Olson DJ, Payne JT. Detailed preliminary analysis of 125iodine implantation for localized prostate cancer using percutaneous approach. *J Urol* 1995;153:1020–1025.

69. Kupelian P, Katcher J, Levin H, Zippe C, Klein E. Correlation of clinical and pathologic factors with rising prostate-specific antigen profiles after radical prostatectomy alone for clinically localized prostate cancer. *Urology* 1996;48:249–260.

70. Sylvester J. Modern permanent prostate brachytherapy, in American Society of Therapeutic Radiology and Oncology 43rd Annual Meeting. San Francisco, 2001

71. Blasko JC, Ragde H, Grimm PD. Transperineal ultrasound-guided implantation of the prostate: morbidity and complications. *Scand J Urol Nephrol Suppl* 1991;137:113–118.

72. Talcott JA, Clark JA, Stark PC, Mitchell SP. Long-term treatment related complications of brachytherapy for early prostate cancer: a survey of patients previously treated. *J Urol* 2001;166:494–499.

73. Wallner K, Lee H, Wasserman S, Dattoli M. Low risk of urinary incontinence following prostate brachytherapy in patients with a prior transurethral prostate resection. *Int J Radiat Oncol Biol Phys* 1997;37:565–569.

74. Stone NN, Ratnow ER, Stock RG. Prior transurethral resection does not increase morbidity following real-time ultrasound-guided prostate seed implantation. *TechniqueUrol* 2000;6:123–127.

75. Zelefsky MJ, Leibel SA, Gaudin PB, et al. Dose escalation with three-dimensional conformal radiation therapy affects the outcome in prostate cancer. *Int J Radiat Oncol Biol Phys* 1998;41:491–500.

76. Kupelian PA, Mohan DS, Lyons J, Klein EA, Reddy CA. Higher than standard radiation doses (> or =72 Gy) with or without androgen deprivation in the treatment of localized prostate cancer. *Int J Radiat Oncol Biol Phys* 2000;46:567–574.

77. Hanks GE, Hanlon AL, Schultheiss TE, et al. Dose escalation with 3D conformal treatment: five year outcomes, treatment optimization, and future directions. *Int J Radiat Oncol Biol Phys* 1998;41:501–510.

78. Kupelian PA, Reddy CA, Klein CA. Factors associated with biochemical relaps after either low-dose external beam radiation, high-dose external beam radiation, or radical prostatectomy for localized prostate cancer: 8 year results [abstr]. *Int J Radiat Oncol Biol Phys* 1999;45(suppl.):219.

79. Pollack A, Zagars GK. External beam radiotherapy dose response of prostate cancer. *Int J Radiat Oncol Biol Phys* 1997;39:1011–1018.

80. Prestidge BR, Bice WS, Prete JJ, et al. A dose-volume analysis of permanent transperineal prostate brachytherapy. *Int J Radiat Oncol Biol Phys* 1997;39(Suppl):289.

81. Ling CC. Permanent implants using Au-198, Pd-103 and I-125: radiobiological considerations based on the linear quadratic model. *Int J Radiat Oncol Biol Phys* 1992;23:81–87.

82. Nag S, Pak V, Blasko J, et al. Prostate brachytherapy, in *Principles and practices of brachytherapy* (Nag S, ed). Armonk, Futura Publishing, 1997; pp. 421–440.

83. Hastak SM, Gammelgaard J, Holm HH. Transrectal ultrasonic volume determination of

the prostate—a preoperative and postoperative study. *J Urol* 1982;127:1115–1118.

84. Paulson DF. Impact of radical prostatectomy in the management of clinically localized disease. *J Urol* 1994;152:1826–1830.

85. Prestidge BR, Prete JJ, Buchholz TA, et al. A survey of current clinical practice of permanent prostate brachytherapy in the United States. *Int J Radiat Oncol Biol Phys* 1998;40:461–465.

86. Zelefsky MJ, Fuks Z, Hunt M, et al. High dose radiation delivered by intensity modulated conformal radiotherapy improves the outcome of localized prostate cancer. *J Urol* 2001;166:876–881.

87. Hanks GE, Hanlon AL, Pinover WH, Horwitz EM, Price RA, Schultheiss T. Dose selection for prostate cancer patients based on dose comparison and dose response studies. *Int J Radiat Oncol Biol Phys* 2000;46:823–832.

88. Pollack A, Smith LG, von Eschenbach AC. External beam radiotherapy dose response characteristics of 1127 men with prostate cancer treated in the PSA era. *Int J Radiat Oncol Biol Phys* 2000;48507–512.

89. Nag S, Orton C, Young D, Erickson B. The American brachytherapy society survey of brachytherapy practice for carcinoma of the cervix in the United States. *Gynecol Oncol* 1999;73:111–118.

90. Nag S, Scaperoth DD, Badalament R, Hall SA, Burgers J. Transperineal palladium 103 prostate brachytherapy: analysis of morbidity and seed migration. *Urology* 1995;45:87–92

91. Grimm PD, Blasko JC, Ragde H, Sylvester J, Clarke D. Does brachytherapy have a role in the treatment of prostate cancer? *Hematol Oncol Clin North Am* 1996;10:653–673.

92. Ling CC, Li WX, Anderson LL. The relative biological effectiveness of I-125 and Pd-103. *Int J Radiat Oncol Biol Phys* 1995;32:373–378.

93. Haustermans KM, Hofland I, Van Poppel H, Oyen R, Van de Voorde W, Begg AC, Fowler JF. Cell kinetic measurements in prostate cancer. *Int J Radiat Oncol Biol Phys* 1997;37:1067–1070.

94. Chu C, Potters L, Ashley R, Waldbaum R, Leibel S. Isotope selection for patients undergoing prostate brachytherapy [abstr]. *Int J Radiat Oncol Phys* 1998;42(Suppl):134.

95. Wallner K. Personal communication, 2001.

96. Merrick G. Personal Communication, 2001.

97. First Advanced Prostate Brachytherapy Workshop, Seattle Prostate Institute, Seattle, Washington, May 15–16, 1998.

98. Sylvester JE, Grimm PD, Blasko JC. Urethral visualization during transrectal ultrasound guided interstitial implantation for early stage prostate cancer, in Annual Meeting of the Radiologican Society of North America. Chicago, IL, 1998.

99. Wallner K, Roy J, Zelefsky M, Fuks Z, Harrison L. Fluoroscopic visualization of the prostatic urethra to guide transperineal prostate implantation. *Int J Radiat Oncol Biol Phys*1994;29:863–867.

100. Prostate brachytherapy seeds to not expose family members to high levels of radiation. *Oncol News Int* 2001;10.

101. Gomella LG, Lotfi MA, Reagan GN. Laboratory parameters following contact laser ablation of the prostate for benign prostatic hypertrophy. *Technique Urol* 1995;1:168–171.

102. Hricak H, Jeffrey RB, Dooms GC, Tanagho EA. Evaluation of prostate size: a comparison of ultrasound and magnetic resonance imaging. *Urol Radiol* 1987;9:1–8.

103. Corn BW, Hanks GE, Schultheiss TE, Hunt MA, Lee WR, Coia LR. Conformal treatment of prostate cancer with improved targeting: superior prostate-specific antigen response compared to standard treatment [see comments]. *Int J Radiat Oncol Biol Phys* 1995;32:325–330.

104. Waterman FM, Yue N, Reisinger S, Dicker A, Corn BW. Effect of edema on the postimplant dosimetry of an I-125 prostate implant: a case study. *Int J Radiat Oncol Biol Phys* 1997;38:335–339.

105. Prestidge BR, Bice WS, Kiefer EJ, Prete JJ. Timing of computed tomography-based postimplant assessment following permanent transperineal prostate brachytherapy [see comments]. *Int J Radiat Oncol Biol Phys* 1998;40: 1111–1115.

106. Kaye KW, Olson DJ, Lightner DJ, Payne JT. Improved technique for prostate seed implantation: combined ultrasond and fluoroscopic guidance. *J Endourol* 1992;6:61–66.

107. Ragde H, Blasko J, Schumacher D, Grimm P. Use of transrectal ultrasound in transperineal I-125 seeding for prostate cancer: methodology. *J Endourol* 1989;3:209–218.

108. Roy JN, Wallner KE, Chiu-Tsao ST, Anderson LL, Ling CC. CT-based optimized planning for transperineal prostate implant with customized template. *Int J Radiat Oncol Biol Phys* 1991;21:483–489.

109. Stock RG, Stone NN, DeWyngaert JK, Lavagnini P, Unger PD. Prostate specific antigen findings and biopsy results following interactive ultrasound guided transperineal brachytherapy for early stage prostate carcinoma. *Cancer* 1996;77:2386–2392.

110. Merrick GS, Wallner K, Butler WM, Galbreath RW, Lief JH, Benson ML. A comparison of radiation dose to the bulb of the penis in men with and without prostate brachytherapy-induced erectile dysfunction. *Int J Radiat Oncol Biol Phys* 2001;50:597–604.

111. Blasko JC, Grimm PD, Ragde H. 6 and 7 year results of permanent seed implantation, in *Transperineal Brachytherapy: Into the Mainstream.* Seattle, WA, Pacific NW Cancer Foundation, 1995.

112. Grier D. Complications of permanent seed implantation. *J Brachytherapy Int* 2001;**17**, 205–210

113. Sylvester JE, Grimm P, Blasko J, Meier RM, Heaney CT, Cavanagh W. Transperineal permanent brachytherapy for local recurrence following external beam radiation for early-stage prostate cancer. *J Brachyther Int* 2001;17:181–188.

114. Sylvester J. Modern Permanent Prostate Brachytherapy, in American Society of Therapeutic Radiology and Oncology. San Francisco, 2001.

115. Blasko J, in Fifth Advanced Prostate Brachytherapy Workshop. Seattle, WA, Seattle Prostate Institute, 2002.

116. Stock RG, Stone NN, DeWyngaert JK. PSA findings and biopsy results following interactive ultrasound guided transperineal brachytherapy for early stage prostate cancer, in Proceedings of the American Radium Society 78th Annual Meeting. Paris, France, 1995; p. 58.

117. Lee WR, Hall MC, McQuellon RP, Case LD, McCullough DL. A prospective quality-of-life study in men with clinically localized prostate carcinoma treated with radical prostatectomy, external beam radiotherapy, or interstitial brachytherapy. *Int J Radiat Oncol Biol Phys* 2001;51:614–623.

118. Davis JW, Kuban DA, Lynch DF, Schellhammer PF. Quality of life after treatment for localized prostate cancer: differences based on treatment modality. *J Urol* 2001;166:947–952.

119. Snyder K, Stock R, Hong S, Lo Y, Stone N. Defining the risk of developing grade 2 proctitis following 125I prostate brachytherapy using a rectal dose-volume histogram analysis. *Int J Radiat Oncol Biol Phys* 2001;50:335–341.

120. Blasko JC, Grimm PD, Sylvester JE, Badiozamani KR, Hoak D, Cavanagh W. Palladium-103 brachytherapy for prostate carcinoma. *Int J Radiat Oncol Biol Phys* 2000;46:839–850.

121. Ragde H, Blasko J, Grimm P. Complications of permanent seed implantation, in *Transperineal Brachytherapy: Into the Mainstream.* Seattle, WA, Pacific NW Cancer Foundation, 1995.

122. Amling C, Bergstralh E, Blute M, Slezak J, Zincke H. Defining prostate specific antigen progression after radical prostatectomy: what is the most appropriate cut point? *J Urol* 2001;165:1146–1151.

123. Oesterling JE, Chan DW, Epstein JI, et al. Prostate specific antigen in the preoperative and postoperative evaluation of localized prostatic cancer treated with radical prostatectomy. *J Urol* 1988;139:766–772.

124. Cavanagh W. Seattle Prostate Institute, 2002.

125. Kupelian PA, Katcher J, Levin HS, Klein EA. Stage T1–2 prostate cancer: a multivariate analysis of factors affecting biochemical and clinical failures after radical prostatectomy. *Int J Radiat Oncol Biol Phys* 1997;37:1043–1052.

126. Han M, Pound CR, Potter SR, Partin AW, Epstein JI, Walsh PC. Isolated local recurrence is rare after radical prostatectomy in men with Gleason 7 prostate cancer and positive surgical margins: therapeutic implications. *J Urol* 2001;165:864–866.

127. Steinberg D, Sauvageot J, Piantadosi S, Epstein J. Correlation of prostate needle biopsy and radical prostatectomy gleason grade in academic and community settings. *Am J Surg Pathol* 1997;21:566–576.

128. Epstein J. Gleason score 2–4 adenocarcinoma of the prostate on needle biopsy. *Am J Surg Pathol* 2000;24:477–478.

129. Stone NN, Stock RG. Prostate brachytherapy: Treatment strategies. *J Urol* 1999;162:421–426.

130. Blasko JC, Grimm PD, Sylsvester JE, Cavanagh W. The role of external beam radiotherapy with I-125/Pd-103 brachytherapy for prostate carcinoma. *Radiother Oncol* 2000;57:273–278.

131. Polascik TJ, Pound CR, DeWeese TL, Walsh PC. Comparison of radical prostatectomy and iodine 125 interstitial radiotherapy for the treatment of clinically localized prostate cancer: a 7-year biochemical (PSA) progression analysis [see comments]. *Urology* 1998;51:884–889; discussion 889–890.

132. Iczkowski KA, Bostwick DG. The pathologist as optimist: cancer grade deflation in prostatic needle biopsies [editorial]. *Am J Surg Pathol* 1998;22:1169–1170.

133. Allsbrook WC Jr, Mangold KA, Johnson MH, et al. Interobserver reproducibility of Gleason grading of prostatic carcinoma: urologic pathologists. *Hum Pathol* 2001;32:74–80.

134. Sylvester J, Blasko J, Grimm P, et al. Neoadjuvant androgen ablation combined with external beam radiation therapy and permanent interstitial brachytherapy boost in localized prostate cancer. *Mole Urol* 1999;3:231–237.

7

Magnetic Resonance Imaging-Guided Interstitial Prostate Brachytherapy

Anthony V. D'Amico, MD, PhD, **Kristin Valentine,** BS,
Ferenc Jolesz, MD, **Lynn Lopes,** RN, **Sanjaya Kumar,** MD,
Clare M. Tempany, MD, **and Robert Cormack,** PhD

INTRODUCTION

Adenocarcinoma of the prostate is currently the most commonly diagnosed cancer in men in the United States and the second leading cause of cancer mortality *(1)*. The natural history of treated clinically localized and potentially curable disease is often protracted. As a result, side effects sustained from the primary treatment may persist for extended periods, often several decades. Therefore, it is important that the treatment, whose goal is to permanently eradicate the disease, also have acceptable complication rates, leaving the patient with an acceptable quality of life after therapy is complete. To this end, efforts aimed at providing a minimally invasive alternative to radical prostatectomy (RP) for the curative treatment of patients with clinically localized prostate cancer have been made.

Brachytherapy is the therapeutic delivery of radiation to a diseased site by the insertion, either temporarily or permanently, of seeds containing radioactive material. The dose distribution around a single source falls off approximately as $1/r^2$, where r is the distance from the source center. The use of brachytherapy exploits the dose fall-off effect by placing sufficient sources within the cancer-bearing volume to deliver the prescription dose to the entire cancer while a rapid decrease in dose beyond the volume containing sources occurs. The rapid dose fall off, therefore, provides the basis on which a high intraprostatic dose can be delivered while maintaining subtolerance doses in the normal juxtaposed (i.e., rectum and neurovascular bundles) and interposed (i.e., urethra) tissues.

The current method of prostate brachytherapy in the United States commonly uses transrectal ultrasound (TRUS) imaging to guide radioactive seed placement *(2)*. Using this approach, nonideal placement of radioactive sources sometimes occurs *(3)*. In the early experience with this approach, inadvertent placement of the radioactive sources lead to complications that included impotence, rectal–prostatic fistula, rectal bleeding, colostomy, superficial urethral necrosis, and urinary incontinence. With modern techniques many of these toxicities are less frequently realized.

From: *Image-Guided Diagnosis and Treatment of Cancer*
Edited by: A. D'Amico, J. S. Loeffler, and J. R. Harris © Humana Press Inc., Totowa, NJ

In an effort to further improve on the advances made in TRUS-guided brachytherapy, a real-time three-dimensional magnetic resonance imaging (MRI)-guided prostate brachytherapy implant technique that uses both real-time MRI and a real-time dose volume histogram analysis program has been designed and implemented (4). Using this technique, the selection of the appropriate seed strength, seed number, and catheter trajectory can be made intraoperatively and then quality assured for accuracy using real-time MRI within seconds. Therefore, in theory this technique is capable of achieving optimized dose distributions in both the prostate gland and normal adjacent structures that may translate into both improved cancer control and quality of life, respectively.

Although the experience with and use of prostate brachytherapy using TRUS guidance is growing, it still lacks long-term follow-up (i.e., 15 yr) (5).Therefore, advancements using a brachytherapy technique that may increase cancer control rates while potentially limiting gastrointestinal, genitourinary, and sexual function morbidity would be critical to the growing number of prostate cancer patients who are choosing prostate brachytherapy as their sole treatment.

METHODS

Patient Selection

Between 1997 and 2002, 184 patients underwent a MRI-guided prostate radiation implant at the Brigham and Women's Hospital under the care of a single physician. The policy for patient selection for prostate brachytherapy alone included men with 1997 American Joint Commission on Cancer (6) clinical category $T_{1c}N_XM_0$ prostate cancer, prostate-specific antigen (PSA) <10 ng/mL, biopsy Gleason score (7) not more than 3 + 4, and T_2 disease on a 1.5 T endorectal coil MR scan. Endorectal MRI evidence of T2 as opposed to T3 disease in this patient population has been shown to be associated with a more favorable PSA outcome (8).

In addition, patients who had urinary daytime frequency less than every 2 h and/or nocturia exceeding 4 that was not medically controlled were not eligible. All patients with a previous history of a transurethral resection of the prostate were excluded. However, patients who had a previous abdominal perineal resection were not excluded because the MRI-guided technique does not require a rectum to guide source placement because the imaging apparatus is extrinsic to the patient (9). Moreover, no patient received androgen suppression therapy before brachytherapy to achieve prostate gland volume reduction because there is no prostate gland volume limit using the MRI-guided technique. The technique permits catheter entry at oblique angles, eliminating the issue of pubic arch interference when implanting the anterior base and midgland in a patient with severe benign prostatic hyperplasia.

Beginning in June 1999, the predictive value of the percent of positive prostate biopsies on PSA outcome after RP in otherwise low-risk patients had been established. Therefore, only patients with <50% positive biopsies was accepted for MRI-guided brachytherapy as mono therapy. The reason patients with biopsy Gleason score 3 + 4 were accepted as candidates for MR guided brachytherapy was because in a low-risk patient population managed with a RP, nearly 50% of these patients were downgraded to prostatectomy Gleason score was 3 + 3 or less when <50% of the biopsy core speci-

Table 1
Clinical Characteristics of the Study Patients, Stratified by the Treatment Received

Clinical characteristic	Implant monotherapy (%) (n = 137)	External beam RT (%) + implant boost (n = 47)
PSA 4 ng/mL or less	34 (25)	4 (8)
PSA >4–10 ng/mL	103 (75)	30 (64)
PSA >10 – 13 ng/mL	0 (0)	13 (28)
Gleason 3 + 3 or less	118 (86)	43 (91)
Gleason 3 + 4	19 (14)	4 (9)
% + biopsies < 50%	115 (84)	34 (72)
% + biopsies 50% or more	22 (16)	13 (28)
Age <60	50 (36)	14 (30)
Age 60–70	67 (49)	23 (49)
Age >70	20 (15)	10 (21)
Prostate Gland Volume 45 cm^3 or less	85 (62)	29 (62)
Prostate Gland Volume > 45–60 cm^3	29 (21)	9 (19)
Prostate Gland Volume > 60 cm^3	23 (17)	9 (19)

% +, Percent positive.

mens contained prostate cancer *(10)*. Patients with either 50% or more positive biopsies, or a PSA >10 to 13 ng/mL or MR evidence of extracapsular extension at the apex or midgland were treated using a combination of external beam radiation therapy (RT) (45.0 Gy) to the prostate and seminal vesicles followed 4 to 6 wk later by a brachytherapy boost. The pretreatment distribution of the clinical characteristics of the 184 patients treated with MRI-guided prostate brachytherapy as monotherapy (n = 137) or as a boost after external beam RT (n = 47) are listed in Table 1.

Preoperative Assessment

Before the procedure, all patients underwent a cystoscopy to assess the integrity of the urethral and bladder mucosa and well as to inspect the bladder neck. The findings of bladder neck contracture, urethral stricture, or muscle invasive bladder or urethral cancer disqualify the patient for MRI-guided prostate brachytherapy. In cases where underlying bladder outlet obstructive symptoms were present, urodynamic studies were performed to determine the etiology of the obstructive symptoms and appropriate medical or surgical intervention is applied prior to the implant procedure. A quality-of-life questionnaire with no patient identifying information developed by Talcott and colleagues *(11)* was completed before therapy and then completed at 3 mo, 1 yr, 2 yr, and 3 yr after completion of therapy. The questionnaire provided the patient the opportunity to report on gastrointestinal, genitourinary, and sexual function in an anonymous setting. Given the limited cardiac monitoring (i.e., single-lead electrocardiogram) possible in the intraoperative magnet, an exercise stress test was obtained on all patients with a cardiac history. If evidence of ischemia was found, then a work up to define and correct the cause of the ischemia was performed. Six months after correction of the cardiac issue, if a stress test was negative for ischemia, then the patient could be reconsidered for MRI-guided prostate brachytherapy.

Medical Management

Patients were started on a selective inhibitor of the α-1a subtype of the α-adrenergic receptors (Tamsulosin) to decrease urethral resistance to urine flow by relaxing the smooth muscle surrounding the urethra. This medication was give by mouth 30 min after supper for 1 wk before treatment using a dose of 0.4 mg and for 1 wk after therapy at a dose of 0.8 mg. Decadron 4 mg by mouth was used 1 d preoperatively and then intravenously intraoperatively and 4 mg by mouth twice daily 1 d postoperatively. This medical intervention was used to limit the edema that can occur within the prostate resulting from its mechanical disruption from source and catheter placement. Concurrent with Decadron use, an H_2-blocker was used for protection of the gastrointestinal mucosa. A prophylactic antibiotic (Ciprofloxacin 500 mg orally every 12 h or Levofloxacin 500 mg orally once a day) was used for 2 d preoperatively, intraoperatively, and then 1 wk postoperatively. Finally, Pyridium at 200 mg by mouth every 8 h was offered for 1 wk after the therapy.

The Magnetic Resonance Therapy Unit

Interstitial prostate radiation was performed using Iodine-125 sources, an MRI-compatible perineal template, a peripheral loading technique, and an intraoperative 0.5 T MRI unit (General Electric Medical Systems, Milwaukee, WI) *(12)*. A standard conventional MRI system consists of a single, long cylindrically shaped magnet with a closed bore and similarly shaped cylindrical imaging coils. This new interventional magnet consists of two shorter cylindrical magnets with imaging coils enclosed. Between these two components, there is a 56-cm gap providing full access to the patient while imaging. Therefore, placement of MRI-compatible (nonferromagnetic) catheters into the perineum can occur simultaneously during patient imaging. Within the center of the 56-cm gap is a 30-cm diameter imaging volume within which the same quality images as obtained in a conventional 0.5 T magnet can be obtained. With the exception of the "open" configuration, the magnet is identical to a conventional unit.

Patient Positioning and Preoperative Imaging

The patient was placed in the lithotomy position and compression stockings and foam-padded boats were used to prevent venous stasis and pressure ulcers. This was followed by the administration of a general anesthetic and neuromuscular blocking agents to prevent motion and a Foley catheter was inserted and clamped. The MRI-compatible template was secured to the MRI table and placed against the patient's perineum. A rectal obturator 3.0 cm in diameter was passed through the template and into the rectum. The rectal obturator was secured to the template using an MRI-compatible screw. Within the central cavity of the rectal obturator was placed a red rubber tube that allowed for the passage of intrarectal gas.

Axial, coronal, and sagittal images were acquired at 5-mm intervals using a MRI pelvic coil in a 0.5 T magnetic field. The images obtained consisted of axial T1-weighted and fast spin echo (FSE) sequences through the prostate. The FSE parameters were TR 5000/TE eff 100, Echo train length 8, field of view 20 × 20 cm, slice thickness 5 mm with a 1-mm interslice gap, and the matrix was 192 with two signal averages. The T1-weighted images had similar fields of view, slice thickness, gap, and matrix;

however, the TR was 500 and TE was 20. FSE images were also obtained in the coronal and sagittal planes.

Preoperative Dosimetry

The peripheral zone (PZ) of the prostate was selected as the clinical target volume (CTV) and was identified and contoured on each axial slice as was the anterior rectal wall and prostatic urethra by an expert MR radiologist as shown in Fig. 1. Based on the CTV and juxtaposed normal tissue volumes, desired minimum peripheral dose, and previously reported normal tissue tolerance (13), a catheter loading was calculated using a previously described dose algorithm (14). The general guidelines for the preplan were to provide approximately a minimum of 150% of the prescription dose to the PZ and higher doses within the MRI-defined tumor within the PZ. The transition zone (TZ) was given approx 100% of the prescription dose. No effort was made to provide full dose to the median lobe when one was present. The goal was to require the maximum dose to any point along the urethra or the anterior rectal wall was kept below reported tolerance doses (13) (400 Gy and 100 Gy, respectively) while dose escalating in the prostate PZ.

Geometric and Dosimetric Feedback

Once the preplan was reviewed and approved by the attending radiation oncologist, source loading would begin followed by placement of each catheter containing the radioactive sources into the designated location on the perineal template and to the predetermined depth. As each catheter was inserted, its position in the coronal, sagittal (Fig. 2), and axial plane was identified in real time and compared with its expected location based on the optimized plan. Adjustments to account for prostate motion, edema, or catheter divergence could be made before source deposition. This process was repeated in an iterative fashion for all planned catheters. The cumulative dose volume histograms for the CTV, anterior rectal wall, and prostatic urethra based on the actual source locations were calculated after each catheter insertion allowing for adjustments intraoperatively if necessary. After all planned sources had been inserted, a review of the dosimetry was performed and additional sources were added to account for regions of inadvertent underdosing that resulted from catheter divergence that could not be corrected intra-operatively. Dose volume histogram analyses were performed intraoperatively in real time for the CTV, anterior rectal wall, and prostatic urethra based on the final source locations. The prescription dose for both implant monotherapy and boost cases were calculated using the recommendations of the American Association of Physicists in Medicine Radiation Therapy Committee Task Force guidelines (15).

Postoperative Instructions

Immediately after the completion of the procedure, our first 100 patients had cystoscopy to assess the integrity of the bladder neck and inspect the bladder lumen for the presence of Iodine-125 seeds. This procedure was discontinued after the first 100 patients because it was determined that the MR guidance system ensured that seed placement into the bladder or urethral lumen was not occurring. The patients were

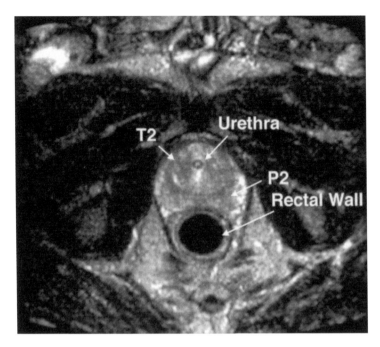

Fig. 1. Axial image through the midgland of the prostate illustrating the prostatic urethra, anterior rectal wall, and PZ and TZ of the prostate gland.

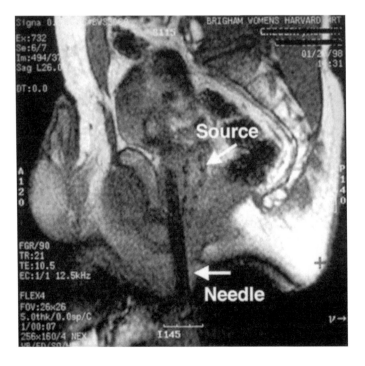

Fig. 2. Real-time intraoperative catheter localization in the sagittal plane. Note that iodine-125 sources from previous catheter insertions can be seen as black voids on the real-time MR images. The catheter appears as black void larger than actual size.

taken to the recovery room and had the Foley catheter removed within 6 to 8 h after extubation. If a voiding trial was unsuccessful, then a Foley catheter was reinserted and the patient was discharged.

All patients were seen 1 wk after the procedure. At that time patients who required reinsertion of the Foley catheter were given a voiding trial. If still unsuccessful then the patient was taught how to perform intermittent self-catheterization and seen weekly in follow up until a successful voiding trial was completed. All patients were instructed to refrain from ejaculation for 1 wk and then to use a condom during sexual intercourse for the first month after the procedure. Although unlikely, this protective measure was used to avoid the inadvertent ejaculation of a radioactive source into the patient's sexual partner. Guidelines used regarding concern about radiation exposure should be based on the growing evidence (Michalski, J., personal communication) that radiation exposure to family members and other close personal contacts is minimal. Therefore, for the first 2 d after the procedure, we asked that children under the age of 13 and pregnant women spend under 30 min within 1 foot of the patient. After 2 d, there were no restrictions.

RESULTS

Dose Volume Histogram Analyses

The percent of the CTV receiving the minimum peripheral dose using the real-time MRI-guided approach in the 184 study patients was 89 to 100% (median 98%). Only two patients (1%) had less than 97% coverage at the end of the procedure. Based on previously described estimate of 400 Gray for urethral tolerance *(13)*, no patient had a point on the urethra exceed tolerance, whereas all patients treated had at least one point on the anterior rectal wall exceed the reported tolerance of 100 Gy. However 28 to 92% (median 64%) of the anterior rectal wall volume remained within the reported dose tolerance of the rectum.

Acute Morbidity

There were no sources found upon inspection of the bladder lumen at the postimplant cystoscopy and only one patient reported passing a source during the first postoperative month. Therefore, postoperative cystoscopy was discontinued after our first 100 patients. Acute urinary retention was noted in 4% of the patients and was related to the volume of the TZ *(16)*. By prostate gland volume, acute urinary retention was noted in 2% (2of 114) , 3% (1of 38), and 34% (10 of 32) patients with prostate gland volume of <45 cm^3, >45 to 60 cm^3, and >60 cm^3, respectively. Minor perineal skin irritation was noted in 15% of patients on postoperative day 1, which resolved in all cases by the first postoperative week. One patient (0.5%) experienced a postoperative urinary tract infection 1 wk after completion of antibiotics that responded to oral antibiotics. Patients returned to work within 1 to 5 d (median 3 d) after the procedure.

Quality of Life

Using the quality-of-life questionnaire developed by Talcott and colleagues *(11)*, a benefit was found to the MRI-guided approach in terms of sexual function and urinary obstructive/irritative symptoms compared with patients treated using TRUS-guided brachytherapy matched for PSA, Gleason score, and clinical T-stage during the same time period. Specifically, there was less urinary frequency, urgency, and leakage after MRI- vs TRUS-guided brachytherapy ($p = 0.06$). There were also more men able to maintain the ability to have an erection after MRI- vs TRUS-guided brachytherapy ($p = 0.02$), although the median age of the MRI (62 yr) vs the TRUS (69 yr) was less. Bowel dysfunction, however, was more common in the MRI- vs TRUS-guided group ($p = 0.01$). This finding is not unexpected given the dose escalating technique up to 150% of prescription dose in the PZ. It is well established that TRUS-guided brachytherapy achieves between 85 to 95% dose coverage of the prostate gland from experienced centers *(3)*, meaning that 5 to 15% of the prostate is not covered to full dose. Perhaps this fact explains the lower rectal injury rate for the TRUS-guided approach.

All 32 cases of radiation induced proctitis, causing rectal bleeding and requiring treatment were documented using colonoscopy ($n = 32$). Rectal bleeding was corrected in all cases either with either cortisone enemas (6 or 32 or 19%) given nightly for 15 min for 3 wk and then every other night in the fourth week or with Argon plasma coagulation delivered endorectally (26 of 32 or 81%). There has been no evidence of rectal injury (i.e., fistula formation or fecal incontinence from damage to the anal sphincter) from either the MRI-guided implant or the Argon plasma coagulation when necessary to treat rectal bleeding. There has been no evidence of urethral stricture or incontinence to date. However 2 and 67% of patients with a prostate gland volume of 60 cm^3 or less vs >60 cm^3, respectively, required the continued use of α-1a blockers to control symptoms related to voiding at 1 yr after the procedure.

Predictive Factors

At a median follow up of 32 (3–64) mo, there have been six PSA failures The definition of PSA failure used was three consecutive increases where each value is separated by 3 mo to help reduce confounding resulting from the PSA bounce phenomenon. Using a Cox regression time to PSA failure analysis *(17)* evaluating the PSA level (>4–10 ng/mL vs 4 ng/mL or less), biopsy Gleason score (3 + 4 vs 3 + 3 or less), and percent positive biopsies (50% or more vs <50%), for predicting time to posttreatment PSA failure. Only the percent positive biopsies of 50% or more approached significance ($p = 0.07$). This finding is similar to what has been noted in a similar patients managed using RP *(19)* or external beam RT *(19)*.

PSA Outcome

The actuarial estimates of PSA failure-free survival (PSA outcome) at 4 yr after prostate brachytherapy were 97% and 84% ($p = 0.07$) as noted in Fig. 3 for patients treated with implant only and with <50% vs 50% or more positive prostate biopsies, respectively. Low-risk patients managed with external beam RT and implant who also had either >50% positive biopsies or a PSA >10 to 13 ng/mL or MRI evidence of extracapsular extension at the apex or midgland had an estimate of 4-yr PSA outcome of 100%. This result was significantly higher (100 vs 84%; $p = 0.03$) than low-risk patients with 50% or greater positive biopsies treated by implant alone as shown in Fig. 4. However as illustrated in Fig. 5, this difference in 4-yr PSA outcome was not significantly different (100 vs 97%; $p = 0.47$) when compared with low-risk patients with

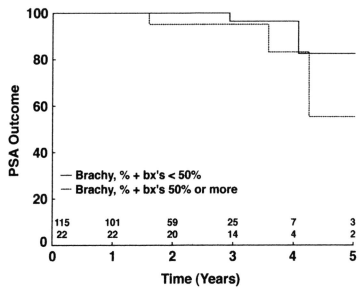

Fig. 3. Estimates of prostate specific antigen failure-free survival (PSA outcome) after full-dose MRI-guided prostate brachytherapy stratified by the percent positive prostate biopsies. Log rank $p = 0.07$.

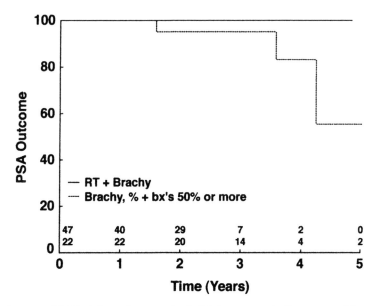

Fig. 4. Estimates of PSA failure-free survival (PSA outcome) after external beam radiation therapy (RT + Brachy) and an MRI-guided prostate brachytherapy boost or full-dose MRI-guided prostate brachytherapy in patients with 50% or more positive biopsies (Brach, % + bx 50% or more). Log rank $p = 0.03$.

<50% positive biopsies treated with implant monotherapy. These results suggest that the addition of external beam RT for low-risk patients with >50% positive biopsies or a PSA >10 to 13 ng/mL or MRI evidence of extracapsular extension at the apex or base

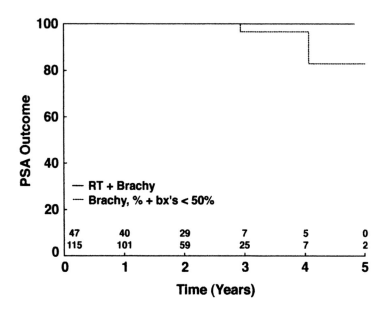

Fig. 5. Estimates of PSA failure-free survival (PSA outcome) after external beam radiation therapy (RT + Brachy) and an MRI-guided prostate brachytherapy boost or full-dose MRI-guided prostate brachytherapy in patients with less than 50% positive biopsies (Brach, % + bx < 50%). Log rank $p = 0.47$.

may be necessary to achieve the best outcome. Longer follow-up will be needed to assess the durability of these results in this select patient cohort.

CONCLUSION

A real-time MRI-guided technique has been developed for the placement of permanent Iodine-125 sources into the prostate gland. This technique used a real-time interactive dosimetry algorithm and was nearly always able to achieve a minimum of 97% coverage of the PZ of the prostate gland while simultaneously respecting the tolerance dose to the prostatic urethra and most of the anterior rectal wall. Urinary morbidity and erectile dysfunction using this technique were significantly less by patient report than that using a TRUS-guided technique. Although rectal toxicity was higher when compared with TRUS-guided placement, all rectal bleeding was correctable. The percent positive biopsies of 50% or greater was predictive of PSA outcome for patients treated using implant monotherapy and is now used as an exclusion criteria. Low-risk patients with this finding are now offered treatment with external beam RT and implant. Although 4-yr results of PSA outcome are excellent, longer follow-up will be needed to assess the durability of these results in this select patient cohort.

REFERENCES

1. Jemal A, Thomas A, Murray T, Thum M. Cancer statistics 2002. *CA Cancer J Clin* 2002;52:23–47.
2. Ragde H, Blasko JC, Grimm PD, et al. (1997) Interstitial iodine-125 radiation without adjuvant therapy in the treatment of clinically localized prostate carcinoma. *Cancer* 1997;80:442–453.

3. Bice WS Jr, Prestidge BR, Grimm PD, et al. (1998) Centralized multiinstitutional postimplant analysis for interstitial prostate brachytherapy. *Int J Radiat Oncol Biol Phys* 1998;41:921–927.

4. D'Amico AV, Cormack R, Tempany CM, et al. (1998) Real time magnetic resonance image guided interstitial brachytherapy in the treatment of select patients with clinically localized prostate cancer. *Int J Radiat Oncol Biol Phys* 1998;42:507–516.

5. Ragde H, Korb LJ, Elgamal AA, Grado GL, Nadir BS. Modern prostate brachytherapy. Prostate specific antigen results in 219 patients with up to 12 years of observed follow up. *Cancer* 2000;89:135–141.

6. *Cancer, Manual for Staging Cancer*, 4th edition. Philadelphia, JP Lippincott, 1997.

7. Gleason DF and the Veterans Administration Cooperative Urological Research Group. Histologic grading and staging of prostatic carcinoma, in *Urologic Pathology* (Tannenbaum M, ed.). Philadelphia, Lea & Febiger; 1977; pp. 171–187.

8. D'Amico AV, Whittington R, Malkowicz SBK, et al. Endorectal magnetic resonance imaging as a predictor of biochemical outcome following radical prostatectomy for men with clinically localized prostate cancer. *J Urol* 2000;164:759–763.

9. D'Amico AV, Cormack RA, Tempany CM. MRI-guided diagnosis and treatment of prostate cancer. *N Engl J Med* 2001;344:776–777.

10. Lee AK, Schultz D, Renshaw AA, Richie JP, D'Amico AV. Optimizing patient selection for prostate monotherapy. *Int J Radiat Oncol Biol Phys* 2001;49:673–677.

11. Talcott JA, Reiker P, Propert KJ, et al. Patient reported impotence and incontinence after nerve-sparing radical prostatectomy. *J Natl Cancer Inst* 1997;89:1117–1123.

12. Jolesz FA. Image-guided procedures and the operating room of the future. *Radiology* 1997;204:601–612.

13. Wallner K, Roy J, Harrison L. Dosimetry guidelines to minimize urethral and rectal morbidity following transperineal I-125 prostate brachytherapy. *Int J Radiat Oncol Biol Phys* 1995;32:465–471.

14. Cormack RA, Tempany CM, D'Amico AV. A clinical method for real-time dosimetric guidance of transperineal I-125 prostate implant using IMRI imaging. *Int J Radiat Oncol Biol Phys* 2000;46:210–217.

15. Nath R, Anderson LL, Luxton G, Weaver K, Williamson JF, Meigooni AS. Dosimetry of interstitial brachytherapy sources: recommendations of the AAPM Radiation Therapy Committee Task Group No. 43. *Med Phys* 1995;22:209–234.

16. Thomas MD, Cormack R, Tempany CM, et al. Identifying the predictors of acute urinary retention following magnetic-resonance image guided prostate brachytherapy. *Int J Radiat Oncol Biol Phys* 2000;47:905–908.

17. Simultaneous inferences and other topics in regression analysis-1, in *Applied Linear Regression models*, 1st ed (Neter J, Wasserman W, and Kutner M, eds.) Homewood, IL: Richard D. Irwin, Inc., 1983; pp. 150–153.

18. D'Amico AV, Whittington R, Malkowicz SB, et al. The clinical utility of the percent of positive prostate biopsies in defining biochemical outcome following radical prostatectomy for patients with clinically localized prostate cancer. *J Clin Oncol* 2000;18:1164–1172.

19. D'Amico AV, Schultz D, Silver B, et al. The clinical utility of the percent of positive prostate biopsies in predicting biochemical outcome following external beam radiation therapy for patients with clinically localized prostate cancer. *Int J Radiat Oncol Biol Phys* 2001;49:679–684.

8

Magnetic Resonance Imaging-Guided Neurosurgery

Hooman Azmi, MD and Michael Schulder, MD

INTRODUCTION

The advent of magnetic resonance imaging (MRI) has had a tremendous impact on medicine and specifically on the field of neurosurgery. Diagnosis of lesions within the central nervous system (CNS), which not so long ago was dependent on such invasive techniques as pneumoencephalography, cerebral angiography, and gas cisternography, has been revolutionized by MRI. MRI provides superb anatomic resolution, the ability to view the lesion in various planes, and the vast capability to localize functional cortex, map white matter tracts, ascertain tissue composition, and to define vascular anatomy. It has supplemented neurosurgical diagnosis and has enhanced the treatment of neoplastic diseases of the CNS. The goal of neurosurgical treatment of neoplastic disease is optimal resection with preservation of essential and viable tissue that may be adjacent to the lesion. MRI has had a tremendous impact toward this end. MRI as we know it today is the culmination of the independent efforts of numerous individuals and later on several commercial interests. Raymond Damadian is credited with the development of the first MRI machine. The notion of using nuclear magnetic resonance (NMR) to differentiate cancerous and noncancerous tissue had been an exciting topic in the late 1960s, and in 1971 Damadian, a physician at the State University of New York at Brooklyn, published an article in *Science* entitled "Tumor Detection by Nuclear Magnetic Resonance" *(1)*. He had been able to detect T1 relaxation times in rats with and without various tumors and had demonstrated a prolonged relaxation time in the rats with tumors.

The possibility of creating images from NMR data was an enticing idea, and both Damadian and Paul Lauterbur had been envisioning it. Lauterbur, a chemist at the State University of New York at Stony Brook, working independently of Damadian, succeeded in producing the first magnetic resonance image. He used capillary tubes filled with water and with deuterium and was able to produce crude but recognizable images using NMR. His work was published in *Nature* in 1973 *(2)*.

Meanwhile in Brooklyn, Damadian, with technical assistance from the Brookhaven National Laboratories and private funds, was working tirelessly on a prototype MR machine large enough to accommodate human subjects (Fig. 1). In July 1977, despite all his critics, he succeeded in creating the first MR image of a human. It was a crude

From: *Image-Guided Diagnosis and Treatment of Cancer*
Edited by: A. D'Amico, J. S. Loeffler, and J. R. Harris © Humana Press Inc., Totowa, NJ

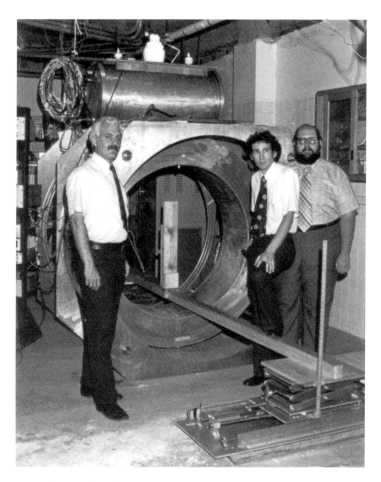

Fig. 1. Drs. Damadian, Minkoff, and Goldsmith and the completed MR scanner Indomitable (property of FONAR Corporation, Dr. Damadian).

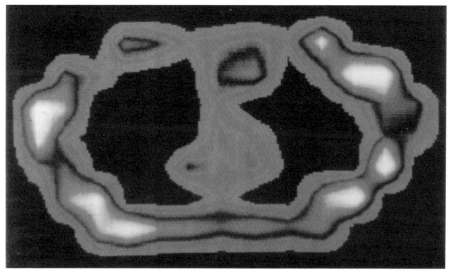

Fig. 2. First MR scan of a live human body. A live cross section of a human chest at the level of the eighth thoracic vertebrae (property of FONAR Corporation, Dr. Damadian).

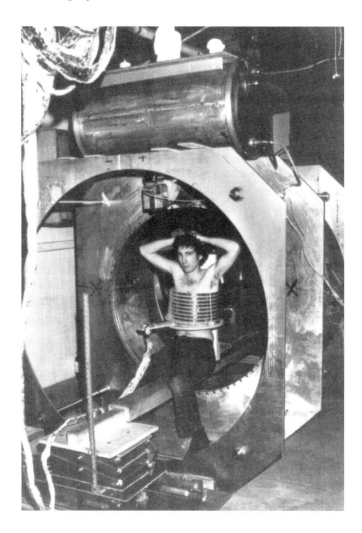

Fig. 3. Larry Minkoff, Damadian's assistant, sitting in the MR scanner for the first scan of the human body (property of FONAR Corporation, Dr. Damadian).

image of the cross section of a chest (Fig. 2). After several attempts with Damadian as the subject, it was determined that his chest diameter was too large for the antenna vest, and one of his assistants volunteered to be used for imaging (Fig. 3). His body was moved along in the magnet through 106 slightly different positions over almost 5 h to produce the rough image *(3)*.

This remarkable breakthrough was followed by many advances in MR technology through the efforts of several institutions and individuals in the United States and in Europe. Richard Ernst and Weston Anderson, both NMR physicists at a private corporation in Palo Alto, California, developed the pulsed Fourier transform technique to enhance the production and quality of images. Ernst later improved on the method developing a two-dimensional Fourier transform method, which was further improved by William Edelstein, a physicist at Aberdeen in the United Kingdom. He called this the spin-warp method *(4)*.

The production of commercial MR units was gaining momentum as the decade of the 1970s was coming to an end. Damadian had left SUNY and had set up the FONAR (Field fOcused Nuclear mAgnetic Resonance) Corporation to develop commercial MR units *(3)*. General Electric (GE) Medical Systems, having recently profited from the new computed tomography (CT) technology and sales, was able to direct resources into the development of magnetic resonance imaging as well.

In 1980, William Edelstein and Paul Bottomley, another NMR physicist, together joined the GE company in Milwaukee. Their efforts at GE culminated in the production of a 1.5 T unit capable of producing high-quality images, and their work was presented at the Radiological Society of North America in 1982. Instrumental to their success was a coil design used in the system termed the "birdcage" coil *(5)*. Both in Europe and the United States, several other companies were also making strides in the advancement of this technology.

The explosion in MRI technology quite remarkably occurred over a relatively short period. It was in 1977 when the first crude image was painstakingly produced in a basement laboratory in New York with essentially homemade material. Just over a decade later, in 1988, Ronald Reagan at the end of his presidency presented the National Medal of Technology to Damadian and Lauterbur for "independent contributions in conceiving and developing the application of magnetic resonance technology to medical uses, including whole body scanning and diagnostic imaging" *(3)*. In just a short few years, MRI had been propelled to the forefront of medicine and had taken its permanent position in the standards of imaging.

IMAGING OF CNS TUMORS

MRI has become the modality of choice for imaging of the CNS. It provides superior tissue contrast, allowing for visualization of lesions in the brain or the spinal cord. It is capable of aiding in the delineation of lesions and their relationship to the surrounding brain structures by providing views in multiple planes. MR also allows imaging of vasculature, not only permitting diagnosis of vascular lesions, but also making it an invaluable tool in the assessment of tumors *(6)*. In addition, the absence of artifacts caused by bone makes it especially useful for imaging the cranial base *(7–10)*. The absence of ionizing radiation, and the type of contrast medium used for MRI make this technique safer than CT.

MR has proven especially useful in the diagnosis of neoplasms. It allows the detection of virtually all kinds of brain tumors, whether primary, metastatic, intra, or extraaxial *(6)*. The breakdown of the blood–brain barrier results in contrast enhancement that distinguishes tumor from edema. In cases of low-grade gliomas where the blood–brain barrier may remain more intact, enhancement is minimal and MR becomes indispensable in diagnosis because of the superior image resolution it offers compared with CT. MR is also better at detecting features associated with tumors such as edema, increased vascularity, or necrosis *(6)*.

The absence of bony artifact makes MR essential for diagnosis of skull base tumors *(11)*, and those of the posterior fossa. Cerebellar tumors and those of the cerebellopontine angle are clearly visualized using MRI *(12)*. Gas cisternograms, not long ago the mainstay of diagnosis for small acoustic neuromas and tumors of the

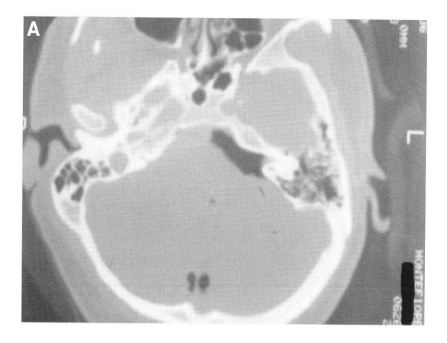

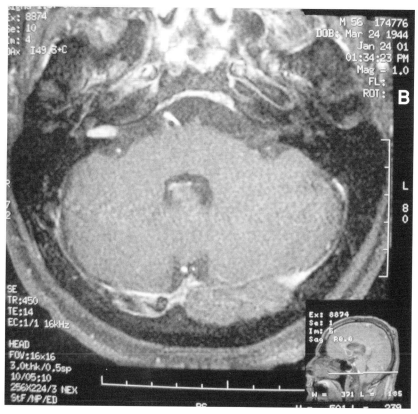

Fig. 4. (A) CT cisternogram obtained after injection of air into the lumbar cistern. **(B)** T1-weighted contrast MR of posterior fossa showing small right-sided enhancing mass.

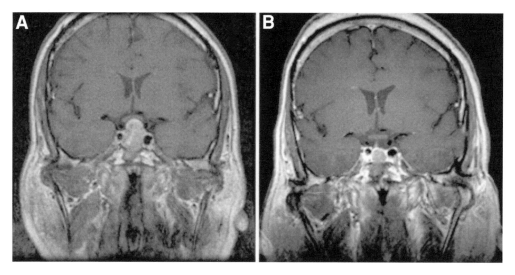

Fig. 5. (A) Preoperative coronal T1-weighted contrast image of optic chiasm pushed up by pituitary mass. **(B)** Postoperative coronal T1-weighted image obtained on a 3 T scanner showing decompression of the optic chiasm.

cerebellopontine angle *(13–16)*, have clearly been replaced by the safer and more specific MR (Fig. 4).

In the assessment of tumors of the suprasellar region as well, MR is also clearly superior. MRI is by far the most efficient technique to establish the diagnosis and evaluate an expansive suprasellar lesion. Its delineation of the origin of the lesion, and the relationship of the lesion to the third ventricle, the optic chiasm and suprasellar vascular structures make it important for the diagnosis and evaluation of primary tumors with extensions into the sella, meningiomas in this region, and craniopharyngiomas (Fig. 5) *(17,18)*.

Outside of the brain, the evaluation of the CNS for tumors has also greatly benefited from MRI. About 20% of CNS tumors occur in the spine *(19,20)*. Spinal cord tumors are best visualized by this imaging modality (Fig. 6) *(21)*. The evaluation of the cord for compression or for edema, the evaluation of the neural foramina for nerve root compromise, the extension into disk space, and the destruction of the vertebral bodies can all be seen with MRI. For most patients, MRI of the spine has obviated the need for CT myelography *(22)*. Not only is it less risky than myelography for assessment of the spine *(23)*, but it is also less likely to miss a tandem lesion and is able to provide more information on the nature of the lesion. For the same reasons, MR has also overtaken radioisotope bone scans in detection of spine tumors. In addition, it is more specific than bone scan in the detection of bone metastases *(24,25)*.

The unique ability to exploit the chemical and paramagnetic quality of tissues, combined with the ability to mathematically manipulate information acquired during imaging, have been essential in the development of the vast diagnostic potential of MRI. Many sequences and protocols have been devised to allow differentiation of specific tissue characteristics, visualization of specific structures, and delineation of task spe-

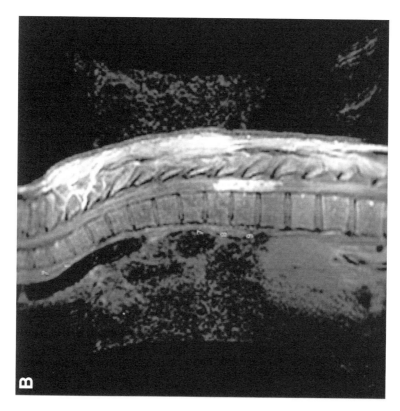

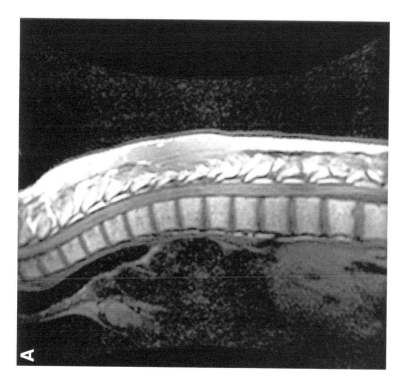

Fig. 6. (**A**) Precontrast T1-weighted image of thoracic spine. (**B**) Postcontrast image showing thoracic cord lesion.

cific functional cortex. Magnetic resonance angiography (MRA), diffusion-weighted MRI, magnetic resonance spectroscopy (MRS), and functional MRI (fMRI) are examples of such applications. The following sections are brief descriptions of these diagnostic modalities.

MAGNETIC RESONANCE ANGIOGRAPHY (MRA)

The diagnosis of brain tumors in the past relied greatly on the recognition of the displacement of vascular structures within the cranium *(26–30)*. With the advent of computer-assisted imaging technology, namely CT and MR, the identification of brain lesions has become safer, easier, and more accurate. The identification of vascular structures, however, still remains an important part of the evaluation and the pretreatment planning of tumors. The relationship of the lesion to surrounding vascular structures and especially the identification of feeding vessels for vascular tumors has important treatment implications.

Since the early 1990s, MRI has been used to demonstrate the cerebral vasculature *(31,32)*. Many sequences have been developed for the assessment of vessels *(33–37)*. There are two broad classes of techniques for MRA. The first, time-of-flight techniques, consists of methods that use the motion of the blood relative to the surrounding tissue, exploiting the difference in signal saturation that exists between flowing blood and stationary tissue. MR methods have also been developed that encode motion into the acquired signal. These form the second class of MRA techniques known as phase-contrast studies *(38)*. In general, all these sequences take advantage of the macroscopic motion of blood to distinguish vessels from surrounding brain *(39,40)*, and the vascular contrast is generated by the difference in saturation between the inflowing spins of the blood and the stationary spins of the tissues in the imaged section *(41)*. Slow moving blood, such as the blood in peripheral arteries, makes visualization of such arteries difficult. This can be overcome by use of contrast agents during the acquisition of the MRAs *(39,42)*.

The relationship of brain lesions to the surrounding vasculature can be depicted using MRA (Fig. 7) *(43–47)*. It may also be possible to demonstrate tumor feeding vessels in some instances *(46)*, as has been shown with AVMs *(48)*.

Using workstations, a cine mode display of the MRA's hemodynamic information could also be obtained *(46)*. The occlusion or encasement of vessels and the demonstration of vessels pushed away by the tumor all have surgical relevance and can be depicted by MRA. In addition, the involvement of dural sinuses *(46)* and their patency can be assessed by this technique *(49–52)*. MRA also provides a safer method for assessment of vasculature as intra-arterial angiography has some inherent and well-known risks *(53)*. In short, MRI is a noninvasive adjunct to the diagnosis and preoperative planning of lesions in the CNS. It helps define vascular anatomy and may assist in the differential diagnosis of tumors *(54,55)*. Moreover, it enhances preoperative planning for neurosurgical procedures by defining the relationship of the lesion to the tumor and the degree of vascular involvement. Further work is needed to compare the sensitivity and specificity of MRI in defining the relationship of tumors and vasculature with the current gold standard, intra-arterial digital subtraction angiography.

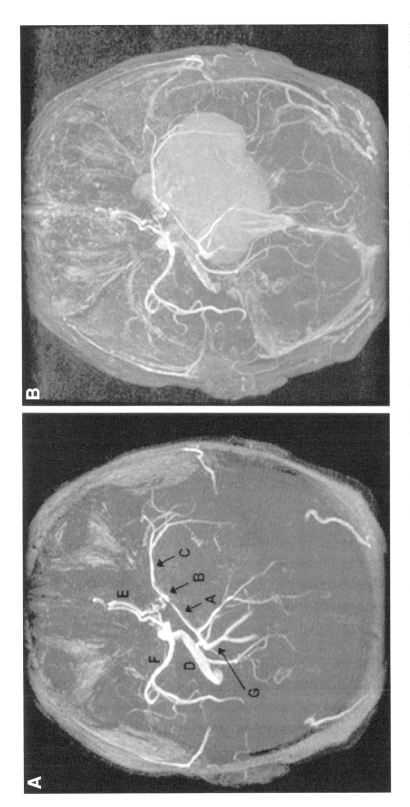

Fig. 7. (**A**) MRA of head showing displacement of vasculature. A: Posterior communicating artery. B: Internal carotid bifurcation. C: Middle cerebral artery. D: Contralateral posterior communicating artery. E: A2s. F: Contralateral middle cerebral artery. G: Basilar artery. (**B**) MRA of same patient with enhancing mass visible.

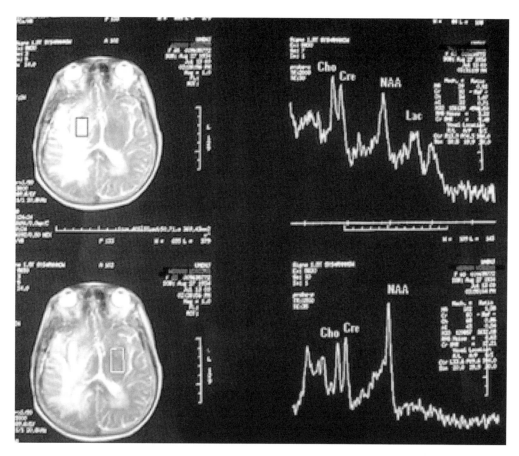

Fig. 8. Top panel, MRS of section including tumor showing elevated levels of choline. Bottom panel, MRS non-neoplastic tissue in same patient showing normal spectroscopic pattern of metabolites.

MAGNETIC RESONANCE SPECTROSCOPY (MRS)

Although tissue diagnosis is the gold standard of diagnosis for neoplastic lesions and is unlikely to be replaced in the near future, successful efforts have been aimed at providing the most accurate noninvasive diagnosis techniques. MRS has been such an endeavor. MRS has allowed the noninvasive evaluation of metabolic patterns in brain tumors *(56–61)*, permitting the differentiation of tumors from normal brain tissue or other intracranial lesions by their unique metabolic "fingerprints."

Metabolites, such as choline, produce a characteristic nuclear magnetic spectrum. It is believed that tissues with high metabolic rates, such as neoplastic lesions, produce these metabolites in a proportion that is higher than that of non-neoplastic brain. Several studies have postulated that elevated choline may reflect an increase in the concentration of the spectroscopically detectable metabolites that are precursors of membrane phospholipids needed to support the increased cell turnover in neoplastic lesions *(62,63)*. Using MRS, this difference can be used to discriminate between cancerous and noncancerous tissue (Fig. 8) *(57,63,64)*.

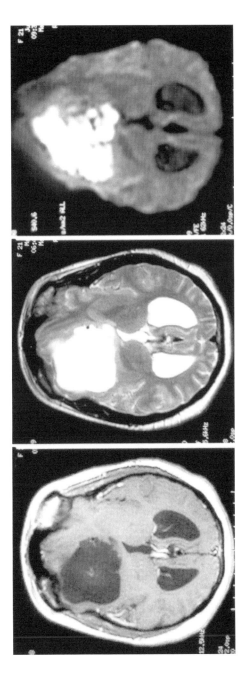

Fig. 9. *From left to right:* T1-weighted image of frontal lesion. T2-weighted image of frontal lesion with lesion showing same signal as cerebrospinal fluid. Diffusion-weighted image of same lesion showing different signal than cerebrospinal fluid.

Furthermore, some studies have suggested that in addition to helping differentiate neoplastic and non-neoplastic lesions, MRS may also be able to assist in the preoperative grading of these lesions. Histological data from a variety of brain tumors have been compared with MRS findings showing that histologically similar tumors exhibit the same spectral pattern *(65)*, allowing preoperative tumor grading *(66–68)*. The ratio of lactate to water and that of choline to water has been shown to differentiate between GBMs, high-grade astrocytomas, and low-grade astrocytomas *(66)*. In addition, low-grade tumors may be distinguished from high grades as well using this technique.

Thus, MRS could be an effective tool in the planning and treatment of CNS lesions. By identifying the most suspect part of a lesion, MRS could aid in selection of a target for stereotactic biopsy and help to reduce sampling error. It can also serve to plan a surgical resection by delineating neoplastic tissue. Another important potential application is the assessment of residual disease after surgery, especially for low-grade gliomas or nonenhancing components of high-grade tumors, assisting to monitor disease progression and to tailor further treatment. Serial monitoring could also be used to assess tumor response to radiation or chemotherapy *(69,70)* and to differentiate tumor recurrence from radiation necrosis.

DIFFUSION-WEIGHTED MRI

The advent of diffusion-weighted MRI has provided an additional instrument in the differentiation of certain space-occupying lesions in the brain. Many intracranial lesions, including some neoplasms, abscesses, and parasitic diseases, may present mainly as cystic or necrotic lesions, and the correct radiologic diagnosis of these lesions is often difficult. Using the translational motion of water, it may be possible to discern these various lesions. Brain abscesses may be distinguished from cystic or necrotic neoplasms *(71,72)*, and epidermoid tumors may be differentiated from arachnoid cysts using this technique (Fig. 9) *(73)*. There may also be some evidence that suggests gliomas may be differentiated from other cystic neoplastic lesions using diffusion-weighted magnetic resonance *(74)*.

In addition to helping in the differentiation of lesions, diffusion-weighted imaging can permit the visualization of fiber bundles in the brain, allowing the study of the course of white matter tracts in vivo *(75)*. The physical phenomenon called diffusion results from the random thermal translational motion of molecules. Diffusion imaging incorporates magnetic field gradients into a standard MR sequence to obtain images that are sensitive to the small displacements of water molecules *(76)*. The diffusion of water is restricted in the cell membranes of cerebral tissue, occurring easily along the direction of fibers but prohibited from crossing them *(77)*. Diffusion-weighted imaging uses this quality to identify a particular fiber tract in the brain (Fig. 10). The identification of these tracts is of great clinical importance in neurosurgery.

Although matter tract fibers can be visualized both in their normal state and in cases where they have been displaced or infiltrated by neoplastic processes *(78)*, diffusion-weighted MRI allows the mapping of large white matter tracts, such as the corticospinal tract *(75,79)*, and the optic radiations. This technique can help reduce the risk of postoperative neurologic deficits by determining the course and integrity of white matter tracts *(80)* preoperatively and providing information indicating the safe border of resection in cases of lesions close to these fibers *(81)*.

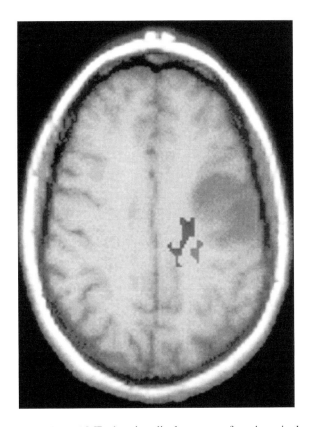

Fig. 10. Axial diffusion-weighted MR showing displacement of corticospinal tracts by the lesion.

FUNCTIONAL MRI (fMRI)

Safe surgical resection of brain tumors near the eloquent areas requires appreciation of eloquent areas of the brain. The introduction of fMRI has brought new perspectives to the study and definition of functional patterns of the human brain *(82–86)*. This technique uses oxygenation levels of blood as a contrast agent. The blood–oxygen level-dependent contrast technique depends on the shifts between concentrations of deoxyhemoglobin and oxyhemoglobin in microvascular networks of the cortex. Oxygenated blood has almost the same magnetic properties as the surrounding tissues. However, deoxygenated hemoglobin molecules are paramagnetic, which means they have a permanent magnetic dipole that partially aligns in the direction of a magnetic field *(87)*. Task performance results in a regional increased blood flow and a decrease in the ratio of deoxyhemoglobin to oxyhemoglobin as the cerebral blood flow increases more than the metabolic oxygen need. This in turn causes an increased signal on T2-weighted imaging sequences *(88)*. The signal change per sequence is on the order of 1 to 3%, hence repeated acquisitions and offline statistical analysis are needed to provide meaningful data. By imaging patients as they repeat specific tasks, this change in signal is amplified and the activated cortex is delineated (Fig. 11).

Using fMRI, it has been possible to noninvasively demonstrate the motor, sensory, and the visual cortices *(85,89–91)*, as well as other eloquent areas of the brain. This information has been used for preoperative planning *(85,92–94)* and intraoperative

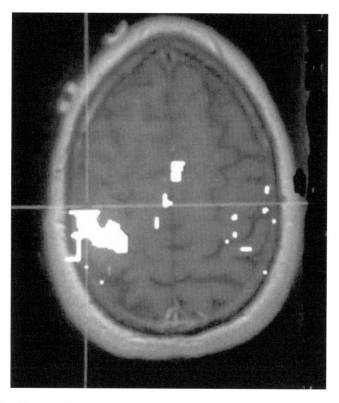

Fig. 11. Functional MR image identifying the motor cortex on the right.

image guidance *(95,96)*. Functional MRI data have been shown to correlate well with intraoperative cortical stimulation *(86,97–99)*, which is the accepted gold standard for identification of eloquent cortex *(100)*. It also offers the advantage of allowing preoperative planning, which is not possible with cortical stimulation. Furthermore, intraoperative cortical stimulation or SSEP may be limited because of the use of muscle relaxation or deep anesthesia *(96)*.

There are also other functional neuroimaging techniques, such as positron emission tomography *(101–103)*, magnetoencephalography *(104–108)*, and angiography with amobarbital infusion (Wada test). Functional MRI has certain advantages over these techniques. Spatial resolution is better than positron emission tomography (PET) *(109)*. In addition, neurosurgeons will most likely have better access to an MR imager than PET or magnetoencephalography devices. An additional advantage of fMRI compared with PET is that the functional and reference anatomic images are acquired simultaneously *(87)*. And, of course, it is completely noninvasive, unlike the Wada test.

Functional MRI does have its limitations, however: It is an indirect indicator of cerebral activation because it measures changes in regional cerebral blood flow and not neuronal activity itself, as is done by magnetoencephalography *(91)*. Thus, the ability of the blood–oxygen-level-dependent contrast technique to localize neuronal activity depends on the anatomic proximity of these vessels to the activated cortex *(109)*. In addition, subcortical functional pathways are not easily identified with this technique

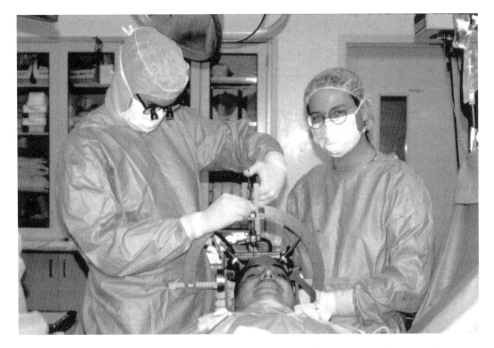

Fig. 12. Example of a frame placed on a patient for a stereotactic procedure.

(110). Changes in blood oxygenation may be affected by dispersions in time and space that cause errors in the accurate localization of activated areas *(111)*.

Despite these limitations, fMRI has provided neurosurgeons with an invaluable tool. To preserve neurologic function controlled by the brain tissue directly adjacent to or involved by the tumor, it is important to be able to identify the anatomic location of this eloquent cortex *(112)*. fMRI mapping has allowed the preoperative identification of sensory, motor, and visual cortices. In addition language mapping and even mapping of memory are afforded by fMRI. As intraoperative guidance systems become more sophisticated, as intraoperative MRI becomes more prevalent in neurosurgical suites, and as more studies validate fMRI data to the accepted standards, this MR modality will prove an integral part of neurosurgical planning and treatment.

IMAGE-GUIDED NEUROSURGERY

The accurate localization and targeting of lesions in the brain has been pursued by neurosurgeons since the 19th century. In 1908, Victor Horsely and Robert Clarke described the use of a stereotactic apparatus in animals *(113)*, and the first stereotactic device designed for human patients was described in 1947 by Spiegel and Wycis *(114)*. Frames and stereotaxis in general were developed for functional neurosurgery. It was not until later, however, that the development of computers, and thus of imaging modalities, provided the technology for major advances in stereotactic neurosurgery and its applicability to tumor surgery.

Currently stereotactic systems include both frame-based and frameless devices, which incorporate preoperatively acquired images to establish a three-dimensional map

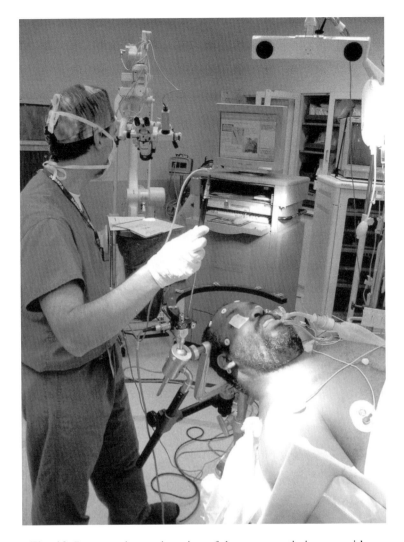

Fig. 13. Preoperative registration of the stereotactic image guidance system.

to guide interventions. Frame-based systems, such as the Brown–Roberts–Wells, *(115,116)* Cosman–Roberts–Wells *(117)*, and Leksell systems *(118)* use externally applied stereotactic frames attached to the patient, with interlocking arcs to generate a coordinate system, and to establish the fiducials for navigation (Fig. 12).

Stereotactic frames register individual points in space. Initially they were used for functional stereotaxy and, with the advent of CT, for biopsies. Modifications were made allowing rotation of the arcs away from the surgical field, which made stereotactic craniotomies possible *(115,119,120)*. But clearly frames had disadvantages. Even though they had proven accurate, they were cumbersome and intruded into the surgical field when used for craniotomies; in addition, they were not designed to provide much feedback to the surgeon *(121)*. Other disadvantages associated with the use of stereotactic head frames include patient discomfort at the time of frame placement, the length of time required to perform the procedure, and the fact that the procedure is performed "blindly" as the needle is passed through the brain toward the target *(122)*.

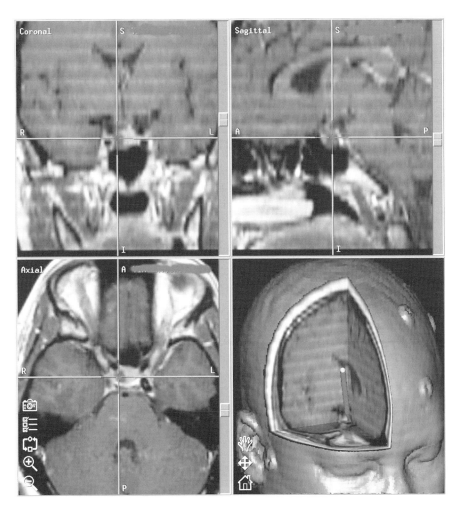

Fig. 14. Intraoperative use of the image guidance system during transsphenoidal resection of a pituitary microadenoma, with cross hairs showing the navigation probe to be just inside the tumor.

Frameless stereotactic devices were developed in the past decade to overcome these obstacles. By obviating the need for frames, these systems have allowed better access to the cranial vault. They have expanded the types of operations that can be performed stereotactically and greatly increased the ability to provide interactive guidance and feed back to the neurosurgeon (123–126). These systems most commonly use anatomic landmarks or markers attached to the scalp as fiducials, which can be identified on preoperative images. The image guidance station then performs a three-dimensional transformation to register the images and the physical space using the markers that have been incorporated into the images. The computer-interfaced optical, electromagnetic, or ultrasound sensors (or alternatively with a mechanical arm) then track the position of surgical instruments relative to the patient's anatomy allowing stereotactic access to the cranial vault and the brain (Figs. 13 and 14) (127–130).

Frameless stereotaxy has allowed a volumetric representation of the lesions as opposed to point stereotaxis and also has permitted an increase in the accuracy and safety of procedures. The constant awareness of vascular and eloquent brain areas also contributes to safer surgical procedures *(131,132)* as does the attention to bony structures associated with the course of cranial nerves *(133)*. Because of the ability to image soft tissue at the skull base and import crucial information, such as fMRI, MRI is the ideal dataset for image-guided navigation.

Image-guided systems are subject to some inaccuracies. These arise from the movement of the fiducials, errors in registration, and errors related to imaging. Inaccuracies as large as 8 mm have been documented *(134,135)*. The major shortcoming of image guided neurosurgery, however, is its dependence on preoperative images. This may render the navigation system inaccurate because it cannot provide a dynamic verification as the surgery proceeds, and the lesion and its surrounding brain tissue change in conformation. These changes, better known as brain shift, can alter stereotactic targets within the cranial vault *(136–138)*.

Brain shift may result from loss of cerebrospinal fluid, brain edema, insinuation of air in the subdural space, and changes in the anatomic lesion after surgical decompression or drainage. It can result in positional changes for both normal neural structures and tumor masses. These spatial changes are also influenced by histological features and sizes of tumors, their locations, patient positioning, the placement of craniotomies, and the use of osmodiuretic agents *(139)*. The brain can settle within the cranial vault and, as tumor resection progresses, can shift in proportion with the degree of resection. As surgery continues, stereotactic targets established on the basis of preoperatively obtained scans become less reliable *(137)*. Shifts of greater than 5 mm have been reported in the literature *(136,140–142)* explaining the limited usefulness of neuronavigation for the assessment of the completeness of tumor resection. This also emphasizes the need of an intraoperative imaging technique to correct for these distortions *(143)*, as only serial imaging or continuous data acquisition can provide consistently accurate image guidance *(144)*.

INTRAOPERATIVE MRI

To date, intraoperative imaging is the only possible approach to obtain information not only on the shifting of the brain surface but also on the deformation of structures beneath the surface, which is much more clinically relevant *(139)*. Intraoperative imaging is not a new concept to neurosurgical procedures. Radiography and fluoroscopy have long been used for imaging during surgeries. However, they provide only two-dimensional information, with no cross-sectional data on brain tissue. Ultrasonography, however, provides real-time three-dimensional information but is useful primarily for cystic lesions, cannot accurately reveal lesions less than 5 mm in size, and cannot adequately define tumor margins *(145)*. Intraoperative CT, introduced by Lunsford and co-workers *(146,147)* in the 1980s, improved tissue resolution compared with ultrasound but provides only uniplanar imaging and may subject the patient and the surgical team to significant radiation exposure *(148)*.

The ability of MRI to provide multiplanar imaging with high resolution of structures *(149)*, in addition to avoiding ionizing radiation team makes this imaging modality desirable for intraoperative imaging in neurosurgical procedures. Intraoperative MRI guidance offers several advantages over other stereotactic image guidance systems. As

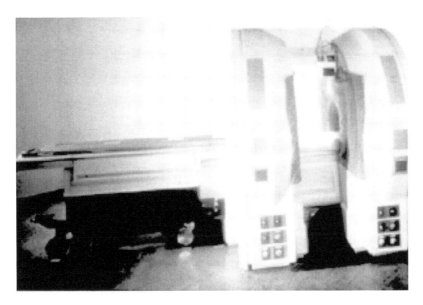

Fig. 15. The GE system. Reprinted with permission from Lippincot Williams and Wilkins.

brain shift occurs, intraoperative MRI allows localization using images that are updated in a dynamic fashion. This has major implications for the ability to obtain accurate biopsies of multiple sites or resections of small and/or deep lesions, in defining the margins of resection, and in identifying the position of normal anatomic structures. Like frameless stereotaxy, intraoperative MRI allows precise preoperative plotting of surgical approaches but with the added benefit of dynamic guidance and verification of the surgical results of the chosen approach. Intraoperative MRI can also help with identification of normal structures, including blood vessels encountered in the surgical field and the relationship of these to the lesion. It also allows surveillance of complications, such as hemorrhage *(150)*. Total removal of all enhancing tumor is made more feasible with intraoperative MRI, improving patient outcome and survival *(96,151–153)*.

There are several intraoperative systems currently in use today. Some have been designed solely as surgical tools, whereas others are diagnostic systems adapted for the operating room (OR). They differ also in their acquisition costs; some systems demand the construction of an entire dedicated operating suite whereas others may require some adaptation of available facilities. Magnetic field strengths are also variable, with some systems permitting acquisition of other MR modalities, such as MRAs and functional MRIs. As experience is gained in the use and applications of intraoperative MR, each design may find a particular niche.

Beginning in 1990, GE and the group of investigators at the Brigham and Women's Hospital *(154,155)* designed a medium field (0.5 T) intraoperative MRI system (Fig. 15). The GE system uses two vertically oriented superconducting magnets in separate but communicating cryostats, with a vertical gap between the coils to permit direct patient access during image acquisition. This system allows for real-time imaging of the patient during surgery because the patient does not have to be moved for imaging *(145)*. The disadvantage of this scanner design is that it requires a dedicated OR and instruments,

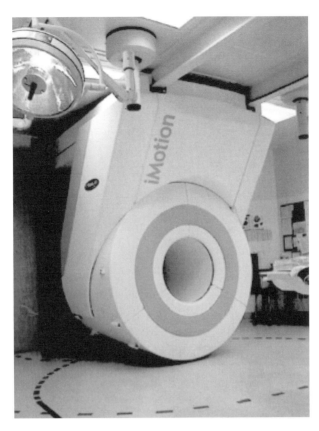

Fig. 16. The Brain lab system at University of Calgary. Reprinted with permission from Lippincot Williams and Wilkins.

and increasing the costs incurred to acquire this technology. The 56-cm gap between magnets also limits surgical access.

Siemens *(156)* and investigators in Germany *(157)* have designed an alternative approach, the Magnetom OPEN scanner. This system utilizes a 0.2-T open configuration magnet installed in a "twin operating theatre." Surgery is performed in a conventional OR, and the patient is moved into the MR unit for imaging. This system allows access to the patient outside the scanner, which provides more room for surgeons than the GE system, and permits the use of non-MR-compatible instruments, helping to reduce costs *(148)*. The disadvantage of this design is the requirement to move the patient intraoperatively for imaging, which incurs potential risks to the patient, and increases operative time. In addition there is a limitation on the use of real time navigation during craniotomies *(145)*.

In contrast with the low-field MRI therapy suites, high-field systems offer complete imaging capabilities, albeit with more limited patient access during scanning. The enhanced imaging capabilities associated with interventional MRI units may provide clear clinical benefits by reducing morbidity or mortality rates. However, this advantage must also be considered in terms of cost *(158)*.

Surgeons at the University of Minnesota have developed a high-field 1.5-T MR scanner in collaboration with Phillips Medical Systems *(158,159)*. This system is integrated

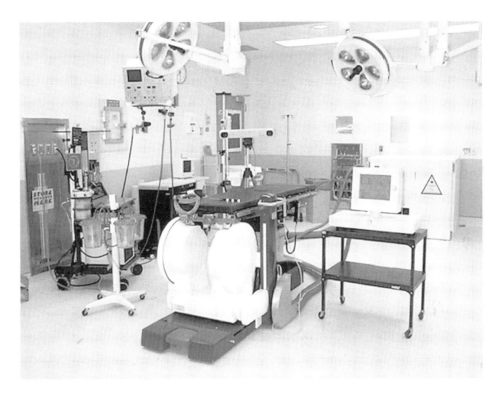

Fig. 17. The PoleStar unit docked under the operating room table in a conventional OR.

into a fully equipped neurosurgical suite. A specially adapted operating table can be attached to the MR system by a docking mechanism that transports the patient along a track for imaging. Surgery may be performed either in or outside of the 5-Gauss line allowing for non-MR instrument use. Biopsies and functional MRI may be performed in the MR unit, but craniotomies require movement in and out of the unit to accommodate standard surgical instrumentation *(145)*. Another high-field unit has been developed by scientists and physicians in Calgary. This mobile ceiling mounted intraoperative MRI system allows the magnet to be moved into and out of the OR using an overhead track (Fig. 16). It allows the use of standard neurosurgical instruments, and the high-field magnet permits better image quality and the possibility to apply other MR modalities such as diffusion, MRA, and fMRI intraoperatively. In addition, elecrophysiological studies are feasible because the magnet can be removed from the operative field *(160,161)*. An important disadvantage of this system are the cost incurred in the installation of the system into a dedicated OR suite.

A unique intraoperative MR system has been developed more recently in conjunction with neurosurgeons in Tel Aviv *(162)*. The PoleStar system is designed as a mobile, compact MR system that can be used in any OR with some updating.

The scanner is made of two vertical parallel, disk-shaped magnets located 25 cm from each other. The magnets are attached together with the gradients and the radiofrequency transmitter coil to a U-shaped arm, which may be displaced in several directions. The arm itself is mounted on a transportable base that can be positioned under a regular OR table (Fig. 17). For scanning, the arm is raised so that the magnets are adjacent to the patient's head, which is held by a specially designed head holder. The opening between the magnets allows enough room for the surgeon to work when the system is in scan position. The system can also be lowered, using a remote control device, to any point and even if required stowed under the OR table. The system is designed so the magnets will remain draped under a sterile field and the magnets can be raised again to the exact former position.

The magnetic field of 0.12 T decays to 0.5 G at a distance of 1.5 m from the magnet isocenter. Therefore, non-MR-compatible instruments can be used when the magnets are lowered, and the system can be installed in a conventional OR with radiofrequency shielding. This shielding can be achieved in a conventional OR by constructing a Faraday cage encompassing the room, using a conductive metal mesh such as copper on the walls. To avoid interference with the images, copper shielding should be used to seal all room openings, including doors, light and power inlets.

The system generates images with a 16-cm × 13-cm field of view, enabling visualization of the lesion and the surrounding areas (Fig. 18). All standard image modes, such as T1-weighted, T2-weighted, and fluid attenuated inversion recovery contrast imaging, are supported by the scanner. Image acquisition, including selection of scan protocol and image orientation, is controlled by the surgeon. Navigation can be performed using images acquired at any time during the operation using an infrared emitting camera and reflective spheres on a wand (similar to the technology in many frameless stereotactic systems) *(163)*.

The low magnetic field allows non-MR-compatible equipment to be used in the OR, including conventional OR tables and microscopes. When the magnets are stowed under the OR table, the magnetic field in the area of the patients head is negligible allowing use of regular instruments, such as standard drills, bipolars, and electrophysiologic recorders. The advantage of this system is that it achieves MRI with maximal surgical access and minimal disruption of the conventional OR. The modular design of the scanner may also permit transport between operating theaters without necessitating dedicated, MR-compatible, shielded operating space, thereby reducing the costs of implementing MRI capabilities.

By helping the surgeon determine the extent of tumor resection, intraoperative MRI may permit safer and more accurate procedures *(158)*. In operations where direct visualization of the tumor and its surrounding are limited due to the approach, such as in transsphenoidal surgery, intraoperative imaging allows real-time assessment of the extent of resection, and of residual disease. Indeed, intraoperative MRI has had a major impact on pituitary surgery *(164)*. In cases of gliomas improved resection is made possible with intaoperative MRI. Intraoperative MRI facilitates greater resection of gliomas by constantly updating the surgeon regarding residual disease and residual enhancement. Even though gliomas may not be cured by complete resection, evidence suggests greater resection may improve survival *(95,96,151–153,165–171)* and that high-grade recurrence may be decreased in patients in whom complete resection has been accomplished *(172)*.

The incorporation of other MR modalities, such as functional MR, diffusion, MRS, and MRA will further promote the role of intraoperative MRI in tumor neurosurgery by providing ever more valuable data to discriminate between tumor and surrounding normal brain tissue. In short, intraoperative MR drastically reduces the guesswork in intracranial tumor surgery.

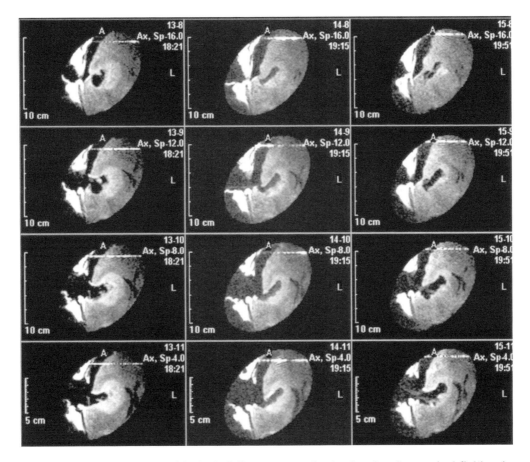

Fig. 18. Images obtained with the PoleStar scanner clearly showing the surgical field and the enhancing lesion.

STEREOTACTIC RADIOSURGERY

A discussion about MRI-guided neurosurgery would be incomplete without considering stereotactic radiosurgery. This technique was first described by Lars Leksell in 1951 *(173)*. Leksell coupled an orthovoltage dental X-ray tube to his first generation stereotactic guiding device to irradiate the gasserian ganglion as a treatment for tic douloureux *(174)*. In subsequent years commercial radiosurgery units using linear accelerators or radiation sources were developed. The indications for radiosurgery have been expanded to include treatment for arteriovenous malformations, vestibular schwannomas, meningiomas, other benign brain tumors, malignant lesions, and even functional procedures.

The essential principle behind the different units is the same. Using a stereotactic frame, a lesion is delineated in a defined three-dimensional space, and a single treatment of focused ionizing radiation is applied to that lesion. It is self-evident that because the surgeon has no direct view of the lesion, he or she relies on the accuracy of the obtained images for directing adequate energy on the lesion to destroy it and to avoid surrounding healthy neuronal tissue. MRI is considered to be the best neurodiagnostic tool for targeting of lesions because of its high resolution and excellent tissue contrast *(173–177)*.

MRI can be used either as the primary imaging modality *(178–180)* where the stereotactic image is obtained using magnetic resonance, or it can be used to supplement a stereotactic CT by fusion *(179,181,182)*. Excellent spatial resolution on MRI facilitates radiosurgical dose planning using either technique.

The use of MRI-based dose planning has decreased the complication rates of radiosurgery. Reduction in facial and trigeminal neuropathies after treatment for vestibular schwannomas, and better preservation of hearing is attributed to the use of better imaging afforded by magnetic resonance *(183,184)*. Indeed Lunsford et al. *(185)*, in a series of 404 patients with vestibular schwannomas treated with radiosurgery, reported a decreased incidence of delayed facial and trigeminal neuropathy (from 28 to 8% and from 34 to 8%, respectively), with preservation of hearing increasing from 39 to 68%, with the use of MRI planning.

MRI-based radiosurgery planning also permits the incorporation of functional data into the planning process *(186,187)* helping to avoid damage to eloquent cortex. Functional data could be co-registered with the stereotactic images providing an additional margin of safety in the radiosurgical treatment of intracranial lesions. Finally, the superior tissue resolution of MR makes it invaluable for serial monitoring after radiosurgery for assessment of the radiobiological effects of radiosurgery and the regression or recurrence of the lesion *(188)*.

CONCLUSION

In the short time since its inception, MR has revolutionized the diagnosis and treatment of intracranial tumors. In just over 20 yr since the first MRI of the human chest was painstakingly obtained in a basement laboratory in Brooklyn, the first intraoperative MRs of the human brain were being obtained in Boston. MR has given us the ability to visualize functionally active cortex and white matter tracts. It has provided us with the capability to noninvasively identify neoplastic tissue, and has allowed us to visualize cerebral vasculature in relation to tumors. All this without the risks of invasive procedures and ionizing radiation.

The incorporation of this imaging technology into the operating room has been a remarkable achievement in the fight against brain tumors. The major goal of surgical treatment, to achieve as complete a resection as possible without causing damage to normal brain tissue, can be facilitated using MRI. Intraoperative imaging with MR allows for specific localization of tumors, delineation of their borders and identification of any residual tumor, all in real time. Contemporary neurosurgery would be unimaginable without the regular use of MRI.

REFERENCES

1. Damadian R. Tumor detection by nuclear magnetic resonance. *Science* 1971;171,1151–1153.
2. Lauterbur PC. Image formation by induced local interaction: examples employing nuclear magnetic resonance. *Nature* 1973;242:190–191.
3. Mattson J, Simon M. (1996) *The Story of MRI: Pioneers of NMR and Magnetic Resonance in Medicine* Jericho, NY, Dean Books, 1996.

4. Edelstein WA, Hutchinson JMS, Johnson G, Redpath T. Spin warp NMR imaging and applications to human whole-body imaging. *Phys Med Biol* 1980;25:751–756.

5. Schenck JF, Foster TH, Henkes JL, et al. High-field surface-coil MR imaging of localized anatomy. *Am J Neuroradiol* 1985;6:181–186.

6. Edelman RR, Warach S. Magnetic resonance imaging (1). *N Engl J Med* 1993;328:708–716.

7. Weber AL. Imaging of the skull base. *Eur J Radiol* 1996;22:68–81.

8. Han JS, Huss RG, Benson JE, et al. MR imaging of the skull base. *J Comput Assist Tomogr* 1984;8:944–952.

9. Meyers SP, Hirsch WL Jr, Curtin HD, Barnes L, Sekhar LN, Sen C. Chordomas of the skull base: MR features. *AJNR Am J Neuroradiol* 1992;13:1627–1636.

10. Meyers SP, Hirsch WL, Jr., Curtin HD, Barnes L, Sekhar LN, Sen C. Chondrosarcomas of the skull base: MR imaging features. *Radiology* 1992;184:103–108.

11. Yoshizumi K, Korogi Y, Sugahara T, et al. Skull base tumors: evaluation with contrast-enhanced MP-RAGE sequence. *Comput Med Imaging Graph* 2001;25:23–31.

12. Jackler RK, Shapiro MS, Dillon WP, Pitts L, Lanser MJ. Gadolinium-DTPA enhanced magnetic resonance imaging in acoustic neuroma diagnosis and management. *Otolaryngol Head Neck Surg* 1990;102:670–677.

13. Oliver TW Jr, Braun IF, Hoffman JC Jr. Gas computed tomographic cisternography: evaluation of small and intracanalicular acoustic neuromas. *J Comput Tomogr* 1984;8:187–190.

14. Solti-Bohman LG, Magaram DL, Lo WW, et al. Gas-CT cisternography for detection of small acoustic nerve tumors. *Radiology* 1984;150:403–407.

15. Pinto RS, Kricheff II, Bergeron RT, Cohen N. Small acoustic neuromas: detection by high resolution gas CT cisternography. *Am J Roentgenol* 1982;139:129–132.

16. Sortland O. Computed tomography combined with gas cisternography for the diagnosis of expanding lesions in the cerebellopontine angle. *Neuroradiology* 1979;18:19–22.

17. Dietemann JL, Cromero C, Tajahmady T, et al. CT and MRI of suprasellar lesions. *J Neuroradiol* 1992;19:1–22.

18. Kucharczyk W, Montanera WJ. The sella and parasellar region, in *Magnetic Resonance Imaging of the Brain and Spine* (Atlas SW, ed.). New York, Raven Press, 1991; pp. 625–627.

19. Osborn AG. *Diagnostic Neuroradiology*. St. Louis, Mosby, 1994.

20. Masaryk TJ. Neoplastic disease of the spine. *Radiol Clin North Am* 1991;29:829–845.

21. Williams MP, Cherryman GR, Husband JE. Magnetic resonance imaging in suspected metastatic spinal cord compression. *Clin Radiol* 1989;40:286–290.

22. Quencer RM. Spine imaging. *AJNR Am J Neuroradiol* 2000;21:2–8.

23. Hollis PH, Malis LI, Zappulla RA. Neurological deterioration after lumbar puncture below complete spinal subarachnoid block. *J Neurosurg* 1986;64:253–256.

24. Frank JA, Ling A, Patronas NJ, et al. Detection of malignant bone tumors: MR imaging vs scintigraphy. *AJR Am J Roentgenol* 1990;155:1043–1048.

25. Gosfield E, III, Alavi A, Kneeland B. Comparison of radionuclide bone scans and magnetic resonance imaging in detecting spinal metastases. *J Nucl Med* 1993;34:2191–2198.

26. Galligioni F, Bernardi R, Mingrino S. Anatomic variation of the height of the falx cerebri. its relationship to displacement of the anterior cerebral artery in frontal space-occupying lesions. *Am J Roentgenol Radium Ther Nucl Med* 1969;106:273–278.

27. Goree JA, Dukes HT. The angiographic differential diagnosis between the vascularized malignant glioma and the intracranial arteriovenous malformation. *Am J Roentgenol* 1963;90:512–521.

28. Blatt ES, McLaurin RL. The arteriographic pattern accompanying centrosylvian mass lesions. *Am J Roentgenol Radium Ther Nucl Med* 1967;101:52–60.

29. Kricheff I. I.Taveras JM. The angiographic diagnosis of suprasylvian space-occupying lesions. *Am J Roentgenol* 1964;82:602–614.

30. Leeds NE, Goldberg HI. Abnormal vascular patterns in benign intracranial lesions: pseudotumors of the brain. *Am J Roentgenol Radium Ther Nucl Med* 118:576–585.

31. Edelman RR, Mattle HP, Atkinson DJ, Hoogewoud HM. MR angiography. *AJR Am J Roentgenol* 1990;154:937–946.

32. el Gammal T, Brooks BS. Conventional MR neuroangiography. *AJR Am J Roentgenol* 1991;156:1075–1080.

33. Dumoulin CL, Cline HE, Souza SP, Wagle WA, Walker MF. Three-dimensional time-of-flight magnetic resonance angiography using spin saturation. *Magn Reson Med* 1989;11:35–46.

34. Dumoulin CL, Souza SP, Walker MF, Wagle W. Three-dimensional phase contrast angiography. *Magn Reson Med* 1989;9:139–149.

35. Pernicone JR, Siebert JE, Potchen EJ, Pera A, Dumoulin CL, Souza SP. Three-dimensional phase-contrast MR angiography in the head and neck: preliminary report. *AJNR Am J Neuroradiol* 1990;11:457–466.

36. Blatter DD, Parker DL, Ahn SS, et al. Cerebral MR angiography with multiple overlapping thin slab acquisition. Part II. Early clinical experience. *Radiology* 1992;183:379–389.

37. Lewin JS. , Laub G. Intracranial MR angiography: a direct comparison of three time-of-flight techniques. *AJNR Am J Neuroradiol* 1991;12:1133–1139.

38. Frayne R, Grist TM, Korosec FR, et al. MR angiography with three-dimensional MR digital subtraction angiography. *Top Magn Reson Imaging* 1996;8:366–388.

39. Marchal G, Michiels J, Bosmans H, Van Hecke P. Contrast-enhanced MRA of the brain. *J Comput Assist Tomogr* 1992;16:25–29.

40. Bosmans H, Wilms G, Marchal G, Demaerel P, Baert AL. Characterisation of intracranial aneurysms with MR angiography. *Neuroradiology* 1995;37:262–266.

41. Laub G. A. Kaiser WA. MR angiography with gradient motion refocusing. *J Comput Assist Tomogr* 1988;12:377–382.

42. Creasy JL, Price RR, Presbrey T, Goins D, Partain CL, Kessler RM. Gadolinium-enhanced MR angiography. *Radiology* 1990;175:280–283.

43. Kadota T, Kuriyama K, Inoue E, Fujita M, Nakagawa H, Kuroda C. MR angiography of meningioma. *Magn Reson Imaging* 1993;11:473–483.

44. Kadota T, Nakagawa H, Kuroda C. Malignant glioma. Evaluation with 3D time-of-flight MR angiography. *Acta Radiol* 1998;39:227–232.

45. Yanaka K, Shirai S, Shibata Y, Kamezaki T, Matsumura A, Nose T. Gadolinium-enhanced magnetic resonance angiography in the planning of supratentorial glioma surgery. *Neurol Med Chir (Tokyo)* 1993;33:439–443.

46. Yoshikawa T, Aoki S, Hori M, Nambu A, Kumagai H, Araki T. Time-resolved two-dimensional thick-slice magnetic resonance digital subtraction angiography in assessing brain tumors. *Eur Radiol* 2000;10:736–744.

47. Wilms G, Bosmans H, Marchal G, et al. Magnetic resonance angiography of supratentorial tumours: comparison with selective digital subtraction angiography. *Neuroradiology* 1995;37:42–47.

48. Tanaka H, Numaguchi Y, Konno S, Shrier DA, Shibata DK, Patel U. Initial experience with helical CT and 3D reconstruction in therapeutic planning of cerebral AVMs: comparison with 3D time-of-flight MRA and digital subtraction angiography. *J Comput Assist Tomogr* 1997;21:811–817.

49. Wang AM. Intracranial venous magnetic resonance angiography, In: Cerebrovascular Disease: Imaging and Interventional Treatment Options *(Rumbaugh CL, Wang AM, Tsai FY, eds.), New York: Igaku-Shoin pp. 346–356.*

50. Ayanzen RH, Bird CR, Keller PJ, McCully FJ, Theobald MR, Heiserman JE. Cerebral MR venography: normal anatomy and potential diagnostic pitfalls. *AJNR Am J Neuroradiol* 2000;21:74–78.

51. Rippe DJ, Boyko OB, Spritzer CE, et al. Demonstration of dural sinus occlusion by the use of MR angiography. *AJNR Am J Neuroradiol* 1990;11:199–201.

52. Liang L, Korogi Y, Sugahara T, et al. Evaluation of the intracranial dural sinuses with a 3D

contrast-enhanced MP-RAGE sequence: prospective comparison with 2D-TOF MR venography and digital subtraction angiography. *AJNR Am J Neuroradiol* 2001;22:481–492.

53. Heiserman JE, Dean BL, Hodak JA, et al. Neurologic complications of cerebral angiography. *AJNR Am J Neuroradiol* 1994;15:1401–1407;discussion 1408–1411.

54. Bullock PR, Mansfield P, Gowland P, Worthington BS, Firth JL. Dynamic imaging of contrast enhancement in brain tumors. *Magn Reson Med* 1991;19:293–298.

55. Ikushima I, Korogi Y, Kuratsu J, et al. Dynamic MRI of meningiomas and schwannomas: is differential diagnosis possible? *Neuroradiology* 1997;39:633–638.

56. Tedeschi G, Lundbom N, Raman R, et al. Increased choline signal coinciding with malignant degeneration of cerebral gliomas: a serial proton magnetic resonance spectroscopy imaging study. *J Neurosurg* 1997;87:516–24.

57. Rand SD, Prost R, Haughton V, et al. Accuracy of single-voxel proton MR spectroscopy in distinguishing neoplastic from nonneoplastic brain lesions. *AJNR Am J Neuroradiol* 1997;18:1695–1704.

58. Sijens PE, Knopp MV, Brunetti A, et al. 1H MR spectroscopy in patients with metastatic brain tumors: a multicenter study. *Magn Reson Med* 1995;33:818–826.

59. Poptani H, Gupta RK, Roy R, Pandey R, Jain VK, Chhabra DK. Characterization of intracranial mass lesions with in vivo proton MR spectroscopy. *AJNR Am J Neuroradiol* 1995;16:1593–1603.

60. Ott D, Hennig J, Ernst T. Human brain tumors: assessment with in vivo proton MR spectroscopy. *Radiology* 1993;186:745–752.

61. Fulham MJ, Bizzi A, Dietz MJ, et al. Mapping of brain tumor metabolites with proton MR spectroscopic imaging: clinical relevance. *Radiology* 1992;185:675–686.

62. Segebarth CM, Baleriaux DF, Luyten PR, den Hollander JA. Detection of metabolic heterogeneity of human intracranial tumors in vivo by 1H NMR spectroscopic imaging. *Magn Reson Med* 1990;13:62–76.

63. Negendank WG, Sauter R, Brown TR, et al. Proton magnetic resonance spectroscopy in patients with glial tumors: a multicenter study. *J Neurosurg* 1996;84:449–458.

64. Preul MC, Caramanos Z, Collins DL, et al. Accurate, noninvasive diagnosis of human brain tumors by using proton magnetic resonance spectroscopy. *Nat Med* 1996;2:323–325.

65. Bruhn H, Frahm J, Gyngell ML, et al. Noninvasive differentiation of tumors with use of localized H-1 MR spectroscopy in vivo: initial experience in patients with cerebral tumors. *Radiology* 1989;172:541–548.

66. Meyerand ME, Pipas JM, Mamourian A, Tosteson TD, Dunn JF. Classification of biopsy-confirmed brain tumors using single-voxel MR spectroscopy. *AJNR Am J Neuroradiol* 1999;20:117–1123.

67. Shimizu H, Kumabe T, Tominaga T, et al. Noninvasive evaluation of malignancy of brain tumors with proton MR spectroscopy. *AJNR Am J Neuroradiol* 1996;17:737–747.

68. Dowling C, Bollen AW, Noworolski SM, et al. Preoperative proton MR spectroscopic imaging of brain tumors: correlation with histopathologic analysis of resection specimens. *AJNR Am J Neuroradiol* 2001;22:604–612.

69. Croteau D, Scarpace L, Hearshen D, et al. Correlation between magnetic resonance spectroscopy imaging and image-guided biopsies: semiquantitative and qualitative histopathological analyses of patients with untreated glioma. *Neurosurgery* 2001;49:823–829.

70. Castillo M. Neuroimaging and cartography: mapping brain tumors. *AJNR Am J Neuroradiol* 2001;22:597–598.

71. Kim YJ, Chang KH, Song IC, et al. Brain abscess and necrotic or cystic brain tumor: discrimination with signal intensity on diffusion-weighted MR imaging. *AJR Am J Roentgenol* 1998;171:1487–1490.

72. Noguchi K, Watanabe N, Nagayoshi T, et al. Role of diffusion-weighted echo-planar MRI in distinguishing between brain brain abscess and tumour: a preliminary report. *Neuroradiology* 1999;41:171–174.

73. Tsuruda JS, Chew WM, Moseley ME, Norman D. Diffusion-weighted MR imaging of the brain: value of differentiating between extraaxial cysts and epidermoid tumors. *AJR Am J Roentgenol* 1990;155:1059–1065;discussion 1066–1068.
74. Park SH, Chang KH, Song IC, Kim YJ, Kim SH, Han MH. Diffusion-weighted MRI in cystic or necrotic intracranial lesions. *Neuroradiology* 2000;42:716–721.
75. Krings T, Coenen VA, Axer H, et al. In vivo 3D visualization of normal pyramidal tracts in human subjects using diffusion weighted magnetic resonance imaging and a neuronavigation system. *Neurosci Lett* 2001;307:192–196.
76. Eriksson SH, Rugg-Gunn FJ, Symms MR, Barker GJ, Duncan JS. Diffusion tensor imaging in patients with epilepsy and malformations of cortical development. *Brain* 2001;124:617–626.
77. Coenen VA, Krings T, Mayfrank L, et al. Three-dimensional visualization of the pyramidal tract in a neuronavigation system during brain tumor surgery: first experiences and technical note. *Neurosurgery* 2001;49:86–92;discussion 92–93.
78. Peled S, Gudbjartsson H, Westin CF, Kikinis R, Jolesz FA. Magnetic resonance imaging shows orientation and asymmetry of white matter fiber tracts. *Brain Res.* 1998;780:27–33.
79. Holodny AI, Ollenschleger MD, Liu WC, Schulder M, Kalnin AJ. Identification of the corticospinal tracts achieved using blood-oxygen-level-dependent and diffusion functional MR imaging in patients with brain tumors. *AJNR Am J Neuroradiol* 2001;22:83–88.
80. Mamata Y, Mamata H, Nabavi A, et al. Intraoperative diffusion imaging on a 0.5 Tesla interventional scanner. *J Magn Reson Imaging* 2001;13:115–9.
81. Inoue T, Shimizu H, Yoshimoto T. Imaging the pyramidal tract in patients with brain tumors. *Clin Neurol Neurosurg* 1999;101:4–10.
82. Bandettini PA, Jesmanowicz A, Wong EC, Hyde JS. Processing strategies for time-course data sets in functional MRI of the human brain. *Magn Reson Med* 1993;30:161–173.
83. Belliveau JW, Kennedy DN, Jr., McKinstry RC, et al. Functional mapping of the human visual cortex by magnetic resonance imaging. *Science* 1991;254:716–719.
84. Kim SG, Ashe J, Hendrich K, et al. Functional magnetic resonance imaging of motor cortex: hemispheric asymmetry and handedness. *Science* 1993;261:615–617.
85. Mueller WM, Yetkin FZ, Hammeke TA, et al. Functional magnetic resonance imaging mapping of the motor cortex in patients with cerebral tumors. *Neurosurgery* 1996;39:515–520;discussion 520–521.
86. Yetkin FZ, Mueller WM, Morris GL, et al. Functional MR activation correlated with intraoperative cortical mapping. *AJNR Am J Neuroradiol* 1997;18:1311–1315.
87. Castelijns JA, Lycklama a Nijeholt GJ, Mukherji SK. Functional MRI: background and clinical applications. *Semin Ultrasound CT MR* 2000;21:428–433.
88. Ogawa S, Menon RS, Tank DW, et al. Functional brain mapping by blood oxygenation level-dependent contrast magnetic resonance imaging. A comparison of signal characteristics with a biophysical model. *Biophys J* 1993;64:803–812.
89. Engel SA, Rumelhart DE, Wandell BA, et al. fMRI of human visual cortex. *Nature* 1994;369:525.
90. Kwong KK, Belliveau JW, Chesler DA, et al. Dynamic magnetic resonance imaging of human brain activity during primary sensory stimulation. *Proc Natl Acad Sci USA* 1992;89:5675–5679.
91. Ogawa S, Tank DW, Menon R, et al. Intrinsic signal changes accompanying sensory stimulation: functional brain mapping with magnetic resonance imaging. *Proc Natl Acad Sci USA* 1992;89:5951–5955.
92. Cosgrove GR, Buchbinder BR, Jiang H. Functional magnetic resonance imaging for intracranial navigation. *Neurosurg Clin North Am* 1996;7:313–322.
93. Gallen CC, Sobel DF, Waltz T, et al. Noninvasive presurgical neuromagnetic mapping of somatosensory cortex. *Neurosurgery* 1993;33:260–268;discussion 268.

94. Pujol J, Conesa G, Deus J, Lopez-Obarrio L, Isamat F, Capdevila A. Clinical application of functional magnetic resonance imaging in presurgical identification of the central sulcus. *J Neurosurg* 1998;88:863–869.

95. Maldjian JA, Schulder M, Liu WC, et al. Intraoperative functional MRI using a real-time neurosurgical navigation system. *J Comput Assist Tomogr* 1997;21:910–912.

96. Schulder M, Maldjian JA, Liu WC, et al. Functional image-guided surgery of intracranial tumors located in or near the sensorimotor cortex. *J Neurosurg* 1998;89:412–418.

97. Puce A, Constable RT, Luby ML, et al. Functional magnetic resonance imaging of sensory and motor cortex: comparison with electrophysiological localization. *J Neurosurg* 1995;83:262–270.

98. Yousry TA, Schmid UD, Jassoy AG, et al. Topography of the cortical motor hand area: prospective study with functional MR imaging and direct motor mapping at surgery. *Radiology* 1995;195:23–29.

99. Jack CR, Jr., Thompson RM, Butts RK, et al. Sensory motor cortex: correlation of presurgical mapping with functional MR imaging and invasive cortical mapping. *Radiology* 1994;190:85–92.

100. Berger MS. , Ojemann GA. Techniques of functional localization during removal of tumors involving cerebral hemispheres, in *Intraoperative Monitoring Techniques in Neurosurgery* (Loftus CM, Traynelis VC, eds.), New York, McGraw-Hill, 1994; pp. 113–127.

101. Fried I, Nenov VI, Ojemann SG, Woods RP. Functional MR and PET imaging of rolandic and visual cortices for neurosurgical planning. *J Neurosurg* 1995;83:854–861.

102. Boling W, Olivier A, Bittar RG, Reutens D. Localization of hand motor activation in Broca's pli de passage moyen. *J Neurosurg* 1999;91:903–910.

103. Bittar RG, Olivier A, Sadikot AF, et al. Localization of somatosensory function by using positron emission tomography scanning: a comparison with intraoperative cortical stimulation. *J Neurosurg* 1999;90:478–483.

104. Rezai AR, Hund M, Kronberg E, et al. The interactive use of magnetoencephalography in stereotactic image-guided neurosurgery. *Neurosurgery* 1996;39:92–102.

105. Baumann SB, Noll DC, Kondziolka DS, et al. Comparison of functional magnetic resonance imaging with positron emission tomography and magnetoencephalography to identify the motor cortex in a patient with an arteriovenous malformation. *J Image Guid Surg* 1995;1:191–197.

106. George JS, Aine CJ, Mosher JC, et al. Mapping function in the human brain with magnetoencephalography, anatomical magnetic resonance imaging, and functional magnetic resonance imaging. *J Clin Neurophysiol* 1995;12:406–431.

107. Ganslandt O, Fahlbusch R, Nimsky C, et al. Functional neuronavigation with magnetoencephalography: outcome in 50 patients with lesions around the motor cortex. *J Neurosurg* 1999;91:73–79.

108. Nakasato N, Seki K, Kawamura T, et al. Cortical mapping using an MRI-linked whole head MEG system and presurgical decision making. *Electroencephalogr Clin Neurophysiol Suppl* 1996;47:333–341.

109. Fandino J, Kollias SS, Wieser HG, Valavanis A, Yonekawa Y. Intraoperative validation of functional magnetic resonance imaging and cortical reorganization patterns in patients with brain tumors involving the primary motor cortex. *J Neurosurg* 1999;91:238–250.

110. Dillon WP, Roberts T. The limitations of functional MR imaging: a caveat. *AJNR Am J Neuroradiol* 1999;20:536.

111. Yousry TA, Schmid UD, Schmidt D, Hagen T, Jassoy A, Reiser MF. The central sulcal vein: a landmark for identification of the central sulcus using functional magnetic resonance imaging. *J Neurosurg* 1996;85:608–617.

112. Holodny AI, Schulder M, Liu WC, Wolko J, Maldjian JA, Kalnin AJ. The effect of brain tumors on BOLD functional MR imaging activation in the adjacent motor cortex: implications for image-guided neurosurgery. *AJNR Am J Neuroradiol* 2000;21:1415–2422.

113. Horsley V. , Clarke RH. The structure and function of the cerebellum examined by new method. *Brain* 1908;31:45–124.

114. Spiegel EA, T. WH, Marks M, Lee AJ. Stereotaxic apparatus for operations on the human brain. *Science* 1947;106:349–350.

115. Brown RA. A computerized tomography-computer graphics approach to stereotaxic localization. *J Neurosurg* 1979;50:715–720.

116. Heilbrun MP, Roberts TS, Apuzzo ML, Wells TH, Jr., Sabshin JK. Preliminary experience with Brown-Roberts-Wells (BRW) computerized tomography stereotaxic guidance system. *J Neurosurg* 1983;59:217–222.

117. Couldwell WT. , Apuzzo ML. Initial experience related to the use of the Cosman-Roberts-Wells stereotactic instrument. Technical note. *J Neurosurg* 1990;72:145–148.

118. Leksell L. Stereotactic radiosurgery. *J Neurol Neurosurg Psychiatry* 1983;46:797–803.

119. Apuzzo M. LSabshin JK. Computed tomographic guidance stereotaxis in the management of intracranial mass lesions. *Neurosurgery* 1983;12:277–285.

120. Kelly PJ, Kall BA, Goerss S, Earnest F.t. Computer-assisted stereotaxic laser resection of intra-axial brain neoplasms. *J Neurosurg* 1986;64:427–439.

121. Paleologos TS, Wadley JP, Kitchen ND, Thomas DG. Clinical utility and cost-effectiveness of interactive image-guided craniotomy: clinical comparison between conventional and image-guided meningioma surgery. *Neurosurgery* 2000;47:40–47;discussion 47–48.

122. Hall WA, Liu H, Martin AJ, Pozza CH, Maxwell RE, Truwit CL. Safety, efficacy, and functionality of high-field strength interventional magnetic resonance imaging for neurosurgery. *Neurosurgery* 2000;46:632–641;discussion 641–642.

123. Golfinos JG, Fitzpatrick BC, Smith LR, Spetzler RF. Clinical use of a frameless stereotactic arm: results of 325 cases. *J Neurosurg* 1995;83:197–205.

124. Gumprecht HK, Widenka DC, Lumenta CB. *Brain*Lab VectorVision Neuronavigation System: technology and clinical experiences in 131 cases. *Neurosurgery* 1999;44:97–104;discussion 104–105.

125. Sipos EP, Tebo SA, Zinreich SJ, Long DM, Brem H. In vivo accuracy testing and clinical experience with the ISG Viewing Wand. *Neurosurgery* 1996;39:194–202;discussion 202–204.

126. Sure U, Alberti O, Petermeyer M, Becker R, Bertalanffy H. Advanced image-guided skull base surgery. *Surg. Neurol.* 2000;53:563–572;discussion 572.

127. Barnett GH, Kormos DW, Steiner CP, Weisenberger J. Intraoperative localization using an armless, frameless stereotactic wand. Technical note. *J Neurosurg* 1993;78:510–514.

128. Roberts DW, Strohbehn JW, Hatch JF, Murray W, Kettenberger H. A frameless stereotaxic integration of computerized tomographic imaging and the operating microscope. *J Neurosurg* 1986;65:545–549.

129. Watanabe E, Watanabe T, Manaka S, Mayanagi Y, Takakura K. Three-dimensional digitizer (neuronavigator): new equipment for computed tomography-guided stereotaxic surgery. *Surg Neurol* 1987;27:543–547.

130. Zinreich SJ, Tebo SA, Long DM, et al. Frameless stereotaxic integration of CT imaging data: accuracy and initial applications. *Radiology* 1993;188:735–742.

131. Chalif DJ, Dufresne CR, Ransohoff J, McCarthy JA. Three-dimensional computed tomographic reconstructions of intracranial meningiomas. *Neurosurgery* 1988;23:570–575.

132. Barnett GH, Steiner CP, Weisenberger J. Intracranial meningioma resection using frameless stereotaxy. *J Image Guid Surg* 1995;1:46–52.

133. Gering DT, Nabavi A, Kikinis R, et al. An integrated visualization system for surgical planning and guidance using image fusion and an open MR. *J Magn Reson Imaging* 2001;13:967–975.

134. Walton L, Hampshire A, Forster DM, Kemeny AA. Accuracy of stereotactic localisation using magnetic resonance imaging: a comparison between two- and three-dimensional studies. *Stereotact Funct Neurosurg* 1996;66(Suppl1):49–56.

135. Walton L, Hampshire A, Forster DM, Kemeny AA. A phantom study to assess the accu-

racy of stereotactic localization, using T1-weighted magnetic resonance imaging with the Leksell stereotactic system. *Neurosurgery* 1996;38:170–176;discussion 176–178.

136. Roberts DW, Hartov A, Kennedy FE, Miga MI, Paulsen KD. Intraoperative brain shift and deformation: a quantitative analysis of cortical displacement in 28 cases. *Neurosurgery* 1998;43:749–758;discussion 758–760.

137. Black PM, Alexander E, III, Martin C, et al. Craniotomy for tumor treatment in an intraoperative magnetic resonance imaging unit. *Neurosurgery* 1999;45:423–431;discussion 431–433.

138. Maurer CR, Jr., Hill DL, Martin AJ, et al. Investigation of intraoperative brain deformation using a 1.5-T interventional MR system: preliminary results. *IEEE Trans Med Imaging* 1998;17:817–825.

139. Nimsky C, Ganslandt O, Cerny S, Hastreiter P, Greiner G, Fahlbusch R. Quantification of, visualization of, and compensation for brain shift using intraoperative magnetic resonance imaging. *Neurosurgery* 2000;47:1070–1079;discussion 1079–1080.

140. Nauta HJ. Error assessment during "image guided" and "imaging interactive" stereotactic surgery. *Comput Med Imaging Graph* 1994;18:279–287.

141. Hill DL, Maurer CR, Jr., Maciunas RJ, Barwise JA, Fitzpatrick JM, Wang MY. Measurement of intraoperative brain surface deformation under a craniotomy. *Neurosurgery* 1998;43:514–526;discussion 527–528.

142. Dorward NL, Alberti O, Velani B, et al. Postimaging brain distortion: magnitude, correlates, and impact on neuronavigation. *J Neurosurg* 1998;88:656–662.

143. Knauth M, Wirtz CR, Tronnier VM, Aras N, Kunze S, Sartor K. Intraoperative MR imaging increases the extent of tumor resection in patients with high-grade gliomas. *AJNR Am J Neuroradiol* 1999;20:1642–1646.

144. Nabavi A, Black PM, Gering DT, et al. Serial intraoperative magnetic resonance imaging of brain shift. *Neurosurgery* 2001;48:787–797;discussion 797–798.

145. Lipson AC, Gargollo PC, Black PM. Intraoperative magnetic resonance imaging: considerations for the operating room of the future. *J Clin Neurosci* 2001;8:305–310.

146. Lunsford LD, Parrish R, Albright L. Intraoperative imaging with a therapeutic computed tomographic scanner. *Neurosurgery* 1984;15:559–561.

147. Lunsford LD. A dedicated CT system for the stereotactic operating room. *Appl Neurophysiol* 1982;45:374–378.

148. Steinmeier R, Fahlbusch R, Ganslandt O, et al. Intraoperative magnetic resonance imaging with the magnetom open scanner: concepts, neurosurgical indications, and procedures: a preliminary report. *Neurosurgery* 1998;43:739–747;discussion 747–748.

149. Jolesz FA. , Blumenfeld SM. Interventional use of magnetic resonance imaging. *Magn Reson Quart* 1994;10:85–96.

150. Black PM, Moriarty T, Alexander E, III, et al. Development and implementation of intraoperative magnetic resonance imaging and its neurosurgical applications. *Neurosurgery* 1997;41:831–842;discussion 842–845.

151. Albert FK, Forsting M, Sartor K, Adams HP, Kunze S. Early postoperative magnetic resonance imaging after resection of malignant glioma: objective evaluation of residual tumor and its influence on regrowth and prognosis. *Neurosurgery* 1994;34:45–60;discussion 60–61.

152. Simpson JR, Horton J, Scott C, et al. Influence of location and extent of surgical resection on survival of patients with glioblastoma multiforme: results of three consecutive Radiation Therapy Oncology Group (RTOG) clinical trials. *Int J Radiat Oncol Biol Phys* 1993;26:239–244.

153. Devaux BC, O'Fallon JR, Kelly PJ. Resection, biopsy, and survival in malignant glial neoplasms. A retrospective study of clinical parameters, therapy, and outcome. *J Neurosurg* 1993;78:767–775.

154. Alexander E, III, Moriarty TM, Kikinis R, Jolesz FA. Innovations in minimalism: intraoperative MRI. *Clin Neurosurg* 1996;43:338–352.

155. Moriarty T, Kikinis R, Jolesz FA, Black PM, Alexander E, III. Magnetic resonance imaging therapy: Intraoperative MR imaging, in *Neurosurgery Clinics of North America: Clinical Frontiers of Interactive Image Guided Neurosurgery* (Maciunas RJ, ed). Philadelphia, W.B. Saunders, 1996; pp. 323–331.

156. Lenz GW. , Dewey C. An open MRI system used for interventional procedures: Current research and initial clinical results, in: *Computer Assisted Radiology* (Lemke HU, Inamura K, Jaffe CC, and Vannier MW, eds.). Berlin, Springer Verlag, 1995; pp. 1180–1187.

157. Wirtz CR, Bonsanto MM, Knauth M, et al. Intraoperative magnetic resonance imaging to update interactive navigation in neurosurgery: method and preliminary experience. *Comput Aided Surg* 1997;2:172–179.

158. Hall WA, Martin AJ, Liu H, Nussbaum ES, Maxwell RE, Truwit CL. Brain biopsy using high-field strength interventional magnetic resonance imaging. *Neurosurgery* 1999;44:807–813;discussion 813–814.

159. Hall WA, Martin AJ, Liu H, et al. High-field strength interventional magnetic resonance imaging for pediatric neurosurgery. *Pediatr Neurosurg* 1998;29:253–259.

160. Sutherland GR, Louw DF. Intraoperative MRI: a moving magnet. *Cmaj* 1999;161:1293.

161. Sutherland GR, Kaibara T, Louw D, Hoult DI, Tomanek B, Saunders J. A mobile high-field magnetic resonance system for neurosurgery. *J Neurosurg* 1999;91:804–813.

162. Hadani M, Spiegelman R, Feldman Z, Berkenstadt H, Ram Z. Novel, compact, intraoperative magnetic resonance imaging-guided system for conventional neurosurgical operating rooms. *Neurosurgery* 2001;48:799–807;discussion 807–809.

163. Schulder M, Liang D, Carmel PW. Cranial surgery navigation aided by a compact intraoperative magnetic resonance imager. *J Neurosurg* 2001;94:936–945.

164. Bohinski RJ, Warnick RE, Gaskill-Shipley MF, et al. Intraoperative magnetic resonance imaging to determine the extent of resection of pituitary macroadenomas during transphenoidal microsurgery. *Neurosurgery* 2001;49:1133–1144.

165. Ammirati M, Vick N, Liao YL, Ciric I, Mikhael M. Effect of the extent of surgical resection on survival and quality of life in patients with supratentorial glioblastomas and anaplastic astrocytomas. *Neurosurgery* 1987;21:201–206.

166. Ciric I, Ammirati M, Vick N, Mikhael M. Supratentorial gliomas: surgical considerations and immediate postoperative results. Gross total resection versus partial resection. *Neurosurgery* 1987;21:21–26.

167. Chandler KL, Prados MD, Malec M, Wilson CB. Long-term survival in patients with glioblastoma multiforme. *Neurosurgery* 1993;32:716–720;discussion 720.

168. Bricolo A, Turazzi S, Cristofori L, et al. Experience in "radical" surgery of supratentorial gliomas in adults. *J Neurosurg Sci* 1990;34:297–298.

169. Obwegeser A, Ortler M, Seiwald M, Ulmer H, Kostron H. Therapy of glioblastoma multiforme: a cumulative experience of 10 years. *Acta Neurochir (Wien)* 1995;137:29–33.

170. Berger MS. Intraoperative MR imaging: making an impact on outcomes for patients with brain tumors. *AJNR Am J Neuroradiol* 2001;22:2.

171. Keles GE, Lamborn KR, Berger MS. Low-grade hemispheric gliomas in adults: a critical review of extent of resection as a factor influencing outcome. *J Neurosurg* 2001;95:735–745.

172. Berger MS, Deliganis AV, Dobbins J, Keles GE. The effect of extent of resection on recurrence in patients with low grade cerebral hemisphere gliomas. *Cancer* 1994;74:1784–1791.

173. Niranjan A. , Lunsford LD. Radiosurgery: where we were, are, and may be in the third millennium. *Neurosurgery* 2000;46:531–543.

174. Leksell L. The stereotactic method and radiosurgery of the brain. *Acta Chir Scand* 1951;102:316–319.

175. Kondziolka D, Dempsey PK, Lunsford LD, et al. A comparison between magnetic resonance imaging and computed tomography for stereotactic coordinate determination. *Neurosurgery* 1992;30:402–406;discussion 406–407.

176. Flickinger JC, Kondziolka D, Niranjan A, Lunsford LD. Results of acoustic neuroma

radiosurgery: an analysis of 5 years' experience using current methods. *J Neurosurg* 2001;94:1–6.

177. Guo WY, Chu WC, Wu MC, et al. An evaluation of the accuracy of magnetic-resonance-guided Gamma Knife surgery. *Stereotact Funct Neurosurg* 1996;66(suppl 1):85–92.

178. Kondziolka D. , Flickinger JC. Use of magnetic resonance imaging in stereotactic surgery. A survey of members of the American Society of Stereotactic and Functional Neurosurgery. *Stereotact Funct Neurosurg* 1996;66:193–197.

179. Gerdes JS, Hitchon PW, Neerangun W, Torner JC. Computed tomography versus magnetic resonance imaging in stereotactic localization. *Stereotact Funct Neurosurg* 1994;63:124–129.

180. Carter DA, Parsai EI, Ayyangar KM. Accuracy of magnetic resonance imaging stereotactic coordinates with the cosman-roberts-wells frame. *Stereotact Funct Neurosurg* 1999;72:35–46.

181. Foote KD, Friedman WA, Buatti JM, Bova FJ, Meeks SA. Linear accelerator radiosurgery in brain tumor management. *Neurosurg Clin North Am* 1999;10:203–242.

182. Cohen DS, Lustgarten JH, Miller E, Khandji AG, Goodman RR. Effects of coregistration of MR to CT images on MR stereotactic accuracy. *J Neurosurg* 1995;82:772–779.

183. Noren G, Greitz D, Hirsch A, Lax I. Gamma knife surgery in acoustic tumours. *Acta Neurochir Suppl (Wien)* 1993;58:104–107.

184. Foote KD, Friedman WA, Buatti JM, Meeks SL, Bova FJ, Kubilis PS. Analysis of risk factors associated with radiosurgery for vestibular schwannoma. *J Neurosurg* 2001;95:440–449.

185. Lunsford LD, Kondziolka D, Flickinger JC. Acoustic Neuroma management: Evolution and revolution, in *Radiosurgery* (Kondziolka D, ed.). Basel, Karger, 1998; pp. 1–7.

186. Kondziolka D. Functional radiosurgery. *Neurosurgery* 1999;44:12–20;discussion 20–22.

187. Witt TC, Kondziolka D, Baumann SB, Noll DC, Small SL, Lunsford LD. Preoperative cortical localization with functional MRI for use in stereotactic radiosurgery. *Stereotact Funct Neurosurg* 1996;66:24–29.

188. Lunsford LD, Kondziolka D, Maitz A, Flickinger JC. Black holes, white dwarfs and supernovas: imaging after radiosurgery. *Stereotact. Funct. Neurosurg.* 1998;70(Suppl1):2–10.

9

Recent Advances in Cancer Imaging as Applied to Radiotherapy

C. Clifton Ling, PhD, John Humm, MD, PhD, Hedvig Hricak, MD, PhD, and Jason Koutcher, MD, PhD,

INTRODUCTION

A century has passed since the discovery of X-rays by Roentgen and of radium by Curie. From those cradles, the use of radiation for disease diagnosis and treatment has steadily grown and expanded to become important branches of medicine, particularly for human cancers. As radiation sciences and their clinical application matured, subspecialties emerged, eventually resulting in diagnostic radiology and radiation oncology developing into distinct entities.

Whereas radiotherapy has always been image-based (in fact, in the beginning radiotherapy and radiological imaging basically used the same equipment), the nature of the "image" has evolved. Until the last three decades of the 20th century, the images were two-dimensional X-ray projections through the patient. The availability of three-dimensional (3D) anatomical data, first provided by computed tomography (CT), ushered in the so-called "image-based" 3D conformal radiation therapy (3D-CRT) (1).

During the last 20 yr, 3D-CRT has become the standard of radiotherapy. In 3D-CRT, the target and nontarget structures are delineated from patient-specific 3D image data sets (at present primarily CT, sometimes supplemented with magnetic resonance imaging [MRI], positron emission tomography [PET], etc.), the treatment portals are designed using beam's eye view (BEV), and the planned dose distributions are calculated by high-speed computers and displayed and evaluated with powerful workstations (2,3). Increasingly, the evaluation of radiotherapy treatment plans include the analysis of structure-specific dose-volume data (dose volume histogram) and consideration of biological indices, for example, and local tumor control probability (TCP) and normal tissue complication probability (NTCP), as surrogates for treatment outcome of local TCP and NTCP, respectively. In the delivery of 3D-CRT, computer-controlled radiation machines, multileaf collimators (MLCs), and treatment verification with electronic portal images are increasingly used (1).

From: *Image-Guided Diagnosis and Treatment of Cancer*
Edited by: A. D'Amico, J. S. Loeffler, and J. R. Harris © Humana Press Inc., Totowa, NJ

Within the past decade, however, an advanced form of 3D-CRT, the so-called intensity-modulated radiotherapy (IMRT), has led to further improvement in the dose distribution conformality using computer-optimized intensity modulation *(4–7)*. In addition, IMRT has the potential of reducing the manual iterative and time-consuming steps in the treatment design phase of 3D-CRT, particularly when the treatment design is complex. In brief, IMRT is an improvement over 3D-CRT because of two key elements: 1) computerized iterative plan optimization, and 2) the use of intensity-modulated radiation beams *(8)*. In terms of delivery methods, intensity modulated radiation fields at fixed gantry angles can be delivered with MLCs, in either the static or dynamic mode *(9,10)*, or using the tomotherapy approach with beams directed from 360° and modulated either with a slit MLC or several MLC-shaped fields *(11,12)*.

COMPUTED TOMOGRAPHY

The primary uses of CT are the following: 1) the delineation of the target volume; 2) the determination of the relative geometry of critical structures; 3) the optimal placement of beams and the shaping of apertures; 4) the calculation of dose distribution; and 5) follow-up evaluation of treatment outcome. The use of CT for radiotherapy treatment planning (the first four items above) began in the early 1980s along with the development of the BEV concept *(2,3)*.

For the proper use of CT, however, there must be correct alignment of the patient in the treatment position on a flat couch. A complete 3D-CT image set is usually obtained, with the number of CT slices and the interslice spacing according to protocols, depending on the size, shape, and location of the target and the treatment technique. However, to produce high-resolution sagittal or coronal images and digitally reconstructed radiographs, the slices are contiguous with interslice spacing of 3 to 5 mm.

Faster and more accurate CT examinations have become possible with the recent introduction of the so-called spiral, or (more appropriately) helical, scanners. This advance was made possible by the slip ring technology, with continuous electrical connections between the rotating and the fixed components of the scanner. Volumetric scan data is acquired by having the table move continuously, relative to the gantry, concomitant with the continuous rotation of the X-ray tube and detector array around the patient. Recently, multislice helical CT has become available, providing high-image quality at a fraction of the previously required time. These scanners can acquire the data for a full set of images in less than 1 min, possibly during one breath hold. For radiotherapy application, however, one must consider the possibility that patient anatomy during a breath hold may not be in its "average" location during radiation treatment.

The advent of high-speed helical scanner has led to the so-called CT simulation, which, by combining the simulation and CT imaging sessions into one, can lead to greater operation efficiency *(13)*. The CT simulator combines the capabilities of spiral (or helical) scanners for volumetric data acquisition and high-speed workstations for rapid image reconstruction and display. This permits the so-called virtual simulation, performed on a computer workstation using the 3D-CT data set (the virtual patient) *(7)*. In this process, a complete 3D-CT data set is first obtained with the patient in the treatment position using 3- to 5-mm slice thickness. Then, corresponding to the specific treatment set-up parameters, patient anatomy are reconstructed from the CT data and displayed in BEV, and simulation fluoroscopic and radiographic images digitally generated for viewing, decision making, and documentation.

Aside from the improved efficiency, CT simulation eliminates or minimizes systematic uncertainties in the registration of simulation films to CT data sets and in set-up errors when transferring the patient from one mechanical coordinate system to another. The disadvantage is the degraded image quality of reconstructed radiographs as compared to conventional simulation films.

MAGNETIC RESONANCE IMAGING

The excellent soft-tissue contrast, based on differences in the T1 and T2 relaxation parameters of normal and pathologic states, underlies the usefulness of MRI as a vital modality for tumor diagnosis and characterization. However, the early promise, based on findings that malignant tissues have higher T1 and T2 values than normal tissue, has been somewhat modulated because of inadequate specificity. Methods for contrast enhancement have been developed to provide images that also yield tumor physiological and micro-environmental information, such as blood flow (perfusion or diffusion), hypoxia, pH, and so on. These parameters may be important prognosticators relative to tumor responsiveness to radiation and other antineoplastic treatment. In addition, it has been suggested that changes in these parameters can be monitored by MRI *(14,15)*. These latter aspects of the potential of MRI are only beginning to be exploited. For radiotherapy treatment, planning MRI images often present unique anatomical information and tumor detail. Although the digital values cannot be directly used in dose calculations, the MRI detail, when correlated with CT attenuation values, can provide a powerful planning tool. The registration of CT and MRI is now widely and effectively used in the treatment planning of brain, head and neck, and pelvic diseases.

The potential importance of tumor oxygenation status for radiotherapy has been a subject of long-standing interest and of recent intensive investigation. In this regard, the use of nuclear magnetic resonance (NMR) techniques for assessing blood flow, angiogenesis, and tumor hypoxia is of relevance to radiation oncology. In the last decade a number of methods to measure perfusion and diffusion in tissues have been developed and many of these are being evaluated in clinical trials. Tissue perfusion and vascular permeability with submillimeter resolution can be estimated from the increase in the T1 signal after the bolus administration of a contrast agent such as gadolinium diethylenetriaminepenta-acetic acid. With faster pulse sequences such as the echo-planar dynamic imaging method, serial images at less than 1 s per frame can be obtained to track the uptake of the contrast agent. The derived parametric image can yield pixel by pixel information on blood volume, blood–brain barrier permeability, blood perfusion, diffusion, and extravascular space. The utility of such techniques to assess tumor grade and type, treatment efficacy, and possibly long-term prognosis as applied to brain, breast, sarcoma, and other sites are being studied. The in vivo mobility of water molecules, that is, diffusion, depends on tissue properties and may provide information on cellular milieu, for example, viscosity, and barriers, such as cell membranes that limit motion *(16)*. Diffusion-weighted images (DWIs) are acquired by applying strong magnetic gradients leading to signal loss from molecules, which increases with their mobility. DWIs may be able to differentiate lesion types because necrotic regions have extensive cell lysis, resulting in higher diffusion coefficients on DWIs. At Memorial Sloan Kettering Cancer Center (MSKCC), diffusion-weighted imaging is used to study bone marrow cellularity and changes in hematopoiesis as the result of chemotherapy in leukemia patients *(17)*.

Another potential application of advance MRI methods is the use of echo planar imaging (EPI) that allows subsecond image acquisition to provide functional locus in the brain, that is, functional MRI. Task activation, associated with increased blood flow, is detected with rapid imaging either by contrast-enhanced method with gadolinium diethylenetriaminepenta-acetic acid, or by the blood oxygenation level-dependent technique *(18)*. Stimulation of the brain by task activation increases blood flow to the stimulated region, resulting in increased oxyhemoglobin and increased signal in T2*-weighted images. These techniques have been used to study a variety of functional and physiological problems, including sensory and motor stimulation, vision, and language *(19,20)*. Variations of these techniques have been used for studying angiogenesis in tumors and wound healing.

Another important potential of NMR is to use the chemical shift in the NMR spectrum to detect the presence and levels of various metabolites. The magnetic resonance spectroscopy (MRS) approach can provide cancel cell signature because of their different chemical moieties. A disadvantage is the large voxel size required to obtain reasonable signal to noise ratio, for example, 0.25 cm^3 for ^{1}H (proton) MRS and more than 2 cm^3 for in vivo ^{31}P MRS, although these can be reduced significantly with further technological advances. ^{1}H MRSI combines the advantages of biochemical data of ^{1}H spectroscopy and spatial localization of ^{1}H imaging. Because of the relative abundance of the ^{1}H nuclei, ^{1}H NMR spectroscopy has better sensitivity, although water and lipid suppression pulse sequences are necessary. Commonly detected compounds that have been detected using ^{1}H NMR spectroscopy, including choline, lactate, and creatine. In the prostate, increased "choline" is regarded as an indicator of enhanced cell membrane phospholipid turnover because of tumor growth *(21)*.

Other compounds that have been detected by in vivo ^{1}H NMR spectroscopy include alanine, glutamate (a major excitatory neurotransmitter and energy source), myo-inositol (involved in intracellular signaling pathways related to growth), γ-aminobutyric acid (a major inhibitory neurotransmitter), and taurine. Lactate is of particular interest because it increases in direct relation to anaerobic glycolysis caused by tumor hypoxia, ischemia, or infection *(22–24)*. ^{1}H NMR has been applied to noninvasive grading and classification of brain tumors, to attempting to characterize metastatic brain tumors from different primary sites, and to monitoring response after treatment with radiation and other modalities. At MSKCC, there is an ongoing study following patients with primary central nervous system lymphoma before, during, and after treatment. The feasibility of discriminating between tumor regrowth and radiation necrosis based on higher choline in tumors and reduction of creatine, choline, and *N*-acetyl-aspartate (NAA) in necrosis has been proposed but requires further study.

In the NMR spectra of ^{31}P, we can detect nucleoside triphosphates, phosphocreatine, inorganic phosphates, phosphocholine, phosphoethanolamine, and can therefore provide information about tumor energy status and phospholipid metabolism *(25)*. ^{31}P NMR, in providing data on energy status, may have prognostic value since hypoxic tumors had a lower energy status compared to well oxygenated tumors *(14)*. Also, changes in ^{31}P spectra have been related to changes in tumor growth fraction, response to therapy and percent necrosis at surgery. With further research in MRSI, other specific chemical spectroscopic markers may be identified to provide a biological rationale for dose painting/sculpting in intensity modulated radiation therapy.

POSITRON EMISSION TOMOGRAPHY

The usefulness and the availability of fluorodeoxy glucose (FDG) as a positron-emitting tracer have propelled the use of and enthusiasm for PET scanning.

The increased glucose metabolism of cancer cells, as compared with normal tissues, underlies the enhanced uptake of FDG in malignant growth. FDG uptake in tumors is most commonly expressed by the standardized uptake value, the ratio of the activity per unit mass in the lesion to the administered activity per unit patient mass. A standardized uptake value of more than 2.5 is generally used to differentiate between benign and malignant lesions.

Clinical studies of many disease sites, including brain, breast, head and neck, colorectal, and ovarian, have shown that PET imaging with FDG has the potential to improve the detection, staging, treatment design, and evaluation *(26–30)*. The efficacy of FDG-PET in diagnosing and staging thoracic lesions is now well established by a large number of clinical studies *(31)*. Its application to CTV definition in radiotherapy of lung cancer has been a subject of several investigations. Several previous studies reported that FDG-PET images may influence the radiation treatment fields in about one-third of the patients *(31–34)*. Our recent prospective study support these data on the ability of FDG-PET in detecting metabolic foci not detected on CT scans *(34)*. Specifically, in seven of 11 patients, the PTV was enlarged, whereas in the remaining four it was decreased.

The ability of FDG-PET to detect small lesions led to its exploratory use for monitoring treatment outcome after radiotherapy of meningioma and colorectal and head/neck tumors *(35,36)*. By and large, the study results have been equivocal, with correlation in some disease sites but not in others. Although in general tumors exhibit enhanced FDG uptake because of increased metabolism, there are other influential factors, including blood flow, tissue inflammation, cellular energy level, and hypoxia. The situation may be even more complex during and subsequent to radiotherapy as the result of radiation-induced reactive changes in both the tumor and the stroma *(37)*. Given the heterogeneous nature of human malignancy and the complexity in radiation-response of both the tumor and normal tissues, it is possible that the usefulness of FDG-PET is disease specific or even patient specific.

Despite the usefulness of FDG in PET imaging, new tracers with different attributes are being developed for cancer detection and characterization. For example, ^{11}C-methionine is a tracer that can differentiate tumor from normal tissue based on different activities of protein synthesis. Although ^{11}C has a half-life of 20 min (even shorted than ^{18}F), ^{11}C-methionine may be superior to FDG for imaging prostate cancers because of the minimal uptake in the bladder *(38)*. However, the high metabolism of methionine in the liver would render this radiotracer suboptimal for the detection of liver metastases. Therefore, the optimum choice of radiotracer for tumor diagnosis depends on the organ site.

Another important PET application is in the detection of tumor hypoxia. The resurgent interest in tumor hypoxia is spurred by results of clinical trials that clearly demonstrated correlations between hypoxia and radiocurability in both metastasis containing lymph nodes in head and neck cancer and in cervical cancer (39,40). Even among the patients who underwent surgery for cancer of the cervix, survival and relapse free survival were poorer for those with hypoxic tumors (40). In high-grade soft tissue sarcomas, Brizel et al. (41) reported an association between tumor hypoxia and the development of metastases after multimodality treatment. Thus, hypoxia may be associated with a more aggressive tumor phenotype, in addition to radioresistance. It follows that an assessment of tumor hypoxia may be of prognostic value, and important for making treatment decisions.

Several groups have demonstrated the imaging of tumor hypoxia using nuclear medicine approaches. The preferential metabolic reduction of nitroimidazoles in hypoxic cells relative to aerobic cells results in the increased retention of bioreductive products in hypoxic cells underlies the efficacy of PET imaging with fluorinated misonidazole (Fmiso) by Rasey et al. (42). Chapman et al. (43) have shown that single-photon emission computed tomography with ^{131}IAZA can also detect tumor hypoxia in both small cell lung and head/neck cancers despite the lower resolution of this imaging method. Other similar efforts include the use of ^{124}IAZG (44), ^{18}F-EF1 (45), and ^{64}Cu-ATSM (46). The enthusiasm, which surrounds hypoxia imaging, is that it provides the opportunity to visualize and localize radioresistant tumor cell populations, and thereby to selectively target these regions by intensity modulated radiotherapy (47).

Lastly, an important recent development in the commercial availability of combination PET/CT units with a common gantry housing both devices, thus allowing patients to be scanned in the same position and imaging session. This will permit accurate anatomical localization of functional PET tracers, which a prerequisite of modern radiotherapy treatment planning

MOLECULAR IMAGING

There are emerging imaging techniques that provide information about molecular processes that underlie various biological functions at the cellular and organ levels (48) in contradistinction to classic diagnostic imaging with its focus on anatomical and structural abnormalities. These methods and the associated probes are often based on molecular biological processes they are designed to assess, and therefore are potentially valuable tools to understand and treat disease processes at the molecular level.

Molecular imaging, in the context of cancer diagnosis and treatment, is to provide spatial and quantitative information concerning DNA, RNA, and proteins that are involved in the disease process. Thus, the imaging methods could be for genotype, gene transcription, post-transcriptional modulation/stabilization of mRNA, protein–protein interactions in signal transduction pathways, and other molecular information that influence tumor phenotype. An example of this is the study of the transcription of report genes at MSKCC (49,50). Clearly, such information would be useful in disease evaluation, treatment planning, and monitoring outcome, so as to improve the clinical management of individual patients.

GROSS, CLINICAL, PLANNING, AND BIOLOGICAL TARGET VOLUMES (GTV, CTV, PTV, AND BTVS)

A common nomenclature for describing the patients disease relative to radiotherapy treatment is useful, and ICRU Reports 50 and 62 have defined the terms of GTVs, CTVs, and PTVs and internal and set-up margins *(51)*. The PTV is essentially derived from the CTV, with appropriate inclusion of the internal and set-up margins. In general, cross-sectional images (CT and MRI) are used to delineate the GTV and CTV, and knowledge on physiological effects and set-up uncertainty incorporated to delineate the PTV. Then, radiation treatment portals are designed to entirely cover the PTV.

Although in conventional radiotherapy a uniform dose distribution within the PTV is usually the goal of treatment planning, there have been suggestions that nonuniformity within the PTV, specifically regions of increased dose, may actually increase the local control. With the ability of IMRT to deliver nonuniform dose patterns by design, there are investigations to evaluate the efficacy of "dose painting" or "dose sculpting" based on information from biological images. For example, the researchers at the University of California, San Francisco, are evaluating the potential clinical gain of using IMRT to deliver a nonuniform dose distribution within the PTV, with a higher dose given to specific regions identified by MRI/MRS as dominant intraprostatic lesions *(52)*. The dominant intraprostatic lesions as identified in the MRI/MRS images are regions of elevated choline/citrate ratio, taken as a surrogate for tumor burden. Another example is the dose painting in head and neck cancers based on tumor hypoxia image obtained with PET *(46)*. Specifically, using the Cu-ATSM that selectively localizes in hypoxic cells, Chao et al *(46)* map the hypoxic regions of the tumor and design an IMRT treatment plan to deliver a higher dose to the regions of low pO_2.

The above discussion advances the concept of IMRT dose painting based on BTVs derived from the new imaging methods. Whereas up to the present, radiological images are largely anatomical, the new imaging techniques can provide biological and mechanistic data, metabolic information from PET-FDG, functional/metabolic data from MRI/MRS, tumor hypoxia distribution from PET, and developing approaches to characterize tumor genotype and phenotype *(48,53–55)*. Thus, we that these "biological images" may yield insights for defining the BTV. For relevance to radiation therapy, characteristics of the BTV should relate to the tumor extent and burden, growth kinetics and factors that influence radiosensitivity and treatment outcome.

REFERENCES

1. Ling CC Fuks Z. Conformal radiation treatment: a critical appraisal. *Eur J Cancer* 1995;5:799–803.
2. Goitein M, Abrams M, Rowell D, Pollari H, Wiles J. Multidimensional treatment planning. II: Beam's eye view, back projection and projection through CT sections. *Int J Radiat Oncol Phys* 1983;9:789–797.
3. McShan DL, Fraass BA, Lichter AS. Full integration of the beam's eye view concept into computerized treatment planning. *Int J Radiat Oncol Phys* 1990;18:1485–1494.
4. Brahme A. Optimization of stationary and moving beam radiation therapy techniques. *Radiother Oncol* 1988;12:129–140.
5. Carol M, Grant WH, Pavord D, et al. Initial clinical experience with the Peacock intensity modulation of a 3-D conformal radiation therapy system. *Stereotactic Functional Neurosurg* 1996;6:30–34.

6. Spirou SV, Chui CS. A gradient inverse planning algorithm with dose-volume constraints. *Med Phys* 1998;25:321–333.

7. Ling CC, Burman C, Chui CS, et al. Conformal radiation treatment of prostate cancer using inversely- planned intensity-modulated photon beams produced with dynamic multileaf collimation [see comments]. *Int J Radiat Oncol Phys* 1996;35:721–730.

8. Burman C, Chui CS, Kutcher G, et al. Planning, delivery, and quality assurance of intensity-modulated radiotherapy using dynamic multileaf collimator: a strategy for large-scale implementation for the treatment of carcinoma of the prostate. *Int J Radiat Oncol Biol Phys* 1997;39:863–873.

9. Spirou S, Chui CS. Generation of arbitrary intensity profiles by dynamic jaws or multileaf collimators. *Med Phys* 1994;21:1031.

10. LoSasso T, Chui CS, Ling CC. Physical and dosimetric aspects of a multileaf collimation system used in the dynamic mode for implementing intensity modulated radiotherapy. *Med Phys* 1998;25:1919–1927.

11. Intensity-modulated radiotherapy: current status and issues of interest. *Int J Radiat Oncol Biol Phys* 51:880–914.

12. Yu CX. Intensity-modulated arc therapy with dynamic multileaf collimation: an alternative to tomotherapy. *Phys Med Biol* 1995;40:1435–1449.

13. Sherouse GW, Bourland JD, Reynolds K, et al. Virtual simulation in the clinical setting: some practical considerations. *Int J Radiat Oncol Phys* 1990;19:1059–1065.

14. Koutcher JA, Alfieri AA, Devitt ML, et al. Quantitative changes in tumor metabolism, partial pressure of oxygen, and radiobiological oxygenation status postradiation. *Cancer Res* 1992;52:4620–4627.

15. Okunieff P, Walsh CS, Vaupel P, et al. Effects of hydralazine on in vivo tumor energy metabolism, hematopoietic radiation sensitivity, and cardiovascular parameters. *Int J Radiat. Oncol Biol Phys* 1989;16:1145–1148.

16. Le Bihan D, Breton E, Lallemand D, Grenier P, Cabanis E, Laval-Jeantet M. MR imaging of intravoxel incoherent motions: application to diffusion and perfusion in neurologic disorders. *Radiology* 1986;161:401–407.

17. Ballon D, Dyke J, Schwartz LH, et al. Bone marrow segmentation in leukemia using diffusion and T (2) weighted echo planar magnetic resonance imaging. *NMR Biomed* 2000;13:321–328.

18. Kim KH, Relkin NR, Lee KM, Hirsch J. Distinct cortical areas associated with native and second languages. *Nature* 1997; 388: 171–174.

19. Kim SG, Ashe J, Hendrich K, et al. Functional magnetic resonance imaging of motor cortex: hemispheric asymmetry and handedness. *Science* 1993; 261: 615–617.

20. Belliveau JW, Kennedy DN Jr, McKinstry RC, et al. Functional mapping of the human visual cortex by magnetic resonance imaging. *Science* 1991; 254:716–719.

21. Kurhanewicz J, Vigneron DB, Nelson SJ, et al. Citrate as an in vivo marker to discriminate prostate cancer from benign prostatic hyperplasia and normal prostate peripheral zone: detection via localized proton spectroscopy. *Urology* 1995;45:459–466.

22. Behar KL, den Hollander JA, Stromski ME, et al. High-resolution 1H nuclear magnetic resonance study of cerebral hypoxia in vivo. *Proc Natl Acad Sci USA* 1983;80:4945–4948.

23. Schwickert G, Walenta S, Sundfor K, Rofstad EK, Mueller-Klieser W. Correlation of high lactate levels in human cervical cancer with incidence of metastasis. *Cancer Res* 1995;55:4757–4759.

24. Walenta S, Salameh A, Lyng H, et al. Correlation of high lactate levels in head and neck tumors with incidence of metastasis. *Am J Pathol* 1997;150:409–415.

25. Koutcher JA, Ballon D, Graham M, et al. 31P NMR spectra of extremity sarcomas: diversity of metabolic profiles and changes in response to chemotherapy. *Magn Reson Med* 1990;16:19–34 .

26. Scheidhauer K, Scharl A, Pietrzyk U, et al. Qualitative [18F]FDG positron emission tomography in primary breast cancer: clinical relevance and practicability. *Eur J Nucl Med* 1996;23:618–623.
27. Rigo P, Paulus P, Kaschten BJ, et al. Oncological applications of positron emission tomography with fluorine-18 fluorodeoxyglucose. *Eur J Nucl Med* 1996;23:1641–1674 .
28. Avril N, Bense S, Ziegler SI, et al. Breast imaging with fluorine-18-FDG PET: Quantitative image analysis. *J Nucl Med* 1997;38:1186–1191.
29. Brock CS, Meikle SR, Price P. Does fluorine-18 fluorodeoxyglucose metabolic imaging of tumours benefit oncology? [see comments]. *Eur J Nucl Med* 1997;24:691–705.
30. Utech CI, Young CS, Winter PF. Prospective evaluation of fluorine-18 fluorodeoxyclucose positron emission tomography in breast cancer for staging of the axilla related to surgery and immunocytochemistry. *Eur J Nucl Med* 1996;23:1588–1593.
31. Mac Manus MP, Hicks RJ, Ball DL, et al. F-18 fluorodeoxyglucose positron emission tomography staging in radical radiotherapy candidates with non-small cell lung carcinoma. *Cancer* 2001;92:886–895.
32. Munley MT, Marks LB, Scarfone C, et al. Multimodality nuclear medicine imaging in three-dimensional radiation treatment planning for lung cancer: challenges and prospects. *Lung Cancer* 1999;23:105–114.
33. Kiffer JD, Berlangieri SU, Scott AM, et al. The contribution of 18F-fluoro-2-deoxy-glucose positron emission tomographic imaging to radiotherapy planning in lung cancer. *Lung Cancer* 1998;19:167–177.
34. Erdi YE, Yorke ED, Erdi AK, et al. Radiotherapy treatment planning for patients with non-small cell lung cancer using poistron emission tomography. *Eur J Nucl Med* 2000;34:861–866.
35. Haberkorn U, Strauss LG, Dimitrakopoulou A, et al. PET studies of fluorodeoxyglufluorodeoxy glucosefluorodeoxy glucosefluorodeoxy glucose;cose metabolism in patients with recurrent colorectal tumors receiving radiotherapy. *J Nucl Med* 1991;32:1485–1490.
36. Minn H, Lapela M, Klemi PJ, et al. Prediction of survival with fluorine-18-fluorodeoxyglucose and PET in head and neck cancer. *J Nucl Med* 1997;38:1907–1911.
37. Fischman AJ, Thornton AF, Frosch MP, Swearinger B, Gonzalez RG, Alpert NM. FDG hypermetabolism associated with inflammatory necrotic changes following radiation of meningioma. *J Nucl Med* 1997;38:1027–1029.
38. Macapinlac HA, Humm JL, Akhurst T, et al. Differential metabolism and pharmacokinetics of C-11 methionine and F-18 fluorodeoxyglucose (FDG) in androgen independent prostate cancer. *Clin Positron Imaging* 1999;2:173–181.
39. Vaupel PW. *Blood Flow, Oxygenation, Tissue pH Distribution, and Bioenergetic Status of Tumors.* Berlin, Hellmich, 1994.
40. Hockel M, Schlenger K, Aral B, Mitze M, Schaffer U, Vaupel P. Association between tumor hypoxia and malignant progression in advanced cancer of the uterine cervix. *Cancer Res* 1996;56:4509–4515.
41. Brizel DM, Scully SP, Harrelson JM, Layfield LJ, Dodge RK, Charles HC. Radiation therapy and hyperthermia improve the oxygenation of human soft tissue sarcomas. *Cancer Res* 1996;56:5347–5350.
42. Rasey JS, Koh WJ, Evans ML, et al. (1996) Quantifying regional hypoxia in human tumors with positron emission tomography of [18F]fluoromisonidazole: a prethera:py study of 37 patients. *Int J Radiat Oncol Phys* 1996;36:417–428.
43. Chapman JD, Engelhardt EL, Stobbe CC, Schneider RF, Hanks GE. Measuring hypoxia and predicting tumor radioresistence with nuclear medicine assays. *Radiother Oncol* 1998;46:229–237.
44. Chapman JD, Schneider RF, Urbain JL, Hanks GE. Single-photon emission computed tomography and positron-emission tomography assays for tissue oxygenation. *Semin Radiat Oncol* 2001;11:47–57.

45. Evans SM, Kachur AV, Shiue CY, et al. Noninvasive detection of tumor hypoxia using the 2-nitroimidazole [18F]EF1. *J Nucl Med* 2000;41:327–336.

46. Chao KS, Bosch WR, Mutic S, et al. A novel approach to overcome hypoxic tumor resistance: Cu-ATSM-guided intensity-modulated radiation therapy. *Int J Radiat Oncol Phys* 2001;49:1171–1182.

47. Ling CC, Humm JL, Larson SM, et al. Towards multidimensional radiotherapy (MD-CRT): biological imaging and biological conformality. *Int J Radiat Oncol Biol Phys* 2000;47:551–560.

48. Weissleder R, Simonova M, Bogdanova A, Bredow S, Enochs WS, Bogdanov A Jr. MR imaging and scintigraphy of gene expression through melanin induction. *Radiology* 1997;204:425–429.

49. Tjuvajev J, Finn R, Watanabe K, et al. Noninvasive imaging of herpes virus thymidine kinase gene transfer and expression: a potential method for monitoring clinical gene therapy. *Cancer Res* 1996;56:4087–4095.

50. Doubrovin M, Ponomarev V, Beresten T, et al. Imaging transcriptional regulation of p53 dependent genes with positron emission tomography in vivo. *Proc Natl Acad Sci USA* 2001;98:9300–9305.

51. ICRU. Dose specification for reporting external beam therapy with photons and electrons. 1993 Report.

52. Pickett B, Vigneault E, Kurhanewicz J, Verhey L, Roach M. Static field intensity modulations to treat a dominant intra-prostatic lesion to 90 Gy compared to seven field 3-dimensional radiotherapy. *Int J Radiat Oncol Biol Phys* 1999;43:921–929.

53. Moore A, Basilion JP, Chiocca EA, Weissleder R. Measuring transferrin receptor gene expression by NMR imaging. *Biochimica Biophysica Acta* 1998;1402:239–249.

54. Kayyem JF, Kumar RM, Fraser SE, Meade TJ. Receptor-targeted co-transport of DNA and magnetic resonance contrast agents. *Chem Biol* 1995;2:615–620.

55. Urbain JL. Oncogenes, cancer and imaging. *J Nucl Med* 1999;40:498–504.

III
Innovations in Imaging

10

Sequential Magnetic Resonance and Response of Breast Cancer to Neoadjuvant Therapy

Gary J. Whitman, MD, Revathy B. Iyer, MD,
Oren H. Lifshitz, MD, and Aman U. Buzdar, MD

INTRODUCTION

Imaging has been shown to be effective and efficacious in detecting and diagnosing breast cancer. Meta-analyses and randomized clinical trials have showed that screening mammography may result in a mortality reduction of 28 to 42% (1,2). A recent report noted that the mortality reduction associated with regular screening mammography might be greater than 60% (3). In addition, studies have noted the benefits of screening sonography in identifying nonpalpable, mammographically occult breast cancers (4). In recent years, the role of imaging has expanded beyond the detection of breast cancers to include monitoring response to preoperative chemotherapy. In this chapter, we discuss the rationale for preoperative chemotherapy and review methods for assessing response to preoperative chemotherapy. Physical examination, mammography, and sonography are examined, with particular emphasis on the role of magnetic resonance imaging (MRI).

PREOPERATIVE CHEMOTHERAPY FOR BREAST CANCER

Preoperative chemotherapy is used as the initial treatment for locally advanced breast cancers as well as for smaller, less advanced malignancies (5,6). Preoperative chemotherapy may afford several benefits. In many cases, preoperative therapy will result in a decrease in tumor size, allowing for breast conservation surgery rather than mastectomy (7,8). Preoperative chemotherapy allows micrometastatic disease to be treated soon after breast cancer is diagnosed, rather than delaying treatment until after surgery has been completed (9).

If one assumes that breast cancer is, or has the potential to be, a systemic disease from the outset, early systemic chemotherapy is appealing. Kuerer et al. (10) studied 191 women with locally advanced breast cancer and cytologically documented axillary lymph node metastases. After doxorubicin-based preoperative chemotherapy, 43 patients (23%) were converted to negative axillary node status at histopathologic examination. The 5-yr disease-free survival rates were 87% in patients with preoperative eradication

From: *Image-Guided Diagnosis and Treatment of Cancer*
Edited by: A. D'Amico, J. S. Loeffler, and J. R. Harris © Humana Press Inc., Totowa, NJ

of axillary metastases and 51% in patients with residual axillary metastases identified after completing preoperative chemotherapy.

Preoperative chemotherapeutic agents can be administered and response to treatment can be assessed in vivo. Preoperative chemotherapy allows for the examination of surrogate biological end points in vivo, and patients not responding to the initial chemotherapeutic regimen may be switched to a more effective agent. Preoperative chemotherapy may inhibit a postsurgical tumor growth spurt. It is possible that the use of preoperative chemotherapy will eventually improve breast cancer survival if effective therapy is offered to patients who do not respond to the initial chemotherapeutic regimen *(5)*.

When preoperative chemotherapy is administered, tumor shrinkage may be dramatic. In some cases, the tumor will no longer be visualized by mammography, sonography, or MRI. At many institutions, metal markers are placed into tumors demonstrating a response to therapy. At The University of Texas M. D. Anderson Cancer Center, platinum embolization coils (Cook Incorporated, Bloomington, IN) are placed into the tumor under sonographic guidance and metal clips (MicroMark II, Ethicon Endosurgery, Cincinnati, OH; or Site Marker Clip, US Surgical, Norwalk, Connecticut) are placed under stereotactic guidance *(11,12)*. In addition, metal pellets may be placed into the center of the tumor under ultrasound guidance *(13)*. Indications for metal marker placement include tumors less than 2 cm in greatest dimension and a decrease in tumor volume of greater than 50% after one cycle of chemotherapy. The metal markers are then used to guide needle localization and breast conservation therapy as well as histopathologic evaluation. If metal pellets are placed into the tumor, MRI may not accurately assess residual tumor size because of susceptibility artifacts from the markers.

ASSESSMENT OF RESPONSE TO THERAPY: CLINICAL EXAMINATION

With the increased use of preoperative chemotherapy, oncologists, surgeons, radiation therapists, and imagers have studied methods for determining response to therapy. Physical examination has been the primary tool, but clinical evaluation becomes less accurate with small (less than 1 cm) and heterogeneous lesions. Physical examination involves inspection and palpation of the breasts. Inspection entails examining the skin and assessing for symmetry. Skin edema, erythema, ulcerations, and nipple discharge should be noted. Palpation involves feeling for masses, noting the consistency of the breast tissues, and identifying areas of tenderness. Although clinical examination is inexpensive, estimates of tumor size based on palpation are subjective and dependent on the size and the consistency of the breasts, the location of the tumor, and the experience of the examiner. In general, estimates of tumor size based on clinical examination are difficult to quantify and difficult to reproduce *(14,15)*.

ASSESSMENT OF RESPONSE TO THERAPY: IMAGING

Imaging techniques offer quantifiable, fairly reproducible methods for assessing response to chemotherapy. At most centers, mammography and sonography have been used to evaluate response to therapy. Imaging protocols continue to evolve, and methods that assess functional tumor activity in addition to morphology are being developed. The same imaging technique should be used to characterize tumors prior to the initiation of chemotherapy and on subsequent follow-up studies.

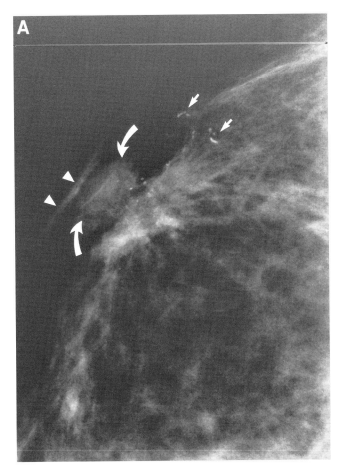

Fig. 1. Invasive ductal carcinoma in a 56-yr-old woman. (**A**) The right craniocaudal tangential mammogram demonstrates a mass (curved arrows), corresponding to the palpable abnormality, and associated skin thickening (arrowheads). Pleomorphic calcifications (straight arrows) are seen adjacent to the mass. Biopsy of the mass under sonographic guidance revealed invasive ductal carcinoma. (**B**) Axial T1-weighted MRI shows a superficial mass (arrows),

A potential pitfall in imaging response to therapy relates to the geometric shape of breast tumors. Although tumor volume determinations are based on the shape of an ellipse, most tumors are not elliptical. Nevertheless, most tumor volume measurements are based on the equation for determining the volume of an ellipsoid:

$$\text{Volume} = d1 \times d2 \times d3 \times 3.14/6 \qquad (1)$$

$$d1 = \text{length}, \ d2 = \text{width, and } d3 = \text{height} \qquad (2)$$

Tumors may appear as irregular, spiculated masses, as masses with poorly defined margins. In many cases, tumor volumes are difficult to measure (Fig. 1). Other potential problems include assessing tumor size in a background of fibrocystic changes, distinguishing tumor margins in dense parenchyma, and differentiating post-treatment fibrosis from viable tumor. Also, there may be operator-dependent variability and differences in machine-based operating parameters.

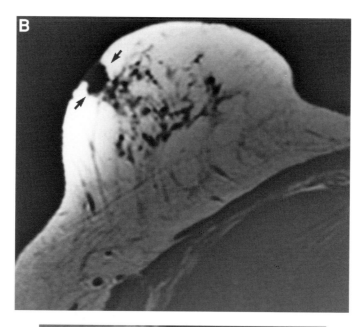

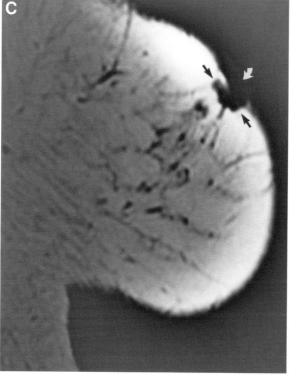

Fig. 1. *(continued)* corresponding to the known malignancy.(**C**) Sagittal T1-weighted MRI demonstrates the mass (straight arrows) and contiguous skin involvement (curved arrow). Preoperative chemotherapy was initiated with adriamycin and taxotere. (**D**) A repeat axial T1-weighted MRI performed 2 mo after the first MRI study shows a decrease in the size of the mass (arrow). (**E**) An axial T1-weighted MRI after the intravenous administration of gadolinium reveals areas of enhancement (arrow) within the residual mass. A right mastectomy was performed 3 wk later, and there was no evidence of residual invasive carcinoma. Ductal

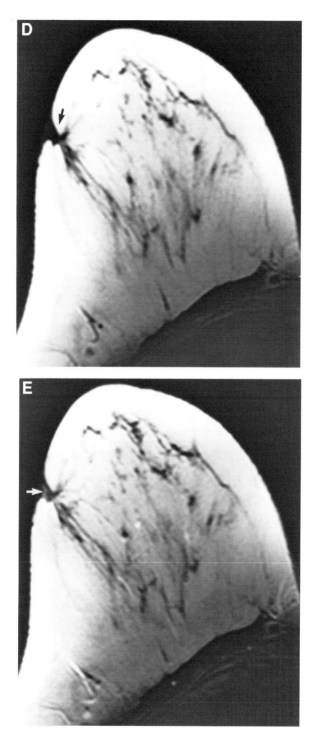

Fig. 1. *(continued)* carcinoma *in situ* was seen along with regions of stromal fibrosis. There was no evidence of tumor involving the skin. Right axillary dissection revealed one out of ten lymph nodes involved with metastatic disease. After surgery, the patient received additional adriamycin and taxotere and then radiation therapy to the right chest wall and the nodal basins. Thereafter, tamoxifen therapy was initiated. Thirteen months after the mastectomy, there was no evidence of residual or metastatic disease.

MAMMOGRAPHY

Mammograms are assessed for the presence of masses, calcifications, areas of architectural distortion, and asymmetric densities. Skin thickening, trabecular thickening, and abnormally dense axillary lymph nodes should be noted along with an assessment of overall parenchymal density. The sensitivity of mammography is related to the parenchymal density of the breast. Nearly all masses and groups of calcifications will be identified in breasts with fatty parenchyma, while extremely dense breast tissue may obscure some masses and make microcalcifications appear less conspicuous *(15)*. Furthermore, the availability of expert mammographers is limited, and some vague masses or subtle areas of architectural distortion may not be identified by inexperienced breast imagers.

Posttreatment mammograms are assessed for the presence of residual cancer. Helvie et al. *(16)* demonstrated that mammography was more sensitive than physical examination in predicting evidence of residual carcinoma after chemotherapy. Mammography is more accurate than sonography in identifying calcifications and in determining the extent of calcifications. Chemotherapy-induced fibrosis may limit mammographic interpretation. It may be difficult to determine what proportion of a residual mass is due to viable tumor vs treatment-induced fibrosis *(14,15,17)*. Mammographic measurements may not be accurate for spiculated or poorly outlined tumors and lesions arising in dense breast parenchyma or fibrocystic tissue *(18)*.

ULTRASOUND

Ultrasound images structures with high frequency sound waves (5–13 mHz) that are reflected, scattered, absorbed, or transmitted through the breast tissues *(18)*. Sonographic measurements may be subjective, and ultrasound is operator-dependent. Furthermore, not all facilities have sonographers and sonologists skilled and experienced in breast ultrasound. Two independent observers may not agree on the borders between a tumor and normal tissue in an ill-defined malignant process. Also, irregular ductal extensions of tumor and small satellite lesions may be difficult to identify with sonography.

To minimize artifacts, ultrasound probes are held orthogonal to the overlying skin, and the longest dimensions of a tumor are measured *(18)*. Sonography is more accurate than palpation and/or mammography for measuring breast cancer size as a result of ultrasound's ability to accurately distinguish the boundaries of the mass from the adjacent peritumoral reaction. Sonography is a valuable tool for evaluating the malignant process in the breast as well as the regional (axillary, infraclavicular, supraclavicular, and internal mammary) lymph nodes.

NUCLEAR MEDICINE

Nuclear medicine techniques that may be used to assess treatment response in the breast include positron emission tomography (PET) and technetium 99m sestamibi imaging. By recording changes in tumor physiology, PET overcomes the limitations of purely anatomically based methods that monitor changes in tumor size. PET can offer a one-stop staging evaluation, and it is anticipated that PET will be validated as a reliable tool for distinguishing fibrosis from viable tumor. PET is limited by inferior spatial resolution capability compared with MRI or computed tomography and partial volume effects. In addition, malignant lesions display varying rates of metabolic activity. Thus, a slow-growing tumor may have little uptake on PET *(19,20)*.

Technetium 99m sestamibi is widely available, and sestamibi scans are less expensive than PET scans. Sestamibi scans are performed with standard gamma cameras, and a cyclotron is not required. The mechanism for increased sestamibi uptake in breast tumors is not well understood; theories include increased blood flow and increased mitochondrial activity. Sestamibi imaging lacks accuracy in demonstrating small (less than 1 cm) tumors, including small areas of residual malignancy after chemotherapy. A potential niche for sestamibi imaging is in identifying patients with multidrug resistance. Absent or reduced sestamibi uptake is suggestive of multidrug resistance *(21,22)*.

MAGNETIC RESONANCE IMAGING (MRI)

MRI of the breast is best accomplished with a dedicated breast phased array coil. High spatial and temporal resolution is important when imaging the breast, as kinetic and morphologic information is necessary for lesion characterization. With currently available MR scanners, spatial resolution of 1 mm is possible.

T1-weighted MR images provide excellent anatomic detail and help to define the morphologic features of breast cancers. For example, masses with irregular shapes and spiculated borders would be considered suspicious for malignancy, while masses with smooth, well-defined margins are likely to represent benign findings. T1-weighted spin echo sequences (TR 500 ms, TE 8 ms) are usually performed in orthogonal planes, typically in the sagittal and the axial projections. T2-weighted images may provide additional information, such as the presence of necrosis within a tumor. T2-weighted images (TR 3000–4000 ms, TE 85 ms) are usually obtained with fat saturation.

Dynamic MRI after intravenous gadolinium administration provides critical information regarding the vascularity of breast tumors. Gadolinium is injected as a rapid intravenous bolus. A three-dimensional volume fat spoiled gradient echo sequence is then performed to image the entire breast in 30 s or less to achieve optimal temporal resolution. Each slice of tissue is imaged over several time points after the administration of contrast material. Time intensity curves are then generated from the dynamic, contrast-enhanced series. Post-processing may be performed to obtain calculated maximal difference and slope images. The maximal difference images indicate the difference between the maximum pixel intensity and the minimum pixel intensity during the entire scan, thereby showing areas of tissue that enhance intensely with the contrast agent, as would be expected with malignant lesions. The slope images are obtained by calculating the slope of the increase in pixel intensity over the time course of the scan. The slope images show areas of tissue that demonstrate rapid enhancement, characteristic of malignant tumors (Fig. 2).

Several studies have shown that breast cancers enhance after gadolinium administration (Fig. 3) *(23)*. This enhancement is related to the preferential accumulation of gadolinium, which shortens T1 relaxation of water protons, and thereby results in increased signal on T1-weighted images. Tumor angiogenesis is defined as the induction of new blood vessels in response to specific mediators. The early signal enhancement typically seen with malignant lesions of the breast after the intravenous administration of gadolinium is likely related to increased or altered vascularity as a

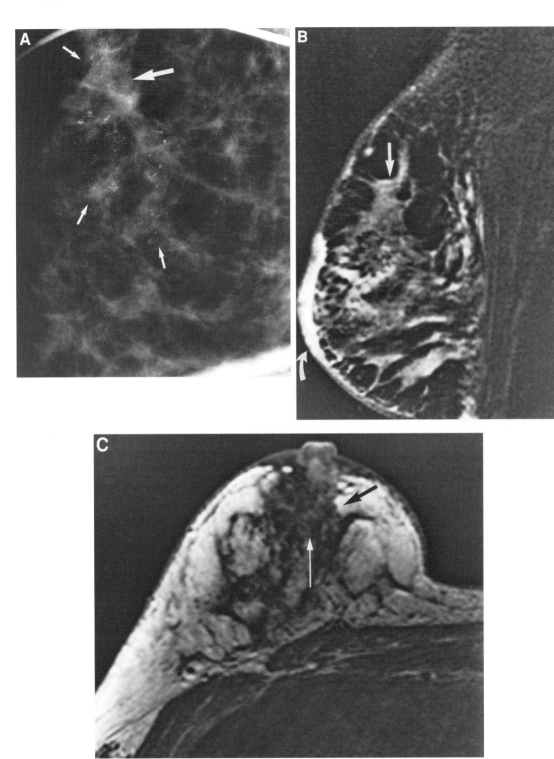

Fig. 2. Locally advanced invasive ductal carcinoma in a 38 yr-old woman. **(A)** The right lateromedial magnified mammogram shows an ill-defined mass (large arrow) and associated pleomorphic calcifications (small arrows) in the upper breast. The mass was palpable, and

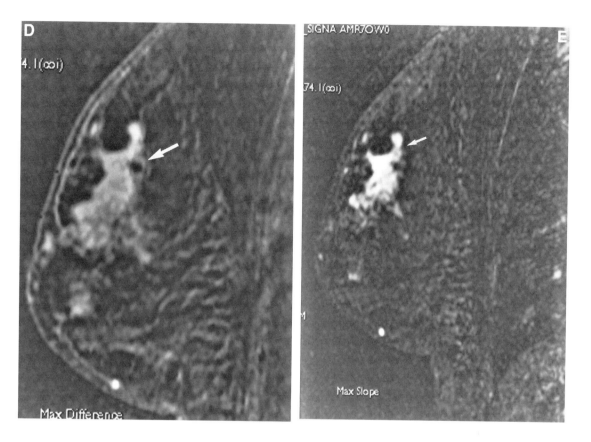

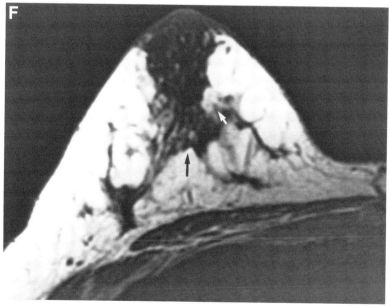

Fig. 2. *(continued)* biopsy revealed invasive ductal carcinoma. (**B**) T2-weighted sagittal MRI taken on the same day as the mammogram showed an ill-defined mass in the upper right breast (straight arrow), with associated skin thickening (curved arrow). (**C**) Axial T1-weighted MRI

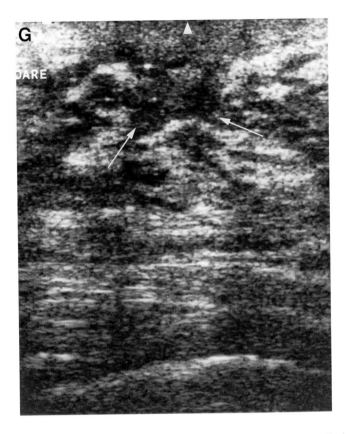

Fig. 2. *(continued)* of the right breast obtained after the intravenous administration of gadolinium shows a retroareolar mass (black arrow) with areas of enhancement (white arrow). (**D**)
Sagittal difference image shows the irregularly shaped mass (arrow) in the upper right breast.
(**E**) Sagittal slope image demonstrates the malignant mass (arrow) in the upper right breast. The
patient then began preoperative chemotherapy with paclitaxel, followed by 5-fluorouracil,
doxorubicin, and cyclophosphamide. (**F**) An axial T1-weighted MRI with intravenous gadolinium, obtained 15 mo after the initial MR examination, shows a decrease in the size of the
right breast mass (black arrow) with residual areas of enhancement noted (white arrow). (**G**)
Transverse right breast sonography performed 3 d after the MR examination revealed an ill-
defined hypoechoic mass (arrows), immediately posterior to the nipple (triangle). Seven days
later, the patient underwent right mastectomy and axillary dissection, revealing invasive ductal
carcinoma with vascular and lymphatic invasion. No tumor was present in the nipple or the
skin. No metastases were identified in 22 axillary lymph nodes.

result of tumor angiogenesis. The increase in T1 signal is proportional to the gadolinium concentration that is delivered to the tumor through these small vessels and to
the accumulated contrast in the interstitial spaces as contrast leaks into the interstitial
tissues. The reported sensitivity for the detection of cancers as small as a few millimeters in size is on the order of 95 to 100%. The difficulty with breast MR arises from the
low to moderate specificity for identifying cancer, ranging between 37 and 97%, as
benign breast lesions may also demonstrate enhancement patterns that cannot be distinguished from malignancy *(24)*.

Microvessel density counts in breast tumors have been evaluated as potential prognostic factors. Microvessel density counts may correlate with long-term survival rates and the risk of metastases in patients with breast cancer *(25)*. Pharmacokinetic studies after intravenous gadolinium are being performed in an attempt to analyze the enhancement behavior of tumors. It is known that microvessels associated with malignant tumors have increased permeability. Using MRI, tumor vascularity can be assessed with uptake curves, and vascular wash-in and wash-out can be analyzed to estimate intratumoral microvessel counts and density *(26)*. Continued research in this area is necessary to gain a greater understanding of changes in tumor vascularity after the initiation of chemotherapy.

Limitations of MRI include the limited availability of scanners and scan time, the need for the intravenous administration of gadolinium, the difficulty in imaging claustrophobic patients, and the lack of experience in breast MRI interpretation. In addition, the capability to perform MRI-guided needle localizations and/or core biopsies for lesions identified only on MRI (and not on mammography or sonography) is limited. Although MRI-guided needle localizations and core biopsies have been performed at several centers, these techniques are not readily available at all breast imaging or all MRI facilities *(27)*.

Davis and McCarty *(17)* noted that MRI could differentiate postchemotherapy residual tumor from fibrosis and glandular tissue. Rieber et al. *(28)* reported that MR demonstrated evidence of therapeutic response after the first or second cycle of chemotherapy with a high degree of accuracy. Abraham et al. *(29)* reported that MRI could be used early in the course of chemotherapy to offer breast conservation to more women without compromising local control or cosmesis.

FUTURE DIRECTIONS IN MRI OF THE BREAST

Magnetic resonance spectroscopy (MRS) is an established research tool for evaluating the metabolism of cancer cells. A spectrum of signals for specific elements can be obtained, and quantitative and qualitative analyses can be performed. MRS is noninvasive, and the metabolic milieu at the tumor site could be studied sequentially during chemotherapy. MRS has yielded valuable information on the effects of substrates and nutrients, drugs, hormones, and growth factors on breast cancer progression. MRS is still in the early stages of development, and further studies are needed to determine how this technique can be integrated into routine clinical practice *(30)*.

MRI-guided focused ultrasound ablation is a procedure in which breast cancer may be treated with heat, rather than surgical excision. MRI can be used to measure the ultrasound-induced temperature in the breast tissue and map the zone of ablation, as several MRI parameters are temperature dependent. The technical feasibility of this approach has been shown in a study in which fibroadenomas were treated with focused ultrasound energy *(31)*. Areas for potential improvement in MRI-guided focused ultrasound ablation include the development of techniques to map organ movement during therapy and the delivery of a sufficient dose of thermal energy throughout the targeted region in a minimum amount of time *(32)*.

In the future, MRI will assume a greater role in assessing response to preoperative chemotherapy. Although MRI units are not as plentiful as mammography units or

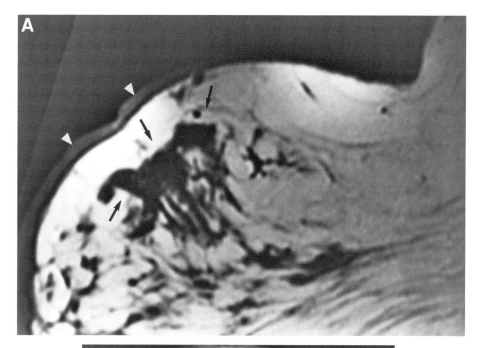

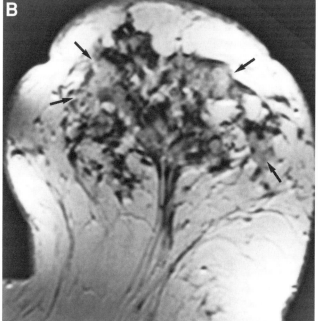

Fig. 3. Locally advanced multicentric invasive ductal carcinoma in a 59-yr-old woman. (**A**) T1-weighted sagittal MRI of the left breast demonstrates an irregular mass (arrows) in the upper breast and associated skin thickening (arrowheads). The mass was biopsied under sonographic guidance, revealing invasive ductal carcinoma. (**B**) T1-weighted axial MRI after the intravenous administration of gadolinium shows an ill-defined enhancing mass (arrows) in the upper central left breast. (**C**) Sagittal difference image shows the mass in the upper left breast (large arrow) along with several satellite lesions (small arrows) and associated skin thickening (arrowheads). Thereafter, the patient began preoperative chemotherapy with paclitaxel

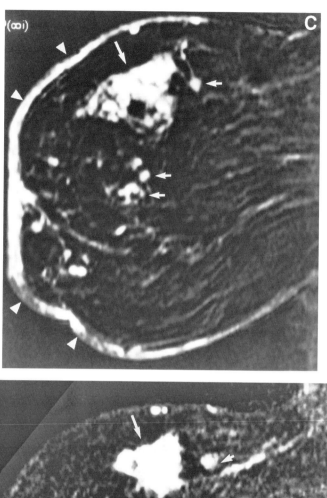

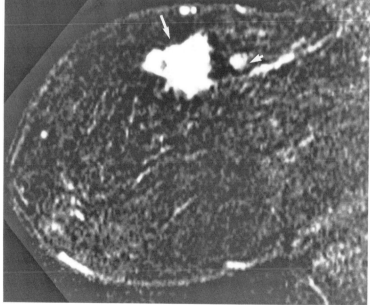

Fig. 3. *(continued)* followed by 5-fluorouracil, doxorubicin, and cyclophosphamide. (**D**) Sagittal difference image obtained 5 mo later demonstrates a decrease in the size of the mass (large arrow), a decrease in the number of satellite lesions (small arrow), and less skin thickening. (**E**) Sagittal left breast sonography performed on the same day as the MRI examination shows a hypoechoic mass in the 12 o'clock region, consistent with residual malignancy. Bilateral mastectomies and bilateral axillary dissections were performed 3 wk later. Pathology revealed invasive

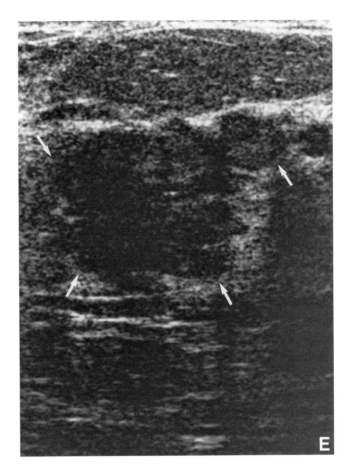

Fig. 3. *(continued)* ductal carcinoma in the left breast, with vascular and lymphatic invasion. Metastatic carcinoma was identified in 3 of 11 left axillary lymph nodes and in 1 of 7 right axillary lymph nodes. The patient underwent radiation therapy to the left chest wall and the left nodal regions. Five months after surgery, there was no evidence of residual or recurrent malignancy.

sonography units, it is thought that clinicians will become more reliant on MRI findings in evaluating women undergoing preoperative chemotherapy. Furthermore, MRI offers the potential to go beyond morphology and provide metabolic and/or functional information about the tumor.

ACKNOWLEDGMENTS

We thank Angela Lynch for secretarial assistance.

REFERENCES

1. Feig SA. Role and evaluation of mammography and other imaging methods for breast cancer detection, diagnosis, and staging. *Semin Nucl Med* 1999;29:3–15.
2. Whitman GJ. The role of mammography in breast cancer prevention. *Curr Opin Oncol* 1999;11:414–418.
3. Tabar L, Vitak B, Chen HH, Yen MF, Duffy SW, Smith RA. Beyond randomized con-

trolled trials: organized mammographic screening substantially reduces breast carcinoma mortality. *Cancer* 2001;91:1724–1731.

4. Kolb TM, Lichy J, Newhouse JH. Occult cancer in women with dense breasts: detection with screening US—diagnostic yield and tumor characteristics. *Radiology* 1998;207,191–199.

5. Meric F, Mirza NQ, Buzdar AU, et al. Prognostic implications of pathological lymph node status after preoperative chemotherapy for operable T3N0M0 breast cancer. *Ann Surg Oncol* 2000;7, 435–440.

6. Fisher B, Brown A, Mamounas E, et al. Effect of preoperative chemotherapy on local-regional disease in women with operable breast cancer: findings from National Surgical Adjuvant Breast and Bowel Project B-18. *J Clin Oncol* 1997;15:2483–2493.

7. Schwartz GF, Birchansky CA, Komarnicky LT, et al. Induction chemotherapy followed by breast conservation for locally advanced carcinoma of the breast. *Cancer* 1994;73:362–369.

8. Kling KM, Ostrzega N, Schmit P. Breast conservation after induction chemotherapy for locally advanced breast cancer. *Am Surg* 1997;63:861–864.

9. Bonadonna G, Valagussa P, Brambilla C, et al. Primary chemotherapy in operable breast cancer: eight-year experience at the Milan Cancer Institute. *J Clin Oncol* 1998;16:93–100.

10. Kuerer HM, Sahin AA, Hunt KK, et al. Incidence and impact of documented eradication of breast cancer axillary lymph node metastases before surgery in patients treated with neoadjuvant chemotherapy. *Ann Surg* 1999;230:72–78.

11. Reynolds HE, Lesnefsky MH, Jackson VP. Tumor marking before primary chemotherapy for breast cancer. *AJR Am J Roentgenol* 1999;173:919–920.

12. Rosen EL, Vo TT. Metallic clip deployment during stereotactic breast biopsy: retrospective analysis. *Radiology* 2001;218:510–516.

13. Edeiken BS, Fornage BD, Bedi DG, et al. US-guided implantation of metallic markers for permanent localization of the tumor bed in patients with breast cancer who undergo preoperative chemotherapy. *Radiology* 1999;213:895–900.

14. Segel MC, Paulus DD, Hortobagyi GN. Advanced primary breast cancer: assessment at mammography of response to induction chemotherapy. *Radiology* 1988;169:49–54.

15. Weatherall PT, Evans GF, Metzger GJ, Saborrian MH, Leitch AM. MRI vs. histologic measurement of breast cancer following chemotherapy: comparison with x-ray mammography and palpation. *J Magn Reson Imaging* 2001;13:868–875.

16. Helvie MA, Joynt LK, Cody RL, Pierce LJ, Adler DD, Merajver SD. Locally advanced breast carcinoma: accuracy of mammography vs clinical examination in the prediction of residual disease after chemotherapy. *Radiology* 1996;198:327–332.

17. Davis PL, McCarty SK Jr. Technologic considerations for breast tumor size assessment. *Magn Reson Imaging Clin N Am* 1994;2:623–631.

18. Tresserra F, Feu J, Grases PJ, Navarro B, Alegret X, Fernandez-Cid A. Assessment of breast cancer size: sonographic and pathologic correlation. *J Clin Ultrasound* 1999;27:485–491.

19. Avril N, Rose CA, Schelling M, et al. Breast imaging with positron emission tomography and fluorine-18 fluorodeoxyglucose: use and limitations. *J Clin Oncol* 2000:18:3495–3502.

20. Wahl RL. Current status of PET in breast cancer imaging, staging, and therapy. *Semin Roentgenol* 2001;36:250–260.

21. Kabasakal L, Ozker K, Hayward M, et al. Technetium-99m sestamibi uptake in human breast carcinoma cell lines displaying glutathione-associated drug-resistance. *Eur J Nucl Med* 1996;23:568–570.

22. Mankoff DA, Dunnwald LK, Gralow JR, Ellis GK, Drucker MJ, Livingston RB. Monitoring the response of patients with locally advanced breast carcinoma to neoadjuvant chemotherapy using [technetium 99m]-sestamibi scintimammography. *Cancer* 1999;85:2410–2423.

23. Heywang SH, Hahn D, Schmidt H, et al. MR imaging of the breast using gadolinium-DTPA. *J Comput Assist Tomogr* 1986;10:199–204.

24. Hylton NM. Vascularity assessment of breast lesions with gadolinium-enhanced MR imaging. *Magn Reson Imaging Clin N Am* 2001;9:321–331.
25. Weidner N, Folkman J, Pozza F, et al. Tumor angiogenesis: a new significant and independent prognostic indicator in early state breast cancer. *J Natl Cancer Inst* 1992;84:1875–1886.
26. Buadu LD, Murakami J, Murayama S, et al. Breast lesions: correlation of contrast medium enhancement patterns on MR images with histopathologic findings and tumor angiogenesis. *Radiology* 1996;200:639–649.
27. Daniel BL, Birdwell RL, Butts K, et al. Freehand iMRI-guided large-gauge core needle biopsy: a new minimally invasive technique for diagnosis of enhancing breast lesions. *J Magn Reson Imaging* 2001;13:896–902.
28. Rieber A, Zeitler H, Rosenthal H, et al. MRI of breast cancer: influence of chemotherapy on sensitivity. *Br J Radiol* 1997;70:452–458.
29. Abraham DC, Jones RC, Jones SE, et al. Evaluation of neoadjuvant chemotherapeutic response of locally advanced breast cancer by magnetic resonance imaging. *Cancer* 1996;78:91–100.
30. Kaplan O, Cohen JS. Metabolism of breast cancer cells as revealed by non-invasive magnetic resonance spectroscopy studies. *Breast Cancer Res Treat* 1994;31:285–299.
31. Hynynen K, Pomeroy O, Smith DN, et al. MR imaging-guided focused ultrasound surgery of fibroadenomas in the breast: a feasibility study. *Radiology* 2001;219:176–185.
32. Huber PE, Jenne JW, Rastert R, et al. A new noninvasive approach to breast cancer therapy using magnetic resonance imaging-guided focused ultrasound surgery. *Cancer Res* 2001;61:8441–8447.

11

Image-Guided Thermal Therapy for Prostate Cancer

Mark D. Hurwitz, MD

BACKGROUND AND RATIONALE

Prostate Cancer

Prostate cancer is the most commonly diagnosed noncutaneous malignancy in the American male population. Since the advent of prostate-specific antigen (PSA) screening, an increasing number of men are diagnosed with potentially curable prostate cancer. The PSA era has led to new predicaments, however, with an increasing number of asymptomatic men with low-risk organ confined disease diagnosed with prostate cancer as a result of a PSA test leading to biopsy. In this population, often difficult choices must be made between radical prostatectomy, external beam radiation, or brachytherapy. Each of these modalities is associated with significant risk of complications for what is typically an asymptomatic and often indolent disease. In men with locally advanced disease, another dilemma arises in regard to maximizing local control in the setting of greater tumor burden and more aggressive biologic behavior.

Current strategies to maximize local control include prostatectomy, radiation dose escalation with either external beam or brachytherapy, or addition of androgen suppression to radiation therapy. Both surgery and radiotherapeutic approaches offer satisfactory outcomes in the low-risk patient but may represent overtreatment if tumor within the prostate could be better localized and targeted for eradication. In a higher-risk population, treatments that address the prostate alone, such as prostatectomy or brachytherapy, may lead to undertreatment of disease with local extension outside of the prostate. Thermal therapy is a strategy with the potential to optimize tumor ablation with minimal impact on quality of life. The term thermal therapy encompasses both hyperthermia, which is the use of mild heating used to enhance the effects of radiation or chemotherapy, and ablation, which is the direct use of high-temperature heating to destroy tissue. In the low-risk patient, thermal ablation may eventually become a primary treatment option, whereas in the higher-risk patient, thermal therapy can be used in combination with additional local and systemic therapies to eradicate tumor.

Hyperthermia

The use of heat in the treatment of malignancies dates back to Hippocrates. In the 19th century, Busch noted the regression of a sarcoma in a patient with erysipelas suffering from high fever (1). Subsequently, Coley described the repeated injection of

From: *Image-Guided Diagnosis and Treatment of Cancer*
Edited by: A. D'Amico, J. S. Loeffler, and J. R. Harris © Humana Press Inc., Totowa, NJ

erysipelas in the treatment of malignancy *(2)*. The use of these bacterial pyrogens, or "Coley's toxins," in the treatment of tumors gained notoriety near the turn of the 20th century. Later work by Westermark *(3)* and Warren *(4)* also suggested a role for heat in the treatment of advanced malignancies.

Thermal therapy may involve both ablative and hyperthermic temperatures. The rationale for use of heat to achieve tissue ablation is readily apparent. Malignant tissue can be destroyed by being heated at high temperatures. Optimal integration of hyperthermia in treatment of malignancies involves a more thorough appreciation for the biology of the cancer cell and the physiology of the tumor microenvironment. Hyperthermia has potential advantageous interplay with both radiation and chemotherapeutic agents. In the treatment of prostate cancer, however, the focus has been on the combination of hyperthermia with radiation. Combination of these two modalities may have complimentary, sensitizing, and synergistic effects. Hyperthermia and radiation are complementary modalities in regard to tumor cell sensitivity to each agent at various points in the cell cycle as well as based on physiologic state. For example, maximum radiation resistance occurs when cells are in late S phase, when they are most sensitive to hyperthermia *(5)*. Likewise, hypoxia, a condition associated with radiation resistance with accompanied low pH and nutritional depletion, is associated with enhanced susceptibility to hyperthermia *(6–8)*. A sensitizing effect may occur via a hyperthermia-induced increase in vascular perfusion, leading to enhanced oxygenation of tumor and greater cell kill when radiation is administered after hyperthermia. Synergism may occur through enhanced induction of apoptosis *(9,10)*.

Hyperthermia has been shown to increase local control, disease-free survival, and overall survival for a variety of malignancies in phase III trials *(11–14)*. The treatment of deep-seated malignancies has proven a greater challenge than treatment of relatively superficial malignancies. A recent report of increased overall survival of patients with locally advanced cervical cancer receiving hyperthermia in a phase III trial, however, indicates that adjuvant hyperthermia can provide a significant benefit to patients with pelvic malignancies *(14)*. With recent literature indicating that radiation dose escalation improves biochemical disease-free survival in prostate cancer *(15–17)*, the complex interplay of hyperthermia and radiation may result in enhanced tumor control without concern for increased radiation related toxicity and have anti-tumor effects beyond radiation induced mechanisms alone. Broad-reaching effects might also be possible through a link between hyperthermia and immune modulation noted both in the laboratory and clinical settings *(18–25)*. Given the central role of heat shock proteins in regulation of cell-mediated immunity, hyperthermia has the potential to effect systemic mechanisms potentially beneficial to the cancer patient at risk for harboring micrometastases *(26,27)*.

Thermal Ablation

Thermal ablation, also referred to as thermal surgery, is a noninvasive or minimally invasive therapeutic approach that is gaining acceptance in treating several types of malignancies. Significant advantages of thermal ablation over surgery may include use of sedation or local anesthesia as opposed to general anesthesia, minimization of patient discomfort, reduced recovery time, decreased risk of complications, and decreased cost.

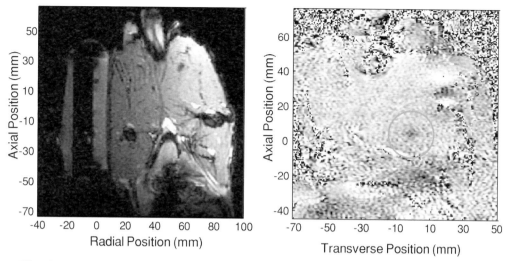

Fig. 1. Example of high-resolution MR thermometry in vivo. The ultrasound probe is positioned to the left of the rabbit muscle in the left figure generated by MRI. A small, less than 1-cm focus of temperature elevation is shown in the right figure (Courtesy of Kullervo Hynynen, Brigham and Women's Hospital, Boston, MA.)

Invasive approaches for thermal ablation include interstitial placement of radiofrequency catheters *(28,29)*, microwave antennae *(30)*, laser fiber *(31,32)*, or thermoconductive seeds *(33)*. Focused ultrasound can be used in a completely noninvasive manner or through a minimally invasive intracavitary approach *(34–41)*. Ultrasound is an attractive modality for thermal ablation because the energy can be deposited into the target in a precise and modifiable manner. Effects of thermal conduction and vascular perfusion can be minimized through use of short sonication times. Short duration, high temperature pulses also result in minimal transfer of thermal energy to surrounding tissues *(42,43)*. A key limitation, however, of ultrasonic energy delivery is the inability to treat through bone or gas. Intracavitary placement of the focused ultrasound applicator, such as intrarectal placement for treatment of prostate cancer can overcome this potential problem and places the target organ in immediate proximity to the applicator

Use of ultrasound allows for a degree of controllable power deposition not possible with use of other methods *(44)*. Another advantage of ultrasound is the short wavelengths at frequencies that can penetrate deep in tissues. Thereby, well-collimated and focused beams can be generated and, from a technical standpoint, transducers can be constructed with minimal size and shape limitations. Although to date clinical studies of use of ultrasound applicators typically have been performed under diagnostic ultrasound guidance, this technique is amenable to magnetic resonance (MR) guidance and also non;invasive MR thermometer (Fig. 1).

Image-Guided Therapy

Image guidance may play a role in several aspects of thermal therapy, including target definition, monitoring of temperature, blood flow, or tumor oxygenation, and ultimately in automated feedback protocols allowing for treatment modification based on real-time data. The need for improved tumor definition has become increasingly important as the ability to focally ablate cancerous areas within the prostate has become possible. Although whole-organ ablation remains an option, the technical challenges of assuring destruction of the prostate without damage to the urethra, bladder, and rectum remain formidable. Improved definition of macroscopic and even microscopic disease through existing and emerging imaging technologies such as optical coherence tomography will complement the technical developments in delivery of ablative energy *(45)*.

Current imaging technologies, including MR, are also being studied as means to monitor treatment. Methods now in widespread use for treatment monitoring leave much to be desired. Thermometry is a fundamental aspect of thermal-treatment monitoring. Temperature within target and normal tissues is now typically monitored by interstitial placement of one or a few thermocouple probes into the tissues of interest. Although multiple thermocouples can be placed along a single probe, even when multiple probes are placed, the resultant temperature profile is merely a sampling of the true overall profile. Inconsistencies in equating thermal profiles with treatment outcomes have been noted in some clinical trials *(14)*, and difficulty in defining predictive thermal parameters likely arise at least in part to thermal sampling error. Another major disadvantage to invasive thermal monitoring is the potential for complications. In fact, several investigators have noted the principal complications with thermal therapy have been related to invasive thermometry as opposed to the treatment itself *(46,47)*. MR thermometry is now evolving as an approach to temperature profiling that will provide for the first time a complete thermal map of treatment in progress in a completely noninvasive manner. Last, once the challenges of target definition and treatment monitoring have been met, advanced treatment delivery mechanisms, perhaps best described as real-time intensity modulated thermal therapy, will be possible.

CLINICAL EXPERIENCE

Hyperthermia

The most widely studied approach to hyperthermia in the treatment of prostate cancer is use of external devices for regional hyperthermia. This strategy is attractive in that it is noninvasive. The limitations on selective deposition of energy into the prostate vs surrounding tissues and organs, however, have been associated with suboptimal patient tolerance and effective prostatic heating. Newer, commercially available phased array devices with enhanced power deposition capabilities and treatment planning algorithms, however, offer more effective thermal targeting and can be MR compatible, allowing for treatment monitoring. A prototype open MR treatment monitoring system is now in commercial development for use with a noninvasive phased array radiofreqency (RF) system (Fig. 2).

Researchers at Duke University reported the results of a phase I/II study of external regional hyperthermia using an RF phased array in combination with radiation therapy for prostate cancer. Hyperthermia was administered after radiation therapy once or twice per week. Intraprostatic thermometry was performed at least once in all patients. Radiation doses were 65 to 70 Gy. In an update of this trial after treatment of 30 patients, patient tolerance was the limiting factor in a majority of hyperthermia sessions. The goal of achieving tumor temperature of greater than or equal to 42.5°C at all measured

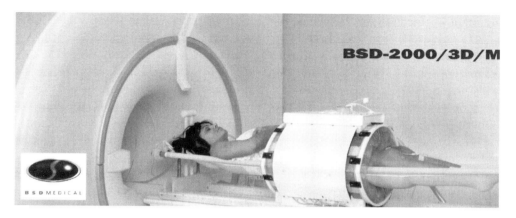

Fig. 2. Integrated RF hyperthermia treatment unit with MR treatment monitoring system The treatment unit is designed to be accomadated within the bore of a standard MRI unit used to monitor temperature and perfusion during treatment. (Courtesy of BSD Medical, Salt Lake City, UT.)

points was achieved in only one treatment and mean CEM T_{90} 43°C, or cumulative equivalent minutes of heating to 43°C as measured by 90% of monitored temperature points within the prostate, was 2.34 min. Twenty one patients, including 18 with newly diagnosed T3 or T4 disease with a pretreatment mean PSA of 69 ng/mL and three with locally recurrent disease, had 36-mo disease-free survival of 25%, which the authors noted compared favorably with historical controls *(48)*.

Stawarz and colleagues *(27)* reported on use of regional hyperthermia in 53 patients with recurrent genitourinary cancer, including 20 patients treated for recurrent prostate cancer. Patients typically received radiation therapy. Complete and partial response was seen most often in patients with prostate or kidney cancer as opposed to other genitourinary malignancies. Treatment was well tolerated.

Interstitial prostate hyperthermia, while invasive and technically demanding, is a site-specific strategy for heat delivery. Similar to radiation dose deposition, "conformal hyperthermia" may be possible with techniques now employed in the performance of interstitial brachytherapy. Stanford University researchers introduced the concept of providing a brachytherapy boost in combination with microwave hyperthermia for the treatment of locally advanced or recurrent prostate cancer *(49)*. A total of 36 patients, including five with locally recurrent prostate cancer after external beam radiation and 31 patients with previously untreated stage B (15 patients) or stage C (16 patients) prostate cancer, received 50 Gy of pelvic radiation followed by an Ir192 interstitial boost with hyperthermia given immediately before and at the completion of the brachytherapy. Treatment was well tolerated with few acute side effects. To date, patient outcomes have not been reported. The authors concluded that interstitial radiofrequency hyperthermia is feasible and that further technical developments were warranted.

A second approach to interstitial hyperthermia is the permanent placement of the hyperthermia source within the prostate in a similar manner to placement of radioactive sources with standard brachytherapy techniques. A system using ferromagnetic

seeds for inductive hyperthermia is currently undergoing early human trials. When
introduced into a magnetic field the seeds are heated to a predetermined temperature
based on their compositional characteristics. In this way, either temperatures sufficient
for hyperthermia or ablation may be achieved.

The transrectal approach to site-specific hyperthermia in an attractive strategy for
prostate cancer treatment. Although not as invasive as interstitial techniques, it nevertheless allows for specific organ targeting. Transrectal technique allows for placement
of the hyperthermia source in close proximity to the prostate including a majority of
the peripheral zone. In the early 1980s, two reports on the use of transrectal microwave
hyperthermia alone in the treatment of patients with locally advanced prostate cancer
suggested good palliative effect and patient tolerance with minimal morbidity *(50,51)*.
Subsequently, in a report of 44 patients with advanced symptomatic disease, researchers at Tel Aviv University found that transrectal microwave hyperthermia provided
palliation of symptoms in a majority of cases *(26)*. Among 11 patients who underwent
subsequent biopsy, nine were negative for malignancy. Only two patients experienced
disease progression with follow-up out to 4 yr, despite the presence of advanced local
disease. Similarly, encouraging palliation was also reported by Stawarz and colleagues
(27) in a series with 15 patients with moderate-to-severe symptoms of progressive prostate cancer refractive to hormonal therapy. Improvement in quality of life was reported
by 73% of patients. The treatment was well tolerated by all patients, with no significant
morbidity.

Transrectal ultrasound hyperthermia is another strategy under investigation. A phase
II study at the Dana-Farber Cancer Institute has recently been completed. In this trial,
an applicator with 16 individually controllable transducer units was used allowing for
targeted heating with fine adjustment capability. All patients underwent multipoint
interstitial thermometry with thermometry probes placed in the prostate under biplanar
diagnostic ultrasound guidance. An initial report of toxicity and patient tolerability in
the first nine patients on study confirmed the findings of a previous phase I study that
the procedure was well tolerated with minimal toxicity *(52–54)*. A more recent assessment of 30 patients has affirmed this conclusion. Temperature data obtained to date
indicate that meaningful hyperthermia can be achieved with the transrectal ultrasound
(TRUS) system used in this study. The mean CEM T_{90} 43°C for the initial 35 patients
was 8.1 min. When assessed by allowable rectal wall temperature, those with a rectal
wall maximum of less than or equal to 40°C had a mean CEM T_{90} 43°C of 5.6 vs 11.2
for patients with an allowable rectal wall temperature greater than 40°C.

Thermal Ablation

The greatest experience with the use of thermal therapy for prostate disease is for
benign prostatic hypertrophy where the aim is to coagulate the prostate tissue around
the urethra. Transurethral microwave hyperthermia has been the most widely used
modality for this indication *(55,56)*, although alternative methods including focused
ultrasound have been used *(57,58)*.

The use of thermal ablation in the treatment of prostate cancer to date is relatively
limited. Strategies explored include interstitial microwave hyperthermia, MR heatable
implanted rods, and high-intensity focused ultrasound (HIFU) therapy. Building upon
their experience with the use of RF thermal ablation for benign prostatic hypertrophy

for which this modality was found to be safe and effective *(59)*, Marberger et al. explored the use of this modality in 14 patients with prostate cancer scheduled to undergo subsequent radical prostatectomy either immediately afterwards (eight patients) or 1 wk later (six patients).

In addition a single patient received RF ablation alone. Both monopolar and bipolar techniques were used. Although the maximum temperature at the active tip of the electrodes was 106°C, when interstitial thermometry was performed the temperature at the posterior prostatic capsule did not exceed 38°C. For all patients the postoperative course was uneventful, and no long-term toxicities were noted. One important limitation noted by the authors was that RF energy can interfere with TRUS imaging, thereby detracting from visualization of the target tissue. Follow-up pathologic assessment confirmed that the ultrasonographic images obtained at the time of the procedure did not correlate accurately with the true thermal lesion. Although other imaging techniques, including MRI, were not assessed, it was concluded that TRUS was inadequate for treatment monitoring *(60)*.

HIFU is the most widely used approach for ablation used to date and the one most amenable to image guidance. The initial study of HIFU for prostate cancer ablation was also performed by Marberger et al. *(61)*. In the initial series, 19 patients with prostate cancer scheduled to undergo radical prostatectomy received HIFU treatment directed at the midline of the prostate irrespective of tumor location to evaluate the impact of various focal lengths and input power levels on the extent of coagulative necrosis. Furthermore, the influence of tissue composition was also evaluated. A second series of 10 patients with unilateral T2a or T2b prostate cancer (fourth edition American Joint Committee on Cancer [AJCC] criteria) with clearly visible hypoechoic areas on ultrasound underwent HIFU ablation of these regions followed by radical prostatectomy.

No technical problems were encountered during HIFU treatment, and the procedure was successfully completed in all 29 cases. At the time of surgery, no gross changes of the prostate capsule or surrounding structures was noted, including the rectal wall, neurovascular bundle, and tissues in the immediate vicinity of the focal zone targeted for ablation. Histologic assessment revealed a zone of sharply delineated intraprostatic coagulative necrosis in all patients. The composition of tissue in the targeted area, either benign or malignant, had no major impact on lesion volume or location. Proctoscopy was routinely performed after transrectal HIFU and consistently revealed an intact rectal wall without signs of mechanical or heat damage. With follow-up exceeding 12 mo in the initial patients on study, no thermal therapy related toxicities were observed.

Although no thermometry was performed in these studies, prior to initiation of treatment, six patients undergoing transrectal HIFU for benign prostatic hypertrophy were enrolled in a thermometry study. Thermocouples were placed with the condom covering the HIFU transducer to measure water temperature, outside the condom in contact with the rectal wall within the HIFU beam path, and inside the prostate at three different sites within the treatment area. During treatment the rectal wall temperature increased to a mean of 39°C. A rise above 45°C was only recorded once with a temperature of 47°C reached for about 5 s. Maximum intraprostatic temperatures ranged from 55.7 to 98.6°C with a mean of 75°C. The heat profile was distinct and dropped sharply outside the focal area in fractions of a second *(62)*.

In the 10 patients in whom TRUS defined lesions were targeted, aiming accuracy was generally satisfactory. In all cases, the TRUS-defined lesions were targeted correctly. In three cases the entire prostate cancer was destroyed whereas in the other seven cases a mean of 53% of tumor was eradicated with a range of 37–78%. A note was made that because there was limited time allowed for thermal ablation as prostatectomy was performed immediately after during the same anesthesia administration, a greater percentage of tumor eradication may have been achieved in some patients if more time was allowed for multiple sonications. Mean tumor volume was 30 mL, and the mean HIFU–lesion volume was 32 mL. In eight, cases a single HIFU-lesion was created whereas in two patients, two adjacent lesions were created, allowing for a cross-section of necrosis of 4.5 cm². The maximum length of the HIFU treatment zone with the device used was 4 cm, allowing for ablation of approx 15 to 20 mL of prostate tissue over 90 to 120 min.

In a study reported by Gelet et al. *(63)*, 50 patients were treated with an average of 24 mo follow-up time. These patients also received radiation therapy. From among these patients, 56% were cancer free (biopsy and PSA) at the follow up. The treatment had 50% complication rate with the first device and a 17% rate with a second generation system that had safety features added. In both of these cancer studies, the treatment time was relatively long as a result of the multiple sonications required to cover the target volume. A subsequent report of 102 patients with T1–T2 disease yielded a 66% freedom from failure rate with median follow-up of 19 mo. Failure was defined by either a positive post-treatment biopsy or three consecutive increases in PSA from nadir *(64)*. At this early point in follow-up patients with PSA less than or equal to 10 (76 vs 50%), Gleason less than or equal to 6 (81 vs. 46%), and sextant biopsy with 1–4 involved cores (68 vs 40%) did significantly better in terms of freedom from failure then patients with adverse risk factors *(64)*.

There are several limitations to HIFU devices used in clinical trials now being addressed. Based on extensive experience with high power sonications of tissues in animal models and in humans *(65–69)*, the temperature elevation induced by ultrasound exposures varies significantly from location to location and adequate tissue coagulation cannot be assured by predetermined power settings. Variability seen in the clinical treatments may potentially be reduced or completely eliminated by real-time noninvasive temperature monitoring. In addition, the single focus transducers used thus far provide a grossly suboptimal heating field for tissue coagulation *(70)* because untreated tissue can be left between sonication locations when the induced temperature distribution is not as high as expected. In addition, the coagulated tissue volume per sonication is small resulting in long procedure times that may be impractical from a clinical standpoint.

Both of these issues can be addressed by using phased arrays. Hynynen and colleagues *(67–69)* have shown that by using a linear transrectal array, the optimal power deposition can be induced to coagulate much larger tissue volumes in a single sonication.

The thermal exposure can be more evenly distributed throughout the exposed volume reducing the risk to unexposed tissues. These optimal power depositions can coagulate the whole prostate within 30 to 60 min. An initial trial for prostate cancer patients utilizing a 62 element transrectal focused array is now in development at the Dana-Farber Brigham and Women's Cancer Institute (Fig. 3).

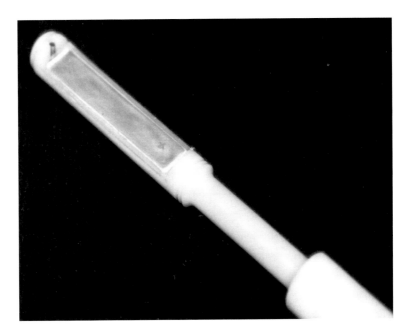

Fig. 3. Prototype transrectal focused ultrasound probe capable of delivering heat for tissue ablation or traditional moderate temperature hyperthermia. (Courtesy of Kullervo Hynynen, Brigham and Women's Hospital, Boston, MA.)

Image-Guided Therapy

Image guidance for therapy has important implications for both hyperthermia and ablation. Although tumor delineation is of greatest importance for ablative procedures and detailed thermal profiles of greatest importance in administration of hyperthermia, both aspects of image guidance are key to provision of optimal thermal therapy regardless of strategy. Presently most hyperthermic procedures and even many ablative procedures are done with no or minimal image guidance. Application of existing and emerging technologies to guide thermal therapy, however, is an active area of research.

Tumor Targeting

Although several techniques, including TRUS, have been used for tumor definition and targeting, magnetic resonance tissue characterization may be the most useful modality to guide thermal therapy of the prostate. To optimize the potential advantage of focused ultrasound tumor obliteration, accurate delineation of cancerous areas of the prostate from noncancerous areas is important. However, a high degree of sensitivity aids in the assurance that regions of greatest tumor burden are identified for obliteration. Improving specificity, however, especially in relation to areas in proximity to the rectum and urethra is desirable in minimizing potential treatment toxicity.

Diagnostic MRI is a noninvasive imaging technique for the detection of focal abnormalities in the prostate gland with sensitivity and specificity each in the range of 60–65%. It is primarily used for staging patients with clinically localized prostate cancer. MRI can clearly depict not only the prostate itself but also its substructure, including the peripheral zone, and on T2-weighted images identify nodules in the peripheral zone. At Brigham and Women's Hospital, an open interventional MRI unit is now being used to perform MRI-guided biopsies *(71)*. This allows for the histologic validation of tumor defined by MRI or other imaging modalities. This information can then be used to guide thermal therapeutic procedures.

Thermometry

There is presently great interest in the hyperthermia community for bringing noninvasive MR thermometry into everyday clinical practice. The concept of noninvasive temperature monitoring has been a topic of research for over 20 yr. Besides MR, computed tomography *(72,73)*, microwave radiometry *(74)*, electrical impedance *(75)*, and ultrasound *(76–79)* have shown promise, but have not yet been developed to a point where they can be used in clinical treatments. Presently, MRI thermometry is the only method that has a significant body of in vivo experiments and now clinical human experience quantifying its performance.

The challenges posed in monitoring lengthy treatments with mild temperature elevations are formidable. As opposed to thermal ablation where very large temperature elevations are induced for brief time periods, issues of accurate temperature definition and patient motion are of greater importance with hyperthermia. If the goal of treatment is ablation that can be achieved at 80°C within approx 1 s, accuracy in temperature definition of 2°C is clinically insignificant. Under 43°C every degree decrease in temperature results in a requirement of four times the length of treatment to achieve an equivalent thermal effect as defined by Sapareto and Dewey *(80)*. Therefore, precision of tenths of degree Celsius may be necessary to guide treatment. Patient and organ motion also become issues in regard to image registration over the time course necessary for hyperthermia that typically ranges between 30 and 90 min.

MR thermometry methods can use the temperature dependence of several physical properties from which the spatial distribution can be visualized. Three tissue properties have been used for this purpose: spin-lattice decay time (T1) *(81,82)*; molecular diffusion of water molecules *(83,84)*; and proton resonance frequency *(85,86)*. A recent study compared the different MR thermometry methods and found the proton resonant frequency shift to be the most sensitive and accurate for therapy monitoring *(87)*.

Changes in the PRF induced by temperature are related to variations in the molecular screening constant of the water molecules. This constant is linearly dependent on temperature *(88)* Results using 1H NMR spectroscopy with swine experiments showed an accuracy of ± 1°C regardless of the physiological changes in the tissue *(89)* Similarly, phase imaging has been used to measure in vivo tumor temperature in dogs *(90)* and in human muscle *(91)*, demonstrating the potential for hyperthermia temperature monitoring. Recent work with intracavitary phased arrays and a commercial noninvasive RF system in human subjects point towards the feasibility of this approach (Fig. 4). The rationale for thermal therapy has been evident for over two decades.

FUTURE DIRECTIONS

The integration of thermal therapy with image guided approaches to target definition and treatment monitoring provides the impetus for advancing this therapeutic strategy towards routine application in the management of prostate cancer. In moving towards this goal, the lessons of the past two decades are instructive. The biologic basis

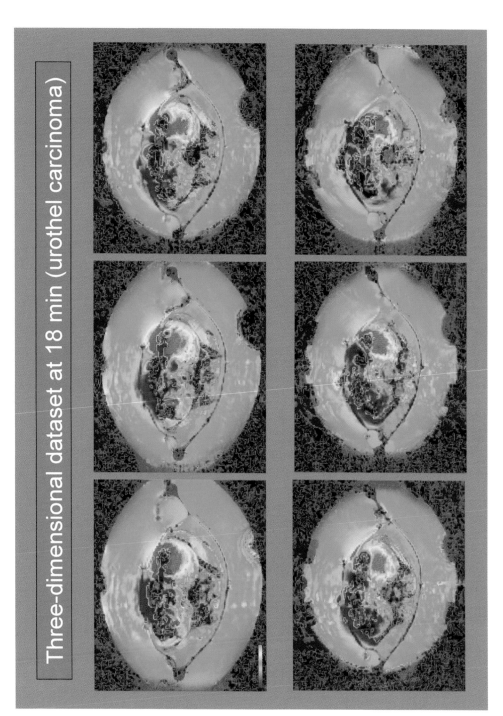

Fig. 4. Volume data set for the PRF temperature in an extended pelvic tumor (recurrence of an urethral carcinoma) after having reached thermal equilibrium (approx 1000 W forward power after 18 min.) Here, a series of artifacts can be seen. The PRF-temperature in the tumor is 5–10°C. (Courtesy of Peter Wust and Johanna Gellermann, Charite Hospital, Humboldt University, Berlin, Germany).

for incorporating hyperthermia with radiation or chemotherapy led to great enthusiasm for this modality in the 1980s. This enthusiasm was tempered, however, by the lag in development of treatment devices capable of delivering sufficient thermal energy to the target tissues with precision and lack of adequate methods and guidelines for treatment monitoring. Over the past decade, the growing use of PSA to detect prostate cancer earlier in its natural history has led to a greater dilemma about the impact of treatment on quality of life. This dilemma coupled with the growing economic pressures on medical care point to the need for new strategies to eradicate prostate cancer that are highly effective yet minimally invasive with a favorable side effect profile. Thermal therapy as applied to prostate cancer is still a way away from becoming a standard treatment option for prostate cancer. Yet, in applying the lessons of the past, both in designing technology and developing new biologically based strategies for application, thermal therapy may yet emerge as an attractive weapon against prostate cancer.

The growing appreciation for the underlying mechanisms of biologic response to heat stress and advances in bioengineering will further the goal of bringing thermal therapy to routine clinical use. Certainly biology plays the greatest role with traditional hyperthermia. Novel new strategies now in translation from the laboratory to the clinic, including heat shock protein response modifiers *(92)*, heat shock protein-based vaccines *(93)*, and thermally inducible gene therapy *(94)*, may play an important part in optimization of thermal therapy.

The greatest needs for thermal therapy, whether heat is used in combination with other therapies or for ablation, are in development of treatment delivery and monitoring systems. Improved tumor delineation is a vital first step in thermal therapy delivery. Moving beyond use of standard MRI, researchers at Brigham and Women's Hospital are assessing how novel magnetic resonance tissue characterization and postprocessing strategies may enhance routine MRI in guiding thermal therapy. These new MR techniques include spectroscopy *(95–101)*, water T2-mapping *(102–104)*, and line scan diffusion imaging *(105,106)*. Other imaging techniques, including immunoscintigraphy with 111-indium-capromab pendetide, also show promise *(107)*.

Once a tumor is identified, state-of-the-art treatment delivery systems are needed to deliver thermal therapy. Widely divergent approaches ranging from noninvasive RF systems to thermoconductive implantable seeds with curie points providing precisely defined temperature profiles likely have a role in the future of thermal therapy. In regards to image-guided therapies, a system that is MR compatible, minimally invasive, precise in energy deposition, capable of fine adjustment, and time efficient is ideal. At present, transrectal ultrasound is perhaps the best available solution for imaged-guided thermal therapy for prostate cancer. Advances in the ability to obtain complete temperature profiles should lead to advances in the understanding of thermal dosimetry. A more complete understanding of how thermal dosimetry equates with treatment outcome will lead to well defined goals for delivery of treatment that is on the one hand efficacious in tumor eradication while on the other hand respectful of normal tissue tolerances. Treatment monitoring should also lead to better understanding of the impact of physiologic mechanisms such as vascular perfusion on the temperature profile within the prostate. With well-defined treatment parameters, future treatment systems now in development allowing for real-time intensity modulated thermal therapy will be able to make automated adjustments to ensure that the therapeutic goals are achieved.

REFERENCES

1. Busch W. Uber den einfluss wlechen heftigere erysipelen zuweilen auf organsierte neubildungenambien. *Verh Naturh Preuss Rheinl* 1866;23:28.
2. Coley W. The treatment of malignant tumors by repeated inncoulations of erysipelas: with a report of 10 original cases. *Am J Med Sci* 1893;105:487.
3. Westermark F. Uber die behandlung des ulcerireneded cerixaccarcinomas. Mittle Kontstanter Warme. *Zentralbl Gynakol* 1898;22:1335.
4. Warren S. Preliminary study of the effect of artificial fever upon hopeless tumor cases. *Am J Roentgenol* 1935;33:75.
5. Westra A, Dewey WC. Variation in sensitivity to heat shock during the cell cycle of Chinese hamster cells in vitro. *Int J Radiat Biol* 1971;19:467–477
6. Dewey WC, Hopwood LE, Sapareto SA, et al. Cellular responses to combinations of hyperthermia and radiation. *Radiology* 1977;123:463.
7. Emami B, Song CW. (199Physiological mechanisms in hyperthermia: A review. *Int J Radiat Oncol Phys* 1984;10:289.
8. Gerweck LE, Steele EL. Metabolic indices for hyperthermia in cancer therapy, in *Biological, Physical, and Clinical Aspects of Hyperthermia*, Medical Physics Monograph No. 16 (Paliwal BR, Jelzel F. W., and Dewhirst NW, eds.). New York, American Association of Physicists in Medicine, 1988; p. 2.
9. Allan DJ, Harmon BV. The morphologic categorization of cell death induced by mild hyperthermia and comparison with death induced by ionizing radiation and cytotoxic drugs. *Scan Electron Microsc* 3:1121–1133.
10. Li WX Franklin WA. Radiation- and heat-induced apoptosis in PC-3 prostate cancer cells. *Radiat Res* 1998;150:190–194.
11. Valdagni R, Amichetti M. Report of long-term follow-up in a randomized trial comparing radiation therapy and radiation therapy plus hyperthermia to metastatic lymph nodes in stage IV head and neck patients *Int J Radiat Oncol Phys* 1994;28:163–169.
12. Vernon CC, Hand JW, Field SB, et al. Radiotherapy with or without hyperthermia in the treatment of superficial localized breast cancer: results from five randomized controlled trials. International Collaborative Hyperthermia Group. *Int J Radiat Oncol Phys* 1996;35, 731–744.
13. Overgaard J, Gonzalez Gonzalez D, et al. Hyperthermia as an adjuvant to radiation therapy of recurrent or metastatic malignant melanoma. A multicentre randomized trial by the European Society for Hyperthermic Oncology. *Int J Hyperthermia* 1996;12:3–20.
14. van der Zee J, Gonzalez Gonzalez D, van Rhoon GC, van Dijk JD, van Putten WL, Hart AA. Comparison of radiotherapy alone with radiotherapy plus hyperthermia in locally advanced pelvic tumours: a prospective, randomised, multicentre trial. Dutch Deep Hyperthermia Group. *Lancet* 2000;355:1119–1125.
15. Hanks GE, Hanlon AL, Schultheiss TE, Pinover WH, Movsas B, Epstein BE, Hunt MA. Dose escalation with 3D conformal treatment: five year outcomes, treatment optimization, and future directions *Int J Radiat Oncol Phys* 1998;41: 501–510.
16. Zelefsky MJ, Leibel SA, Gaudin PB, et al. Dose escalation with three-dimensional conformal radiation therapy affects the outcome in prostate cancer. *Int J Radiat Oncol Phys* 1998;41:491–500.
17. Pollack A, Zagars GK, Starkschall G, et al. Prostate cancer radiation dose response: Results of the M.D. Anderson phase randomized trial. *Int J Radiat Oncol Biol Phys* 2002;53(5):1097–1105.
18. Przepiorka D, Srivastava P. Heat shock protein-peptide complexes as immunotherapy for human cancer. *Mol Med Today* 1998;4:478–784.
19. Menoret A, Chandawarkar R. Heat-shock protein-based anticancer immunotherapy: an idea whose time has come. *Semin Oncol* 1998; 25:654–660.

20. Srivastava P, DeLeo A, Old L. Tumor rejection antigens of chemically induced sarcomas of inbred mice. *Proc Natl Acad Sci USA* 1986; 83:3407–3411.

21. Ullrich S, Robinson E. A mouse tumor-specific transplantation antigen is a heat shock-related protein. *Proc Natl Acad Sci USA* 1986;83:3121–3125.

22. Blachere N, Udono H, Janetzki S, et al. Heat shock protein vaccines against cancer. *J Immunother* 1993;14:352–356.

23. Udono S, Srivastava P. Heat shock protein 70-associated peptides elicit specific cancer immunity. *J Exp Med* 1993;178:1391–1396.

24. Udono S, Srivastava P. Comparison of tumor-specific immunogenicities of stress induced proteins gp96:hsp 90:and hsp 70. *J Immunol* 1994;152:5398–5403

25. Udano S. Levy D, Srivastava P. Cellular requirements for tumor-specific immunity elicited by heat shock proteins: tumor rejection antigen gp96 primes CD8+ T cells in vivo. *Proc Natl Acad Sci USA* 1994;91:3077–3081.

26. Sevadio C, Leib Z. Local hyperthermia for prostate cancer. *Urology* 1991;38:307–309.

27. Stawarz B, Zielinski H. Szmigielski S, et al. Transrectal hyperthermia as Palliative treatment for advanced adenocarcinoma of prostate and studies of cell-mediated immunity. *Urology* 1993;41:548–553.

28. Farahani K, Mischel PS, Black KL, De Salles AAF, Anzai Y, Lufkin B. Hyperacute thermal lesions: MR imaging evaluation of development in the brain *Radiology* 1995;196:517–520.

29. Neal DE. Evaluation and results of treatments for prostatism *Urol. Res.* 1994;22:61–66.

30. Sato M, Watanabe Y, Udeda S, et al. Microwave coagulation therapy for hepatocellular carcinoma. *Gastroenterology* 1996;110,1507–1514.

31. Vogl TJ, Mack MG. Percutaneous MR imaging-guided laser-induced thermotherapy of hepatic metastases. *Eur Radiol* 1997;7:1156.

32. Mumtaz H, Hall-Craggs MA, Wotherspoon A, et al. Laser therapy for breast cancer: MR imaging and histophatologic correlation. *Radiology* 1996;200:651–658.

33. Tucker RD, Huidobro C, Larson T, Platz CE. Use of permanent interstitial temperature self-regulating rods for ablation of prostate cancer. *J Endourol* 2000;14:511–517

34. Fry WJ, Barnard JW, Fry FJ, Krumins RF, Brennan JF. Ultrasonic lesions in the mammalian central nervous system. *Science* 1955;122:517–518.

35. Frizzell LA, Linke CA, Carstensen EL, Fridd CW. Thresholds for focal ultrasonic lesions in rabbit kidney, liver and testicle. *IEEE Trans Biomed Eng* 1977;24:393–396.

36. Lizzi FL. High-precision thermometry for small lesions. *Eur Urol* 1993;23(suppl. 1):23–28.

37. Coleman DJ, Lizzi FL, Driller J, et al. Therapeutic ultrasound in the treatment of glaucoma. *Ophthalmology* 1985;92:339–346.

38. Sanghvi NT, Hawes RH. High-intensity focused ultrasound. *Exp Invest. Endosc* 1994;4:383–395.

39. Cain CA, Umemura SA. Concentric-ring and sector vortex phased array applicators for ultrasound hyperthermia therapy. *IEEE Trans Microwave Theory Tech* 1986;34:542–551.

40. Ebbini ES, Cain CA. A spherical-section ultrasound phased array applicator for deep localized hyperthermia. *IEEE Trans Biomed Eng* 1991;38:634–643.

41. Bednarski MD, Lee JW, Callstrom MR, King CP. In vivo target-spesific delivery of macromolecular agents with MR-guided focused ultrasound. *Radiology* 1997;204:263–268.

42. Billard BE, Hynynen K, Roemer RB. Effects of physical parameters on high temperature ultrasound hyperthermia. *Ultrasound Med Biol* 1990;16:409–420.

43. Hunt JW, Lalonde R, Ginsberg H, Urchuk S, Worthington A. Rapid heating: critical theoretical assessment of thermal gradients found in hyperthermia treatments. *Int J Hyperthermia* 1991;7:703–718.

44. Field SB, Hand JW, eds. *An Introduction to the Practical Aspects of Clinical Hyperthermia*. London, Taylor & Francis, 1990.

45. Fujimoto JG, Pitris C, Boppart SA, Brezinski ME. Optical coherence tomography: an emerging technology for biomedical imaging and optical biopsy. *Neoplasia* 2000;2:9–25.

46. van der Zee J. Peer-Valstar JN, Rietveld PJ, de Graaf-Strukowska L, van Rhoon GC. Practical limitations of interstitial thermometry during deep hyperthermia. *Int J Radiat Oncol Phys* 1998;40:1205–1212.

47. Wust P, Gellermann J, Harder C, et al. Rationale for using invasive thermometry for regional hyperthermia of pelvic tumors. *Int J Radiat Oncol Phys* 1998;41:1129–1137.

48. Ascher MS, Samulski TV, Dodge R, et al. Combined external beam irradiationand external regional hyperthermia for locally advanced adenocarcinoma of the prostate. *Int J Radiat Oncol Phys* 1997;37:1059–1065.

49. Prionas S, Kapp D, Goffinet D, et al. Thermometry of interstitial hyperthermia given as an adjuvant to brachytherapy for the treatment of carcinoma of the prostate. *Int J Radiat Oncol Phys* 1994;28:151–162.

50. Mendecki J, Friedenthal E, Botstein C, et al. Microwave applicators for localized hyperthermia treatment of cancer of the prostate. *Int J Radiat Oncol Phys* 1980;6:1583–1588.

51. Yerushalmi A, Servadio C, Leib Z, et al. Local hyperthermia for treatment of carcinoma of the prostate: a preliminary report. *Prostate* 1982;3:623–630.

52. Fosmire H, Hynynen K, Drach GW, Stea B, Swift P, Cassady JR. Feasibility and toxicity of transrectal ultrasound hyperthermia in the treatment of locally advanced adenocarcinoma of the prostate. *Int J Radiat Oncol Biol Phys* 1993;26:253–259

53. Algan O, Fosmire H, Hynynen K, et al. External beam radiotherapy and hyperthermia in the treatment of patients with locally advanced prostate carcinoma. *Cancer* 2000;89:399–403.

54. Hurwitz MD, Kaplan ID, Svensson GK, Hynynen K, Hansen MS. Feasibility and patient tolerance of a novel transrectal ultrasound hyperthermia system for treatment of prostate cancer. *Int J Hyperthermia* 2001;17:31–37.

55. Yerushalmi A, Fishelovitz Y, Singer D, et al. Localized deep microwave hyperthermia in the treatment of poor operative risk patients with benign prostatic hyperplasia. *J Urol* 1985;133:873–876.

56. Francisca EA, Keijzers GB, d'Ancona FC, Debruyne FM, de la Rosette JJ. Lower-energy thermotherapy in the treatment of benign prostatic hyperplasia: long-term follow-up results of a multicenter international study. *World J Urol* 1999;17:279–284.

57. Madersbacher S, Kratzik C, Szabo N, Susani M, Vingers L, Marberger M. Tissue ablation in benign prostatic hyperplasia with high-intensity focused ultrasound. *Eur Urol* 1993;23(Suppl 1):39–43.

58. Gelet A, Chapelon JY, Margonari J, et al. High-intensity focused ultrasound experimentation on human benign prostatic hypertrophy. *Eur Urol* 1993;23(Suppl 1):44–47.

59. Madersbacher S, Kratzik C, Marberger M. Prostatic tissue ablation by transrectal high intensity focused ultrasound: histological impact and clinical application. *Ultrason Sonochem* 1997;4: 175–179.

60. Zlotta AR, Djavan B, Matos C, et al. Percutaneous transperineal radiofrequency ablation of prostate tumour: safety, feasibility and pathological effects on human prostate cancer. *Br J Urol* 1998;81:265–275.

61. Madersbacher S, Pedevilla M, Vingers L, Susani M, and Marberger M. Effect of high-intensity focused ultrasound on human prostate cancer in vivo. *Cancer Res* 1995;55:3346–3351.

62. Bursa B, Wammack R, Djavan B, et al. Outcome predictors of high-energy transurethral microwave thermotherapy. *Tech Urol* 2000;6:262–266.

63. Gelet A, Chapelon JY, Bouvier R, Pangaud C, Lasne Y. Local control of prostate cancer by transrectal high intensity focused ultrasound therapy: preliminary results. *J Urol* 1999;161:156–162.

64. Gelet A, Chapelon JY, Bouvier R, Rouviere O, Lyonnet D, Dubernard JM. Transrectal high intensity focused ultrasound for the treatment of localized prostate cancer: factors influencing the outcome. *Eur Urol* 2001;40:124–129.

65. Dorr LN, Hynynen K. The effect of tissue heterogeneities and large blood vessels on the thermal exposure induced by short high power ultrasound pulses. *Int J Hyperthermia* 1992;8:45–59.

66. Chung A, Jolesz FA, Hynynen K. Thermal dosimetry of a focused ultrasound beam in vivo by MRI. *Med Phys* 1999;26:2017–2026.

67. Hynynen K, Vykhodtseva NI, Chung A, Sorrentino V, Colucci V, Jolesz FA. Thermal effects of focused ultrasound on the brain: determination with MR Imaging. *Radiology*, 1997;204:247–253.

68. Hynynen K, Shimm D, Anhalt D, et al. Temperature distributions during clinical scanned, focussed ultrasound hyperthermia treatments. *Int J Hyperthermia* 1990;6:891–908.

69. Hynynen K, Freund W, Cline HE, et al. A clinical noninvasive MRI monitored ultrasound surgery method. *RadioGraphics* 1996;16:185–195.

70. Hutchinson EB Hynynen K. Intracavitary phased arrays for non-invasive prostate surgery. *IEEE Trans Ultrason Ferroelectr Freq Contr* 1996;43:1032–1042.

71. Hata N, Jinzaki M, Kacher D, et al. MR imaging-guided prostate biopsy with surgical navigation software: device validation and feasibility. *Radiology* 2001;220:263–268

72. Fallone BG, Moran PR, Podgorsak EB. Non-invasive thermometry with clinical X-ray CT scanner. *Med Phys* 1982;9:715–721.

73. Jenne JW, Bahner M, Spoo J, et al. CT on-line monitoring of HIFU therapy. *IEEE Ultrasonics Symp* 1997;2:1377–1380.

74. Leroy Y, Bocquet B, Mamouni, A. Non-invasive microwave radiometry thermometry. *Physiol Meas* 1998;19:127–148.

75. Moskowitz MJ, Paulsen KD, Ryan TP, Pang D. Temperature field estimation using electrical impedance profiling methods. II. Experimental system description and phantom results. *Int J Hyperthermia* 1994;10:229–245.

76. Seip R, VanBaren P, Cain CA, Ebbini ES. Noninvasive real-time multipoint temperature control for ultrasound phased array treatments. *IEEE Trans Ultrason Ferroelectr Freq Contr* 1996;43:1063–1073.

77. Simon C, VanBaren P, Ebbini, ES. Two-dimensional temperature estimation using diagnostic ultrasound. *IEEE Trans Ultrason Ferroelectr Freq Contr* 1998;45: 1088–1099.

78. Maas-Moreno R, Damianou CA. Noninvasive temperature estimation in tissue via ultrasound echo-shifts. Part I. Analytical model. *J Acoust Soc Am* 1996;100:2514–2521.

79. Maas-Moreno R, Damianou CA, Sanghvi NT. Noninvasive temperature estimation in tissue via ultrasound echo-shifts. Part II. In vitro study. *J Acoust Soc Am* 100:2522–2530.

80. Sapareto S, Dewey W. Thermal dose determination in cancer therapy. *Int J Radiat Oncol Phys* 1984;10:787–800.

81. Parker DL. Applications on NMR imaging in hyperthermia: an evaluation of the potential for localized tissue heating and noninvasive temperature monitoring. *IEEE Trans Biomed Eng* 1984;31:161–167.

82. Dickinson RJ Hall AS, Hind AJ, Young IR. Measurement of changes in tissue temperature using MR imaging. *J. Comp. Asst. Tomogr.* 1996;10:468–472.

83. Delannoy J, Chen CN, Turner R, Lewin RL, Le Bihan D. Noninvasive temperature imaging using diffusion MRI *Magn. Reson. Med.* 1991;19:333–339.

84. Zhang Y, Samulski TV, Joines WT, Mattiello J, Levin RL, LeBihan D. On the accuracy of noninvasive thermometry using molecular diffusion magnetic resonance imaging. *Int J Hyperthermia* 1992;8:263–274.

85. Hall LD, Talagala SL Mapping of PH and temperature distribution using chemical-shift-resolved tomography. *J Magn Reson* 1985;65:501–505.

86. De Poorter J, De Wagter C, De Deene Y, Thomsen C, Stahlberg F, Achten E. The proton resonance frequency shift method compared with molecular diffusion for quantitative measurements of two dimensional time dependent temperature distributions in a phantom. *J Magn Reson* 1994;103: 234–241.

87. Wlodarczyk W, Hentschel M, Wust P, et al. Comparison of four magnetic resonance methods for mapping small temperature changes. *Phys Med Biol* 1999;44:607–624.

88. Hindman JC. Proton resonance shift of water in the gas and liquid states. *J Chem Phys* 1966;44:4582–4592.

89. Corbett RJT, Laptook AR, Tollefsbol G, Kim B. Validation of a noninvasive method to measure brain temperature in vivo using 1HNMR spectroscopy. *J Neurochem* 1995;64:1224–1230.

90. MacFall JR, Prescott DM, Charles HC, Samulski TV. 1H MRI phase thermometry in vivo in canine brain, muscle, and tumor tissue. *Med Phys* 1996;23:1775–1782.

91. De Poorter J, De Wagter C, De Deene Y, Thomsen C, Stahlberg F, Achten E. Noninvasive MRI thermometry with the proton resonance frequency (PRF) method: In vivo results in human muscle. *Magn Reson Med* 1995;33:74–81.

92. Asea A, Ara G, Teicher BA, Stevenson MA, Calderwood SK. Effects of the flavonoid drug quercetin on the response of human prostate tumours to hyperthermia in vitro and in vivo. *Int J Hyperthermia* 2001;17:347–356.

93. Janetzki S, Palla D, Rosenhauer V, Lochs H, Lewis JJ, Srivastava PK. Immunization of cancer patients with autologous cancer-derived heat shock protein gp96 preparations: a pilot study. *Int J Cancer* 2000,88:232–238.

94. Lohr F, Hu K, Huang Q, et al. Enhancement of radiotherapy by hyperthermia-regulated gene therapy. *Int J Radiat Oncol Phys* 2000;48: 1513–1518.

95. Garcia-Segura JM, Sanchez-Chapado M, Ibarburen C, et al. In vivo proton spectroscopy of diseased prostate: spectroscopic features of malignant versus benigh pathology. *Magn Reson Imaging* 1999;17:755–765.

96. Kurhanewicz J, Dahiya R, Macdonald JM. Citrate alterations in primary and metastatic human prostatic adenocarcinomas: ^{1}H magnetic resonance spectroscopy and biochemical study. *Magn Reson Med* 1993;29:149–157.

97. Schiebler ML, Miyamoto KK, White M, Maygarden SJ, Mohler JL. In vitro high resolution ^{1}H spectroscopy of the human prostate: benign prostatic hyperplasia, normal peripheral zone and adenocarcinoma. *Magn Reson Med* 1993;29:285–291.

98. Kurhanewicz J, Vigneron DB, Hricak H, Narayan P, Carroll P, Nelson SJ. Three-dimensional H-1 MR spectroscopic imaging of the in situ human prostate with high (0.24–0.7-cm^3) spatial resolution. *Radiology* 1996;198:795–805.

99. Van der Graaf M, van den Boogert HJ, Jager GJ, Barentsz JO, Heerschap A. Human prostate: multisection proton MR spectroscopic imaging with a single spin-echo sequence-preliminary experience. *Radiology* 1999;213:919–925.

100. Schick F, Bongers H, Kutz S, Jung W.-I., Pfeffer M, Lutz O. Localized proton MR spectroscopy of citrate in vitro and of the human prostate in vivo at 1.5 T. *Magn Reson Med* 1993;29:38–43.

101. Lowry M, Liney GP, Turnbull LW, Manton DJ, Blackband SJ, Horsman A. Quantification of citrate concentration in the prostate by proton magnetic resonance spectroscopy: zonal and age related differences. *Magn Reson Med* 1996;36:352–358.

102. Liney GP, Lowry M, Turnbull LW, et al. (1996) Proton MR T2 maps correlate with the citrate concentration in the prostate. *NMR Biomed* 9:59–64.

103. Liney GP, Turnbull LW, Lowry M, Turnbull LS, Knowles AJ, Horsman A. In vivo quantitation of citrate concentration and water T2 relaxation time of the pathologic prostate gland using ^{1}H MRS and MRI. *Magn Reson Imaging* 1997;15:1177–1186.

104. Liney GP, Knowles AJ, Manton DJ, Turnbull LW, Blackband SJ, Horsman A. Compari-

son of conventional single echo and multi-echo sequences with a fast spin-echo sequence for quantitative T2-mapping: application to the prostate. *J. Magn Reson Imaging* 1996;6:603–607.

105. Chenevert TL, McKeever PE, Ross BD. Monitoring early response of experimental brain tumors to therapy using diffusion magnetic resonance imaging. *Clin Cancer Res* 1997;3:1457–1466

106. Galons JP, Altbach MI, Paine-Murrieta GD, Taylor CW, Gillies RJ. Early increases in breast tumor xenograft water mobility in response to paclitaxel therapy detected by non-invasive diffusion magnetic resonance imaging. *Neoplasia* 1999;1:113–117

107. Ellis RJ Kim EY, Conant R, et al. Radioimmunoguided imaging of prostate cancer foci with histopathological correlation. *Int J Radiat Oncol Phys* 2001;49:1281–1286.

12

Molecular Imaging of Cancer Using Fluorescent Probe Technology

Farouc A. Jaffer, MD, PhD, Vasilis Ntziachristos, PhD, and Ralph Weissleder, MD, PhD

INTRODUCTION

Clinical imaging is the traditional cornerstone of cancer diagnosis. Detailed anatomic, physiologic, and metabolic information can be obtained by conventional techniques, such as X-ray, computed tomography (CT), ultrasound, nuclear, and magnetic resonance imaging (MRI). In our opinion, the next major advance in clinical imaging will be the ability to image specific molecules and molecular function, broadly encompassed in the field of molecular imaging. Molecular imaging couples sensitive clinical imaging systems with "smart" probes that interact with specific molecules. With this approach, image contrast can be directly ascribed to the presence or function of a target molecule. Ultimately, molecular imaging of tumor receptors and enzyme function is expected to have a major impact in the diagnosis and treatment of cancer, as well as in the field of cancer biology (1).

Although molecular imaging approaches have been applied in nuclear and MR imaging, recent developments in optical imaging instrumentation and activatable fluorescent probes have led to rapid growth in optical molecular imaging. Optical molecular imaging, like all molecular imaging methods, requires several key characteristics: 1) sensitive, fast, and high-resolution imaging techniques; 2) the availability of high-affinity probes with reasonable pharmacological behavior; 3) the ability of the probes to overcome biological delivery barriers (vascular, interstitial, cell membrane); and 4) use of signal amplification strategies. Compared with nuclear imaging, optical imaging has a number of unique advantages, such as the lack of radioactivity, stable compounds, and activatable compounds. Given the armamentarium of novel fluorescent probes and sophisticated imaging systems under development, optical imaging is expected to play a leading role in the future diagnosis and treatment of cancer. Although a discussion of the entire field of medical optical imaging is beyond the scope of this chapter, the interested reader is encouraged to review discussions of endogenous fluorescence imaging (autofluorescence), absorption imaging, and spectral imaging (2–4). In this chapter, we provide a brief overview of optical molecular imaging, with a focus on proteases that are implicated in cancer. We begin with a discussion of smart fluorescent probes, followed by an overview of the required instrumentation, and then provide relevant examples in cancer diagnosis and therapy.

From: *Image-Guided Diagnosis and Treatment of Cancer*
Edited by: A. D'Amico, J. S. Loeffler, and J. R. Harris © Humana Press Inc., Totowa, NJ

FLUORESCENT PROBES

Near Infrared Fluorochromes

Noninvasive and minimally invasive in vivo imaging with light photons represents an intriguing avenue for extracting relevant biological information. Although light in the visible range is routinely used for intravital microscopy, imaging of deeper tissues (>500 nm to tens of cm) requires the use of near infrared fluorescent (NIRF) light. Hemoglobin and water, the major absorbers of visible and infrared light, respectively, have their lowest absorption coefficient in the NIR region around 650–900 nm (Fig. 1). Light photons can be used to measure different native parameters of tissue through which they travel for example absorption, scattering, polarization, spectral characteristics, and fluorescence. Many of these parameters, however, are fairly nonspecific with regards to specific molecular abnormalities *(5)*. The major impact for imaging molecular information in vivo has come from the recent development of targeted NIR fluorochromes *(6,7)*, activatable NIR fluorochromes *(8)*, red-shifted fluorescent proteins *(9)*, and red-shifted bioluminescent probes *(10)*.

Nonspecific NIRF Probes

A number of nontargeted NIRF probes have been used for biomedical applications. The most common fluorochrome is indocyanine green (ICG), which is FDA approved for ophthalmic retinal angiography. ICG has been used in tens of thousands of patients with reported side effects of <0.15%, which is an extremely favorable index when compared with other reporter agents *(11)*. In addition to retinal angiography, ICG has also been used as a compartmental contrast agent to facilitate breast cancer detection *(12)*. The biodistribution of ICG reflects initial vascular distribution (through binding to plasma proteins) and subsequent hepatobiliary excretion *(13)*. Similar to other nonspecific contrast agents used routinely in CT and MRI, these agents provide arbitrary primarily physiologic information (e.g., blood volume, extravasation kinetics) and have been used to detect tumors *(12)*.

Targeted NIRF Probes

A number of different approaches to image molecular targets using fluorescent probes are available, most of them relying on targeting specific molecules (affinity ligands). After intravenous injection, NIRF imaging is performed after a fraction of the agent has bound to its target and the remainder of nonbound agent has been cleared *(7,14)*. These approaches have been particularly useful for imaging receptors and other cell surface expressed molecules. Affinity ligands have primarily included monoclonal antibodies *(6,15)*. The more recent use of peptide ligands may well represent a step towards smaller, more penetrable reporter probes and may have particular applications in unique clinical situations where nuclear imaging is not an option, e.g., for reasons of resolution, during endoscopy or in surgery. The concept of tagging NIR fluorochromes can potentially be extended to a myriad of other peptide/small molecule receptor systems. The technology may also be useful for in vivo screening of limited peptide libraries and/or for identifying structure-activity relationships. Other small molecules attached to NIR fluorochromes, for example, diphosphonates for bone imaging *(16)* are also being developed.

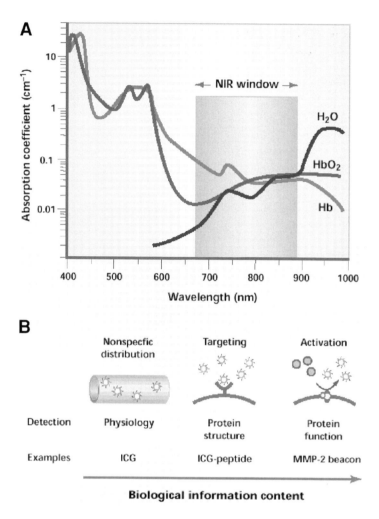

Fig. 1. (**A**) Absorption spectrum showing the NIR window. (**B**) Strategies for improving specificity and informational content of NIR reporters. (Reprinted with permission from ref. 5.)

Activatable NIRF Probes

Fluorescent probes offer several pathways for signal amplification and suppression of signals emanating from nonspecific uptake by using activation techniques (quenching-dequenching), wavelength-shifting techniques, and by loading multiple fluorochromes on the same delivery molecule. A number of different designs of optical smart agents have been described, two of which will briefly be discussed here (Fig. 2). The first agent *(17)* has pioneered detection of complementary DNA strands. These molecular beacons contain a stem-loop structure with a fluorochrome at one terminus and (4-[4'-dimethylaminophenylazo] benzoic acid) as a universal quencher at the other. The probe DNA sequence is in the center of the molecule and the bases at both termini are self-complementary, yielding a 5- to 8-nucleotide stem with a loop. Once duplex formation occurs, the fluorochrome and quencher become spatially separated and fluorescence resonance energy transfer and/or fluorescence direct energy transfer is no

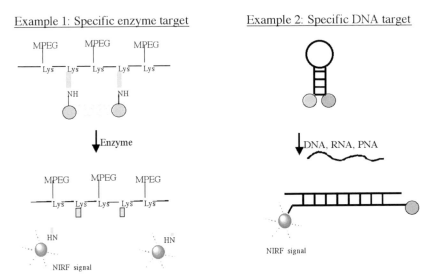

Fig. 2. Examples of large MW activatable enzyme-specific (left) and DNA/RNA-specific (right) imaging probes. Note that the fluorochromes are excited in the near infrared.

longer possible. The fluorochrome then emits light of the appropriate wavelength when excited. Several investigators have demonstrated that molecular beacons can be used to directly demonstrate DNA duplex formation in living cells. More recently, wavelength-shifting molecular beacons that fluoresce in a variety of different colors, yet are excited by a common monochromatic light source have been developed. Wavelength-shifting molecular beacons are reported to be substantially brighter than conventional molecular beacons that contain a fluorophore that cannot efficiently absorb energy from the available monochromatic light source *(18)*. Although DNA/RNA molecular beacons are of tremendous value for in vitro applications, their in vivo use is not without problems, primarily because of intracellular delivery barriers, circulating DNAses and competing elimination.

The second type of probe ("activatable probe") described here can de designed to report on specific enzyme activities. The activatable probe is based on the following principle: enzyme cleavage of a baseline quenched probe, leading to dequenching and amplification of the otherwise "optically silent" fluorochrome (Fig. 2) *(8)*. The probe has two key structural features: 1) baseline quenching and 2) a peptide substrate specific for the enzyme of interest. Quenching of the probe occurs by exploiting fluorescence resonance energy transfer in one of two schemes: autoquenching, where identical fluorochromes with overlapping excitation and emission spectra are placed in close physical proximity; or absorption, where a quencher molecule is placed in close proximity to a fluorochrome. In either case, a peptide substrate serves as the linkage between the fluorochromes and/or quenchers. Furthermore, the peptide substrate is constructed be specific for a target enzyme. After cleavage of the peptide substrate, the fluorochromes and/or dequenchers are physically separated, leading to elimination of baseline quenching and amplification of the NIRF signal. The release of the NIRF probes results in a fluorescent signal that can be detected in vivo at depths sufficient for experimental or clinical imaging depending on the NIRF image acquisition technique *(19)*. This approach has four major advantages over other methods where single fluorochromes are attached to affinity molecules: 1) a single enzyme can cleave multiple fluorochromes, thus resulting in one form of signal amplification; 2) reduction of background "noise" by several orders of magnitude is possible; 3) very specific enzyme activities can potentially be interrogated; and 4) multiple probes can be arranged on delivery systems to simultaneously probe for a spectrum of enzymes. These activatable NIRF probes are currently being used to detect disease at their earliest stage, (e.g., small cancers, vulnerable plaque, rheumatoid arthritis, and thrombosis), to image transgenes or to test the in vivo efficacy of enzyme inhibitors within hours after administration (*see* section on Applications of Optical Molecular Imaging in Cancer) *(22)*.

A specific example of an activatable probe targeted to cysteine protease cathepsin B is shown in Fig. 2. The peptide sequence lysine–lysine serves as the proteolytic substrate. Other examples of activatable probes include cathepsin D, which cleaves two phenylalanine peptides *(23)*, matrix metalloproteinase 2 (MMP-2)-specific probes *(22)* or caspase-3-specific probes. In general, any peptide cleavage substrate can be incorporated into the molecule, thus providing a potentially powerful tool to studying protease activity.

The biodelivery vehicle is another important component of the activatable probe. In general, two types of carrier vehicles exist: large molecular weight (MW) compounds and small MW compounds. As shown in Fig. 2, one example of a large MW probe uses a novel long circulating synthetic graft copolymer (PGC). This copolymer has recently been tested in clinical trials *(24)* and accumulates in tumors by slow extravasation through permeable neovasculature reaching up to 2–6% injected dose/g tissue in mice within 24 to 48 h after injection in some tumor models *(25)*. Uptake of the polymer into tumor cells occurs by pinocytosis and is comparable in magnitude to that of tumor-specific internalizing monoclonal antibodies. Large MW compounds have long intravascular half-lives, which may be advantageous for vascular imaging applications, but in general result in slower tissue and tumor uptake, leading to longer imaging delays. However, this approach has been well tested, with excellent results in vivo *(8,20,22)*.

However, small MW compounds have the advantages of simpler construction and faster tissue uptake and consequent imaging. An example of a small MW activatable probe using a quencher-fluorochrome paradigm is shown in Fig. 3. At present, our laboratory is exploring both large molecular weight and small molecular weight activatable and targeted probes for cancer diagnosis and therapy.

DETECTION TECHNOLOGY

A number of different optical imaging approaches can be used for imaging fluorescence in vivo. Traditionally, optical methods have been used to look at surface and subsurface events using confocal imaging *(26,27)*, multiphoton imaging *(28–30)*, microscopic imaging by intravital microscopy *(31,32)*, optical coherence tomography *(33,34)*, or spectral imaging *(35)*. Recently, however, light has been used for in vivo interrogations deeper into tissue using photographic systems with continuous light *(14,36)* or with intensity-modulated light *(37)*, as well as tomographic systems *(38)*. Potentially, phased-array detection *(39)* can be also applied. In the following section,

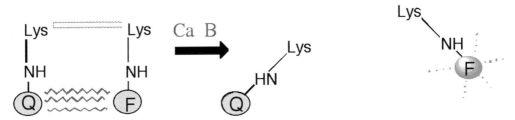

Fig. 3. Example of small MW cathepsin-B activatable enzyme-specific imaging probe. The Lys–Lys bond is a substrate for the protease cathepsin B. Q = quencher, F = NIR Fluorochrome. Lys = lysine, Ca B = cathepsin B.

we discuss imaging techniques that use the diffuse component of light-detecting fluorochromes deep in tissue. Specifically, we focus on fluorescence reflectance imaging (FRI) and fluorescence-mediated molecular tomography (FMT) because these approaches are most commonly used. We further predict the capacity of near-infrared fluorescent signals to propagate through human tissue for noninvasive medical imaging and address feasibility issues for clinical studies.

Fluorescence Reflectance Imaging

Simple "photographic methods" of tissue whereas the light source and the detector reside on the same side of the animal imaged, are generally referred to using the term "reflectance imaging." The term encompasses but is not limited to imaging NIRF probes, imaging of fluorescent proteins, or even bioluminescence, even if in the latter case no excitation light is used. Near infrared fluorescence reflectance imaging, in particular, operates on light with a defined bandwidth as a source of photons that encounters a fluorescent molecule. After this interaction, the emitted signal has different spectral characteristics that can be resolved with an emission filter and can be captured by a high-sensitivity charge-coupled device (CCD) camera.

A typical reflectance imaging system is shown in Fig. 4. The light source can be either a laser at an appropriate wavelength for the fluorochrome targeted or white light sources using appropriate low-pass filters (a bioluminescence system works identically except does not require an excitation light source). For FRI, laser sources are preferable because they offer higher power delivery at narrower and better-defined spectral windows (typically ±3 nm for laser diodes vs ±20 nm or more for filtered white light sources). The laser beam is expanded on the animal surface with an optical system of lenses (not shown). Narrow wavelength selection is important, especially in the NIR, whereas the excitation and emission spectra overlap and it is likely that excitation photons can propagate into the fluorescent images. The CCD camera is usually a high-sensitivity camera because fluorescent signals are of low strength. On the other hand, since the targeted measurement is a diffuse-light measurement, emanating from a virtually flat surface, CCD chip resolution and dynamic range are not crucial factors in these types of systems. The fluorescence sensitivity is primarily set by the tissue autofluorescence and extrinsic background fluorescence because of the administered probe.

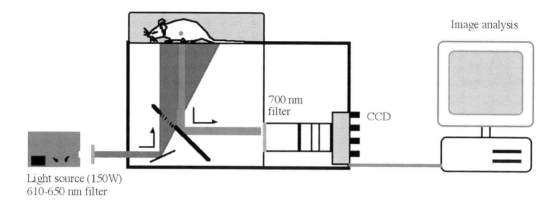

Fig. 4. A typical reflectance imaging system. The construction is usually encased in a photon-sealing box (black box). *See* section on Fluorescence Reflectance Imaging for details.

Such approaches have been used to evaluate activatable probes *(8,20,22)* or peptide-nearinfrared dye conjugates *(7,14,16)*. Reflectance imaging can also be used to image endogenous gene products by using fluorescent (e.g., green fluorescent protein) or bio-luminescent (e.g., luciferases from firefly, coral or jellyfish) proteins *(10)*.

Advantages and Limitations

As FRI or similar technology combined with endoscopic systems are commercially available, the most immediate applications of activatable and targeted NIRF probes to detect human cancers will be using FRI-coupled endoscopic detection of various cancers (e.g., colorectal *(40)*, bronchial, esophageal, gastric, urological, gynecological, and oropharyngeal, laryngeal). Another important application will be to identify dermatological cancers (e.g., malignant melanoma, squamous cell carcinoma). FRI is also an ideal tool for high throughput imaging, screening of animals, evaluating excised tissues, or imaging structures near the surface (skin or subcutaneous). It offers simplicity of operation and high sensitivity for molecular events that are close to the surface. Typical acquisition times range from a few seconds to a few minutes. For laboratory settings, multiple animals can be simultaneously imaged. Hardware development and implementation is also straightforward and relatively inexpensive. Reflectance systems do not use ionizing radiation or safe laser powers, can be made portable, and can attain small space requirements to be ideal for the laboratory bench.

However, reflectance imaging has fundamental limitations both as a research or clinical tool. The technique attains only small penetration depths and lack of quantification. Indeed, a small structure of high fluorochrome concentration that is deeper into tissue could yield the same appearance on the surface as a larger structure of low fluorochrome concentration that is closer to the surface. This results from the nature of propagation of diffuse photon density waves into tissue. In practice, the surface-detected photon count of a lesion at a position within the body depends on the lesion depth, the lesion volume and the optical properties of both the lesion and the surrounding tissue. Therefore, images from different subjects or from the same animal at different time points are generally insufficient of yielding quantitative insights.

Fluorescence-Mediated Molecular Tomography

To resolve and quantify fluorochromes deep in tissue, tomographic approaches are necessary. The general framework of reconstruction techniques, combined with technological advancements in photon sources and detection techniques, has made possible the application of tomographic principles to imaging with diffuse light *(41–45)*. This technique, generally termed Diffuse Optical Tomography (DOT) uses multiple projections and measures light around the boundary of the illuminated body. It then effectively combines all measurements into an inversion scheme that takes into account the highly scattered photon propagation to deconvolve the effect of tissue on the propagating wave, even though high-frequency components are generally significantly attenuated. DOT has been used for quantitative imaging of absorption and scattering *(46,47)*, as well as fluorochrome lifetime and concentration measurements *(48,49)*. Recently, DOT has been applied clinically for imaging tissue oxy- and deoxy-hemoglobin concentration and blood saturation *(50–52)*, as well as contrast agent uptake *(12)*.

A particular class of these techniques was developed specifically for molecular interrogations of tissue in vivo and is termed FMT *(53)*. To perform FMT, tissue has to be illuminated at different projections and multiple measurements collected from the boundary of the tissue of investigation. The method is by definition a volumetric method that produces quantified three-dimensional reconstructions of fluorescence concentration. In its optimal implementation, FMT uses measurements at both emission and excitation wavelengths to offer significant advantages for in vivo imaging. The basic concept has been described in the past for a normalized Born expansion *(49)*, but the method can be applied to different mathematical constructions for the forward problem, including numerical approaches. The main advantage of using both intrinsic and fluorescence contrast lies in that no absolute photon-field measurements are required, yet absolute fluorochrome concentrations can be reconstructed. Furthermore, the method does not require any measurements obtained before contrast agent administration. In the following paragraphs we describe in more detail these unique characteristics and present key features of FMT performance and imaging examples.

Figure 5 shows a prototypical FMT system for mouse imaging. In theory, an FMT imaging can be scaled up to perform fluorescence imaging in human-sized subjects *(54)*. The light source (A) is generally comprised of a laser diode at the appropriate wavelength to excite the targeted fluorochrome. Multiple laser diodes at different wavelengths can be combined in the same system (either by time-sharing or spectral separation) to simultaneously excite multiple fluorochromes. The light from the laser diode can be directed to an optical switch (D) for time-sharing one input to many outputs and directed with optical fibers (E) at different points around the body of investigation or a specially designed "optical bore" (F). The optical bore contains the body of examination similar to a CT or MRI scanner. Typically, this implementation requires the animal to be immersed into a "matching fluid," such as a water solution of a scatterer (e.g., TiO_2 particles) and an absorber (e.g., India Ink) that matches the optical properties of the tissue under investigation. The matching fluid serves virtually the same function as gel to ultrasound. Fiber bundles (G) can be used to collect photons through the turbid medium and then direct them onto the CCD chip (J) either by direct fiber coupling or by an appropriate positioning arrangement (H), so that the fiber output can be imaged

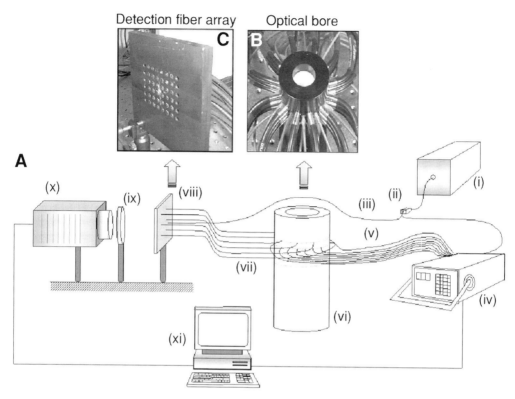

Fig. 5. FMT system. *See* section on Fluorescence Mediated Molecular Tomography for details. (Reprinted with permission from reference *53.*)

via a lens system (as depicted in Fig. 5). Appropriate filters (I) are necessary to reject intrinsic or fluorescence light according to the measurement performed and background noise. A reference measurement can also be introduced to account for temporal variations in laser intensity. This approach has been realized using a beam-splitter (B) to direct part of source light directly onto the CCD chip via an optical fiber (C). The use of an optical bore and matching fluid is mainly for illustration purposes and by no means limiting. Different schemes including direct fiber positioning on the tissue surface, at arbitrary geometries, including geometries that could be used by endoscopic probes, could also be devised.

To assess clinical feasibility of FMT, we recently simulated the ability of the near-infrared light to propagate through large human organs *(54)*. Using our prototypical FMT system, we characterized the fluorescence strength of a NIR fluorochrome, and then extrapolated the experimental results to simulated human tissue. Figure 6 shows the potential of NIR photons to pass through tens of centimeters of breast and lung and several centimeters through muscle and brain, assuming a two-order improvement in detection technology. With further advancements in photon detection, for example, direct fiber coupling to the CCD chip *(54)*, even deeper detection of NIR light in human tissue may be possible. Ultimately, next-generation FMT systems may allow for true noninvasive screening of cancer and quantification of protease activity with the human body.

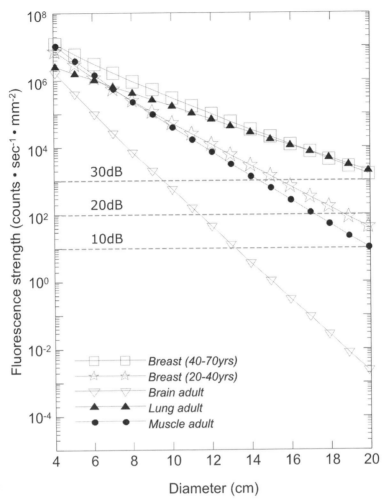

Fig. 6. Estimation of fluorescence penetration in human tissues as a function of depth. The graph shows the expected fluorescence at the margin of each organ, assuming an NIR fluorochrome (100 mL volume at concentration of 100 n*M*) situated in the center of the organ. The three horizontal lines indicate different signal-to-noise ratio of the measurements achieved for signal shot-noise limited systems and can be interpreted as detection thresholds in the absence of background fluorescence. (Reprinted with permission from ref. *54.*)

APPLICATIONS OF OPTICAL MOLECULAR IMAGING IN CANCER

Although current methods to image cancer are of tremendous clinical value, early detection of small (less than submillimeter) tumors remains a significant diagnostic challenge. Because cancer remains a leading cause of death worldwide, more sensitive and high-resolution diagnostic imaging modalities, such as fluorescence imaging, are urgently needed. Imaging of cancer using fluorescent technology has already been performed in the clinical arena to successfully diagnose cancer and guide cancer therapy. These detection schemes rely on endogenous autofluorescence (e.g., bronchoscopy, endoscopy) or use nontargeted flow-based fluorescent reporters (e.g., ICG). Although of clinical value, the dependence on autofluorescence or nontargeted probes leads to low target-to-background imaging ratios for many cancers. Furthermore, these methods have largely relied on FRI and are therefore unable to resolve fluorescence within deep tissues, limiting their use in cancer detection.

Recently, several groups have employed activatable and targeted near-infrared fluorescent probes to increase the biological specificity of a probe for its target *(7,8,14)*. This approach results in an enhanced target-to-background imaging ratio, permitting detection of cancer and dysplastic lesions of less than 100 microns in diameter. Furthermore, very recent data suggests that noninvasive detection of cancers by fluorescence-mediated tomography is achievable several centimeters deep into tissue *(53)*. Although these results are in largely preclinical studies, both activatable and targeted probes, as well noninvasive fluorescent sensing in deep tissues (FMT), can be adapted for human studies. With ongoing advancements in both probe and detection technology, we anticipate that near-infrared fluorescence imaging of tumor proteases and receptors will play an important role in both diagnosis and therapy of human cancers within this decade. In this section, we present the current status of NIRF imaging of cancer using activatable and targeted probes, as well as of novel NIRF signal detection technology, such as FMT.

Tumor Detection by FRI

FRI has been the basis for most approaches to detect tumors. Recently, we have described the use of activatable NIRF probes with FRI to successfully image tumor-associated protease activity in vivo *(8)*. In this study, our laboratory synthesized a novel NIRF activatable probe that was sensitive to cleavage by enzymes with lysine-lysine sensitivity, such as cathepsin B (Fig. 2). We hypothesized that tumor lysosomal endopeptidases might serve to activate the NIRF probe. Cell cultures using a human cancer cell line (LX-1 small cell lung carcinoma) confirmed rapid probe activation that was easily detectable with fluorescence microscopy. Furthermore, analysis of the subcellular fractions showed that probe activation was suppressed by inhibitors of cysteine proteases (e.g., cathepsins B and L), such as E64 *(55)*, as well as trypsin, and trypsin-like serine protease inhibitors. We concluded that the activation of the probe within tumor was a result of lysosomal cysteine/serine protease activity.

Following these in vitro results, a series of in vivo FRI experiments were performed using the cathepsin B activatable probe. In this model, LX-1 tumor cells were implanted into the mammary fat pad of nude mice. After tumor growth to less than 3 mm in diameter, the mice were injected with the tumor-protease activatable NIRF probe. At baseline imaging before and immediately after probe injection, tumors remained undetectable. However, by 24 h, all tumors had generated enough NIRF signal to be easily detectable by an FRI system. Tumors less than 300 mm were detectable and generated up to 12-fold increases in the baseline (quenched) NIRF signal (Fig. 7). The large target-to-background ratio was produced by the synergistic effects of the activatable probe and the inherent sensitivity of fluorescent signal detection (to nanomolar fluorochrome concentrations). To further confirm tumor activation of the probe, lesions were excised and subjected to histological processing and correlative fluorescence microscopy. These studies showed that the NIRF signal emanated from the tumor cells with minimal signal from the interstitium or necrotic cells (Fig. 7), confirming the ability to obtain high-quality images of submillimeter tumors in vivo.

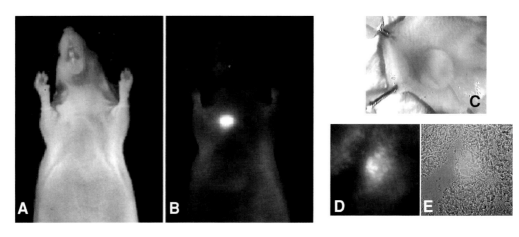

LIGHT IMAGE   NIRF IMAGE

Fig. 7. NIRF imaging of tumor-associated cathepsin B activity in LX-1 tumor cells implanted into the mammary pad of a mouse. The animal shown here was anesthetized with an intraperitoneal injection of ketamine (90 mg/kg) and xylazine (9 mg/kg). FRI was performed on custom-built surface imaging system *(36).* (**A**) The tumor is not visible on the light image. (**B**) After injection of the cathepsin-B activatable probe (2 nmol iv), the tumor brightly fluoresces in the NIR range and is easily detectable by FRI (image acquisition time 10 s). (**C**) Excision of the tumor followed by (**D**) fluorescence microscopy and (**E**) histology reveals that the NIRF signal emanates from within the tumor cells. (Reprinted with permission from ref. *8.*)

Recently, our group has further elucidated the mechanism of cellular activation of the cathepsin B activatable NIRF probe. Using two-photon confocal microscopy, we have found that the strongest activation of this probe occurs in tumor-recruited host cells, rather than the tumor cells *(56).* Furthermore, these host cells have been found to be CD45 and MAC3 cell marker positive, suggesting that the probe was degraded by the monocyte/macrophage population of the cells residing in tumor. In addition to elucidating the mechanism of NIRF probe activation, these results suggests that antiprotease anticancer therapy may in large part be targeting host cells rather than tumor cells.

Finally, targeted, nonactivatable NIRF probes have also recently been used to improve detection of tumors by FRI. Becker et al. *(14)* conjugated a near-infrared cyanine fluorochrome to a peptide analogue of somatostatin. This target was chosen because several tumors overexpress the somatostatin receptor *(57).* In several elegant experiments using dual-channel confocal microscopy, the group demonstrated that only RIN38/SSTR2 tumor cells expressing the somatostatin receptor internalized the targeted NIRF probe. In subsequent in vivo experiments using FRI, the authors demonstrated that the tumor cells brightly fluoresced within hours, generating a three-fold increase in the tumor-to-background ratio by 24 h. In a similar approach, Achilefu et al. *(7)* conjugated a derivative of ICG to a somatostatin-specific peptide, octreotate. Using rats bearing a somatostatin receptor-expressing pancreatic acinar carcinoma (CA20948), the authors used an in vivo FRI system to detect tumor cells containing the targeted NIRF probe. The ex vivo tumor-to-background ratios of pooled organ samples ranged from 2 to10.

Tumor Detection by FMT

Although clinically and scientifically useful, FRI systems are heavily surface-weighted, only semi-quantitative, and unable to resolve fluorescence from deep tissues. FMT, described earlier, attempts to address these issues. In a preclinical system in our laboratory, FMT has been recently used for imaging of cathepsin B activity in murine gliosarcomas deep within the body *(53)*. Importantly, cathepsin B has been implicated in glioma invasion *(58)*. Figure 8 shows a representative experiment of the results obtained from 9-L gliosarcomas stereotactically implanted into unilateral brain hemispheres of nude mice. All animals were subjected to correlative MRI to determine the presence and location of tumors before the FMT imaging studies. For coregistration purposes, we used special water-containing fiducials and body marks that facilitated matching of the MRI and FMT orientation and animal positioning. The in vivo imaging data correlated well with surface-weighted fluorescence reflectance imaging of the excised brain (Fig. 8). Cathepsin B expression in the tumors was further confirmed by immunohistochemistry, Western blotting and reverse transcription polymerase chain reaction. The above results confirm that cathepsin B can be used as a cancer-imaging marker *(8)*, as this protease is produced in considerable amounts by tumor cells and by recruited host cells *(56)*.

As demonstrated in the above examples, tumors containing activatable and targeted NIR fluorescent molecular imaging probes can be rapidly imaged in vivo by using fluorescent imaging technology systems, and provide excellent tumor-to-background imaging ratios. This combination makes fluorescent imaging of human cancers with NIRF probes a potentially viable clinical diagnostic tool. As FMT evolves, the ability to detect human cancers in deep tissue may also become a reality. Of course, to utilize this powerful technology requires the development of appropriate targeted and activatable NIRF probes. As implied by its name, the field of molecular imaging is intimately related to molecular biology, and thus advances in fluorescent imaging will likely parallel fundamental advances in tumor biology.

Proteases as Biomarkers for Detection of Preneoplastic Lesions

Identification of precancerous lesions is a major goal of cancer screening. In particular, removal of colonic adenomatous polyps has been shown to decrease the incidence of colorectal cancers *(59)*. With this background, our group has recently shown that the cathepsin B activatable NIRF probe *(8)* can be used to detect dysplastic intestinal adenomas in a murine model of colorectal cancer *(60)*. This probe was chosen as cathepsin B is upregulated in invasive colorectal carcinoma *(61)* and in dysplastic adenomas *(62)*. In this study, we used mice heterozygous for a germ-line mutation in the mouse homologue of the human adenomatous polyposis coli gene, a model that recapitulates many of the features of dysplastic human colorectal adenomas *(63)*.

Using the cathepsin-B activatable NIRF probe, we identified intestinal adenomas as small as 50 microns in diameter using a FRI system. Mice that were injected with a nonspecific, nontargeted fluorescent dye (ICG) exhibited minimal NIRF signal increases above background. We further confirmed adenomatous localization of the cathepsin B probe by immunohistochemistry, Western blotting, and reverse-transcription polymerase chain reaction.

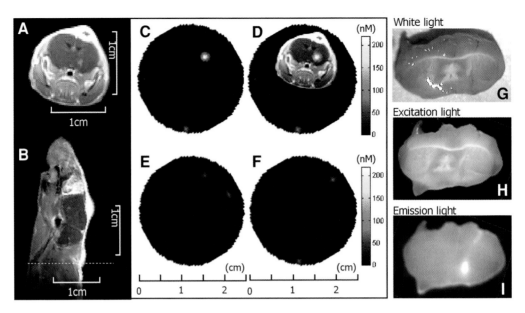

Fig. 8. In vivo FMT of cathepsin B expression levels in 9-L gliosarcomas stereotactically implanted into unilateral brain hemispheres of nude mice. (**A**) Axial and (**B**) sagittal MR slices of an animal implanted with a tumor, which is shown in green after gadolinium enhancement. (**C,E,F**) Consecutive FMT slices obtained from top to bottom from the volume of interest shown on (**B**) by thin white horizontal lines. (**D**) Superposition of the MR axial slice passing through the tumor (**A**) onto the corresponding FMT slice (**C**) after appropriately translating the MR image to the actual dimensions of the FMT image. (**G–H**) Axial brain section through the 9-L tumor imaged with white light and with monochromatic light at the excitation wavelength (675 nm), respectively, and (**I**) fluorescence image of the same axial brain section demonstrating a marked fluorescent probe activation, congruent with the tumor position identified by gado-linium-enhanced MRI and FMT. (Reprinted with permission from reference *53*.)

This exciting result demonstrates the ability of activatable NIRF probes to detect pre-malignant tumors in vivo. As FRI technology is already available endoscopically, this approach could be incorporated in routine screening colonoscopy. Adjunctive FRI of cathepsin B-rich adenomatous polyps could significantly increase the sensitivity of screening colonoscopy *(40)*. Furthermore, as tomographic imaging methods such as FMT evolve, noninvasive colorectal cancer screening might become a viable clinical tool.

Molecular Imaging of Protease Inhibitor Treatment in Cancer

In addition to detecting tumors with FRI and FMT, imaging of protease activity has also been used to study protease inhibition in vivo. We have recently applied this approach to study the MMP inhibitor, prinomastat (AG3340) *(22)*. MMPs are overexpressed in many cancers and are associated with advanced tumor stage *(64)*, invasiveness *(65)*, metastasis *(66)*, and angiogenesis *(67)*. In particular, MMP-2 (gelatinase), which degrades type-IV collagen, the major component of basement mem-branes *(68)*, is thought to be a key MMP involved in aggressive tumor behavior. Con-sequently, MMP inhibitors have been developed and are undergoing clinical testing for

Table 1
Applications and Peptide Substrates That Have Been Used
for the Development of NIRF Probes at the Center for Molecular Imaging Research

Protease target	Disease	Substrate
Cathepsin B	Cancer, inflammation	KK
Cathepsin D	Breast ca more than others	PIC(Et)FF
Cathepsin K	Osteoporosis	GGPRGLPG
Prostate-specific antigen	Prostate ca	HSSKLQG
MMP-2	Metastases	P(L/Q)G(I/L)AG
CMV protease	Viral	GVVQASCRLA
HIV protease	HIV	GVSQNYPIV
Thrombin	Cardiovascular	dFPipR
Caspase 3	Apoptosis	DEVD

Note: Table courtesy of Dr. Chiang-Hsuan Tung

cancer therapy. However, the ability to image the efficacy of MMP protease inhibition is limited, often requiring weeks to reach statistical significance if tumor growth rates are used as a surrogate marker for treatment efficacy *(69)*. We therefore postulated that fluorescent imaging of MMP activity and its inhibition might offer a rapid, sensitive method to assess MMP inhibitor efficacy.

In this study, a novel NIRF MMP-2 molecular beacon was used. In vitro results demonstrated that probe was specific for MMP-2 (compared with MMP-1, MMP-7, MMP-8, and MMP-9). Using nude mice, MMP activity and inhibition was investigated using either HT1080 fibrosarcomas, which are known to express high levels of MMP-2, or BT20 mammary adenocarcinomas, which are known to lack MMP-2. In HT1080-bearing mice, the MMP-2 probe group produced a significantly higher NIRF signal than both the control probe group and the BT20-bearing mice group. To demonstrate the ability to image MMP inhibition in vivo, a group of HT1080-bearing mice was pretreated with prinomastat 150 mg/kg twice a day or a control vehicle for 2 d. After injection of the MMP-2 activatable probe, there was nearly a three-fold reduction in the NIRF signal in the prinomastat pretreatment group ($p < 0.0001$). These findings were confirmed using correlative fluorescence microscopy and cathepsin B immuno-histochemistry.

Imaging of Other Proteases

In addition the activatable probes described above, our laboratory has synthesized and investigated a number of activatable probes for use in cancer as well as other fields (Table 1). Recently, for example, we have used this approach to diagnose thrombosis by employing a novel thrombin-sensitive activatable probe *(21)*. Thrombin is a serine protease responsible for fibrin generation, the scaffolding of thrombus *(70)*. In a murine model of ferric chloride induced venous thrombosis, we have demonstrated rapid activation of the probe in vivo (Fig. 9) *(71)*. Using human blood, we have shown that this probe is specific for the protease thrombin. As the link between cancer and thrombosis has been well appreciated for many years, the thrombin probe may also have potential clinical relevance in cancer, as well as vascular biology *(72)* and angiogenesis *(73)*.

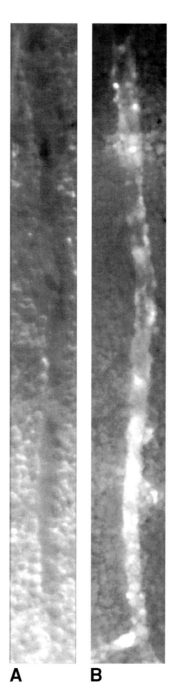

A   **B**

Fig. 9. In vivo activation of a thrombin-sensitive NIRF probe by endogenous thrombin activity within thrombosis. A femoral vein thrombosis was induced by topical ferric chloride. One hour later, the thrombin probe (2 nmol) was injected intravenously and images were acquired 15 min later. (**A**) The light image shows a venous segment with thrombus throughout the vessel (findings were confirmed on histology). (**B**) The FRI image demonstrates focal NIRF signal enhancement in microthrombi throughout the vessel. The images have been windowed individually.

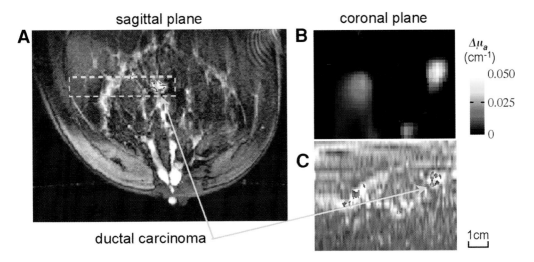

Fig. 10. DOT of a ductal carcinoma. (**A**)The precontrast sagittal MR slice shows the carcinoma in grayscale and the relative signal increase caused by Gadolinium contrast superimposed in color (functional MRI) The color image is obtained by subtracting the corresponding pre-Gadolinium from the post-Gadolinium slice and thresholding the resulting image to 40% of the maximum. The rectangle (dotted yellow) surrounding the carcinoma indicates the volume imaged by NIRF-DOT. (**B**) Coronal DOT image showing a marked absorption increase in the upper right of the image, congruent with the position of a later-proven carcinoma. The local absorption coefficient increase of this lesion was approx 0.05 cm^{-1} at 830 nm, corresponding to an ICG concentration of approx 0.1 mg/L (approx 130 pmol/tumor) (**C**) Functional MR coronal re-slicing of the volume with the same dimensions as (**B**). (Reprinted with permission from ref. *12*.)

Clinical Applications

The capacity of light to propagate through human tissues and the ability to model and reconstruct the native optical properties has been demonstrated in patients with breast cancers *(12)*. This particular study obtained quantitative optical images of human breast in vivo following intravenous administration of ICG, a nonspecific contrast agent as described previously. The optical examination was performed concurrently with an MRI exam on patients scheduled for excisional biopsy or surgery so that accurate image co-registration and histopathological information of any suspicious lesions was available. The ICG-enhanced optical images co-registered accurately with gadolinium-enhanced MR images, validating the ability of DOT, an analog of FMT, to image breast tissue. Figure 10 shows the results from one of the patients with an infiltrating ductal carcinoma of approx 1 cm in size *(12)*. There was a marked absorption increase in the upper right of the NIRF-DOT image, which was congruent with the position of a later-proven carcinoma. There was another lesion towards the left part of the NIRF image, congruent with enhancements seen on the MR images, albeit with a different size and shape than the MRI lesions. The full width at half maximum of the DOT-resolved carcinoma was comparable with the carcinoma size seen on the MRI. Overall, this study demonstrates that noninvasive NIRF-DOT can be performed in a clinical environment to resolve fluorescence in large healthy and diseased organs *in situ*.

CONCLUSIONS

As outlined in this chapter, the future of fluorescence imaging of cancer appears bright (no pun intended). The coupling of NIRF reflectance and tomographic imaging systems to activatable and targeted fluorescent probes has yielded important advances in cancer diagnosis and therapy, as well as cancer biology. As diagnostic fluorescent imaging is still in its infancy, we expect that advances in NIRF probe and detection technology will ultimately revolutionize clinical imaging of cancer.

REFERENCES

1. Weissleder R. Scaling down imaging: molecular mapping of cancer in mice. *Nat Rev Cancer* 2001;2:11–18.
2. Andersson-Engels S, Klinteberg C, Svanberg K, Svanberg S. In vivo fluorescence imaging for tissue diagnostics. *Phys Med Biol* 1997;42:815–824.
3. Ramanujam N. Fluorescence spectroscopy of neoplastic and non-neoplastic tissues. *Neoplasia* 2000;2: 89–117.
4. Shah N, Cerussi A, Eker C, et al. Noninvasive functional optical spectroscopy of human breast tissue. *Proc Natl Acad Sci USA* 2001;98:4420–4425.
5. Weissleder R. A clearer vision for in vivo imaging. *Nat Biotechnol* 2001;19:316–317.
6. Ballou B, Fisher GW, Waggoner AS, et al. Tumor labeling in vivo using cyanine-conjugated monoclonal antibodies. *Cancer Immunol Immunother* 1995;41:257–263.
7. Achilefu S, Dorshow RB, Bugaj JE, Rajagopalan R. Novel receptor-targeted fluorescent contrast agents for in vivo tumor imaging. *Invest Radiol* 2000;35:479–485.
8. Weissleder R, Tung CH, Mahmood U, Bogdanov A. In vivo imaging of tumors with protease-activated near-infrared fluorescent probes. *Nat Biotech* 1999;17:375–378.
9. Gross LA, Baird GS, Hoffman RC, Baldridge KK, Tsien RY. The structure of the chromophore within DsRed, a red fluorescent protein from coral. *Proc Natl Acad Sci USA* 2000;97:11990–11995.
10. Contag CH, Spilman SD, Contag PR, et al. Visualizing gene expression in living mammals using a bioluminescent reporter. *Photochem Photobiol* 1997;66:523–531.
11. Hope-Ross M, Yannuzzi LA, Gragoudas ES, et al. Adverse reactions due to indocyanine green. *Ophthalmology* 1994;101:529–533.
12. Ntziachristos V, Yodh AG, Schnall M, Chance B. Concurrent MRI and diffuse optical tomography of breast after indocyanine green enhancement. *Proc Natl Acad Sci USA* 2000;97:2767–2772.
13. Licha K, Riefke B, Ntziachristos V, Becker A, Chance B, Semmler W. Hydrophilic cyanine dyes as contrast agents for near-infrared tumor imaging: synthesis, photophysical properties and spectroscopic in vivo characterization. *Photochem Photobiol* 2000;72: 392–398.
14. Becker A, Hessenius C, Licha K, et al. Receptor-targeted optical imaging of tumors with near-infrared fluorescent ligands. *Nat Biotechnol* 201;19:327–331.
15. Neri D, Carnemolla B, Nissim A, et al. Targeting by affinity-matured recombinant antibody fragments on an angiogenesis associated fibronectin isoform. *Nat Biotechnol* 1997;15:1271–1275.
16. Zaheer A, Lenkinski RE, Mahmood A, Jones AG, Cantley LC, Frangioni JV. In vivo near-infrared fluorescence imaging of osteoblastic activity. *Nat Biotechnol* 2001;19:1148–1154.
17. Tyagi, S, Kramer FR. Molecular beacons: probes that fluoresce upon hybridization. *Nat Biotechnol* 1996;14:303–308.
18. Tyagi S, Marras SAE, Kramer FR. Wavelength-shifting molecular beacons. *Nat Biotechnol* 2000;18: 1191–1196.
19. Weissleder, R, Mahmood U. Molecular imaging. *Radiology* 2001;219:316–333.

20. Tung C, Mahmood U, Bredow, S, Weissleder R. In vivo imaging of proteolytic enzyme activity using a novel molecular reporter. *Cancer Res* 2000;60:4953–4958.

21. Tung CH, Gerszten RE, Jaffer FA, Weissleder R. A novel near infrared fluorescence sensor for detection of thrombin activation in blood. *ChemBiochem* 2002;3:207–211.

22. Bremer C, Tung C, Weissleder R. Imaging of metalloproteinase inhibition in vivo. *Nat Med* 201;7:743–748.

23. Tung CH, Bredow S, Mahmood U, Weissleder R. Preparation of a cathepsin D sensitive near infrared fluorescence probe for imaging. *Bioconjug Chem* 1999;10:892–896.

24. Callahan RJ, Bogdanov A, Fischman AJ, Brady TJ, Weissleder R. Preclinical evaluation and phase I clinical trial of a 99mTc-labeled synthetic polymer used in blood pool imaging. *AJR Am J Roentgenol* 1998;71:137–143.

25. Marecos E, Weissleder R, Bogdanov A Jr. Antibody-mediated versus nontargeted delivery in a human small cell lung carcinoma model. *Bioconjug Chem* 1998;9:184–191.

26. Korlach J, Schwille P, Webb WW, Feigenson GW. Characterization of lipid bilayer phases by confocal microscopy and fluorescence correlation spectroscopy. *Proc Natl Acad Sci USA* 1999;96:8461–8466.

27. Rajadhyaksha M, Grossman M, Esterowitz D, Webb RH, Anderson RR. In vivo confocal scanning laser microscopy of human skin: melanin provides strong contrast. *J Invest Dermatol* 1995;104:946–952.

28. So PT, Konig K, Berland K, et al. New time-resolved techniques in two-photon microscopy. *Cell Mol Biol* 1998;44:771–793.

29. Masters BR, So PT, Gratton E. Multiphoton excitation fluorescence microscopy and spectroscopy of in vivo human skin. *Biophys J* 1997;72:2405–2412.

30. Brown EB, Campbell RB, Tsuzuki Y, Xu L, Carmeliet P, Fukumura, D, Jain RK. In vivo measurement of gene expression, angiogenesis and physiological function in tumors using multiphoton laser scanning microscopy. *Nat Med* 2001;7:864–868.

31. Dellian M, Yuan F, Trubetskoy VS, Torchilin VP, Jain RK. Vascular permeability in a human tumour xenograft: molecular charge dependence. *Br J Cancer* 2000;82:1513–1518.

32. Monsky WL, Fukumura D, Gohongi T, et al. Augmentation of transvascular transport of macromolecules and nanoparticles in tumors using vascular endothelial growth factor. *Cancer Res* 1999;59:4129–4135.

33. Tearney GJ, Brezinski ME, Bouma BE, et al. In vivo endoscopic optical biopsy with optical coherence tomography. *Science* 1997;276:2037–2039.

34. Fujimoto JG, Pitris C, Boppart SA, Brezinski ME. Optical coherence tomography: an emerging technology for biomedical imaging and optical biopsy. *Neoplasia* 2000;2:9–25.

35. Farkas DL, Becker D. Applications of spectral imaging: detection and analysis of human melanoma and its precursors. *Pigment Cell Res* 2001;14:2–8.

36. Mahmood U, Tung C, Bogdanov A, Weissleder R. Near infrared optical imaging system to detect tumor protease activity. *Radiology* 1999;211:866–870.

37. Reynolds JS, Troy TL, Mayer RH, et al. Imaging of spontaneous canine mammary tumors using fluorescent contrast agents. *Photochem Photobiol* 1999;70:87–94.

38. Ntziachristos V, Hielscher AH, Yodh AG, Chance B. Diffuse optical tomography of highly heterogeneous media. *IEEE Trans Med Imaging* 2001;20:470–478.

39. Chance B, Kang K, He L, Weng J, Sevick E. Highly sensitive object location in tissue models with linear in-phase and anti-phase multi-element optical arrays in one and two dimensions. *Proc Natl Acad Sci USA* 1993;90:3423–3427.

40. Pasricha PJ, Motamedi M. Optical biopsies, "bioendoscopy," and why the sky is blue: the coming revolution in gastrointestinal imaging. *Gastroenterology* 2002;122:571–575.

41. Schotland J-C Continuous wave diffusion imaging. *J Opt Soc Am* 1997;A-14:275–279.

42. Yodh AG, Chance B. Spectroscopy and Imaging with Diffusing Light. *Physics Today* 1995;48:34–40.

43. Barbour R, Graber H, Chang J, Barbour S, Koo P, Aronson R. MRI-guided optical tomog-

raphy: Prospects and computation for a new imaging method. *IEEE Comp Sci Eng* 1995;2:63–77.

44. Colak S, van der Mark M, Hooft G, Hoogenraad J, van der Linden E, Kuijpers F. Clinical optical tomography and NIR spectroscopy for breast cancer detection. *IEEE J Selected Topics Quantum Electronics* 1999;5:1143–1158.

45. Arridge SR. Optical tomography in medical imaging. *Inverse Problems* 1999;15:R41–R93.

46. Jiang H, Paulsen K, Osterberg U, Patterson M. Improved continuous light diffusion imaging in single- and multi-target tissue-like phantoms. *Phys Med Biol* 1998;43:675–693.

47. Ntziachristos V, Ma XH, Chance B. Time-correlated single photon counting imager for simultaneous magnetic resonance and near-infrared mammography. *Rev Sci Instru* 1998;69:4221–4233.

48. Chernomordik V, Hattery D, Gannot I, Gandjbakhche AH. Inverse method 3-D reconstruction of localized in vivo fluorescence—Application to Sjogren syndrome. *IEEE J Selected Topics Quantum Electronics* 1999;5:930–935.

49. Ntziachristos V, Weissleder R. Experimental three-dimensional fluorescence reconstruction of diffuse media using a normalized Born approximation. *Optics Lett* 2001;26:893–895.

50. Pogue B, Poplack S, McBride T, Wells W, Osterman K, Osterberg U. Hemoglobin imaging of breast tumors with near-infrared tomography. *Radiology* 2000;214:G05H.

51. Hillman EMC, Hebden JC, Schweiger M, et al. Time resolved optical tomography of the human forearm. *Phys Med Biol* 2001;46:1117–1130.

52. Benaron DA, Hintz SR, Villringer A, et al. Noninvasive functional imaging of human brain using light. *J Cerebral Blood Flow Metab* 2000;20:469–477.

53. Ntziachristos V, Tung C-H, Bremer C, Weissleder R. Fluorescence-mediated tomography reslves protease activity in vivo. *Nat. Med*, 2002;8:757–760.

54. Ntziachristos V, Ripoll J, Weissleder R. Would near-infrared fluorescence signals propagate through large human organs for clinical studies? *Opt Lett* 2002;27:333–335.

55. Hashida S, Towatari T, Kominami, E, Katunuma N. Inhibitions by E-64 derivatives of rat liver cathepsin B and cathepsin L in vitro and in vivo. *J Biochem (Tokyo)* 1980;88:1805–1811.

56. Bogdanov A, Lin C, Matuszewski L, Weissleder R. Cellular activation of self-quenched fluorescent reporter probe in tumor microenvironment. *Neoplasia*, 2002;4:228–236.

57. Reubi JC, Lang W, Maurer R, Koper JW, Lamberts SW. Distribution and biochemical characterization of somatostatin receptors in tumors of the human central nervous system. *Cancer Res.* 1987;47:5758–5764.

58. Demchik LL, Sameni M, Nelson K, Mikkelsen, T, Sloane BF. Cathepsin B and glioma invasion. *Int J Dev Neurosci* 1999;17:483–494.

59. Winawer SJ, Fletcher RH, Miller L, et al. Colorectal cancer screening: clinical guidelines and rationale. *Gastroenterology* 1997;112:594–642.

60. Marten K, Bremer C, Khazaie K, et al. Detection of dysplastic intestinal adenomas using enzyme-sensing molecular beacons in mice. *Gastroenterology* 2002;122:406–414.

61. Emmert-Buck MR, Roth MJ, Zhuang Z, et al. Increased gelatinase A (MMP-2) and cathepsin B activity in invasive tumor regions of human colon cancer samples. *Am. J. Pathol* 1994;145:1285–1290.

62. Herszenyi L, Plebani M, Carraro P, et al. The role of cysteine and serine proteases in colorectal carcinoma. *Cancer* 1999;86:1135–1142.

63. Shoemaker AR, Gould KA, Luongo C, Moser AR, Dove WF. Studies of neoplasia in the Min mouse. *Biochim Biophys Acta* 1997;1332:F25–F48.

64. Stearns ME, Wang M. Type IV collagenase (M(r) 72,000) expression in human prostate: benign and malignant tissue. *Cancer Res.* 1993;63:878–883.

65. Davies B, Waxman J, Wasan H, et al. Levels of matrix metalloproteases in bladder cancer correlate with tumor grade and invasion. *Cancer Res* 1993;53:5365–5369.

66. Moses MA, Wiederschain D, Loughlin KR, Zurakowski D, Lamb CC, Freeman MR. Increased incidence of matrix metalloproteinases in urine of cancer patients. *Cancer Res* 1998;58:1395–1399.
67. Fang J, Shing Y, Wiederschain D, et al. Matrix metalloproteinase-2 is required for the switch to the angiogenic phenotype in a tumor model. *Proc Natl Acad Sci USA* 2000;97:3884–3889.
68. Morgunova E, Tuuttila A, Bergmann U, et al. Structure of human pro-matrix metalloproteinase-2: activation mechanism revealed. *Science* 1999;284:1667–1670.
69. Koivunen E, Arap W, Valtanen H, et al. Tumor targeting with a selective gelatinase inhibitor. *Nat Biotechnol* 1999;17:768–774.
70. Coughlin SR. Thrombin signalling and protease-activated receptors. *Nature* 2000;407:258–264.
71. Jaffer FA, Tung CT, Gerszten RE, Weissleder R. In vivo imaging of thrombolin activity in experimental thrombi using a thrombin-sensittive near-infrared molecular probe. *Arterioscler Thromb Vasc Biol* 2002;22:1929–1935.
72. Patterson C, Stouffer GA, Madamanchi N, Runge MS. New tricks for old dogs: nonthrombotic effects of thrombin in vessel wall biology. *Circ Res* 2001;88:987–997.
73. Griffin CT, Srinivasan Y, Zheng YW, Huang W, Coughlin SR. A role for thrombin receptor signaling in endothelial cells during embryonic development. *Science* 2001;293:1666–1670.

Index